DIFFERENTIAL DIAGNOSIS IN PHYSICAL THERAPY

Musculoskeletal and Systemic Conditions

DIFFERENTIAL DIAGNOSIS IN PHYSICAL THERAPY

Musculoskeletal and Systemic Conditions

Catherine Cavallaro Goodman, M.B.A., P.T.
Formerly, Visiting Assistant Professor, Clinical Director,
University of Montana
Missoula, Montana
Private Practice, Missoula, Montana

Teresa E. Kelly Snyder, R.N., M.N.
Associate Professor of Nursing,
Montana State University
Bozeman, Montana

1990

W.B. SAUNDERS COMPANY
Harcourt Brace Jovanovich, Inc.
Philadelphia London Toronto Montreal Sydney Tokyo

W. B. SAUNDERS COMPANY
Harcourt Brace Jovanovich, Inc.

The Curtis Center
Independence Square West
Philadelphia, PA 19106

Library of Congress Cataloging-in-Publication Data

Goodman, Catherine Cavallaro.
Differential screening in physical therapy: musculoskeletal and systemic conditions / Catherine Cavallaro Goodman, Teresa E. Kelly Snyder.
p. cm.
ISBN 0-7216-4159-8
1. Physical therapy. 2. Diagnosis, Differential. I. Snyder, Teresa E. Kelly. II. Title.
[DNLM: 1. Diagnosis, Differential. 2. Physical Therapy. WB 460 G853d]
RM701.G66 1990 616.07'5--dc20 90-8005

Editor: Margaret M. Biblis
Developmental Editor: Shirley Kuhn
Designer: Joan Wendt
Production Manager: Peter Faber
Manuscript Editor: Marjory Fraser
Illustrators: Elizabeth Strausbaugh and Sharon Iwanczuk
Illustration Coordinator: Ceil Kunkle
Indexer: Kathleen Cole

Differential Diagnosis in Physical Therapy:
Musculoskeletal and Systemic Conditions ISBN 0-7216-4159-8

Printed in the United States of America.

Last digit is the print number: 9 8 7 6 5 4 3 2 1

To Cliff, Ben, and Guy without whom this book would have been finished much sooner . . . and to Jane

C.C.G.

To my husband, R.C.; my son, James; and my daughter, Deann, who fill my life with laughter and enthusiasm

T.E.K.S.

Preface

Differential Diagnosis in Physical Therapy: Musculoskeletal and Systemic Conditions developed as a result of my own experience as a physical therapist in the United States Army Reserves. In all branches of the military, physical therapists have traditionally functioned as independent practitioners. In the military environment, physical therapists have screened thousands of troops annually without the benefit of having the results of a physician's evaluation. Because an increasing number of states are passing direct access laws to provide for evaluation and treatment of a patient without referral, this quick reference book would likely be most helpful to the physical therapist.

The goal is to provide the therapist (both students and clinicians) with a systematic approach in the use of a physical therapy interview and to recognize systemic disease that may mimic neuromusculoskeletal problems. Throughout the text, the therapist is encouraged to correlate all of the findings from the patient's Personal/Family History, the physical therapy interview, and the objective evaluation. The therapist must be able to recognize when a patient may be exhibiting signs and symptoms of systemic disease that require medical referral.

We do not intend to teach physical therapists how to diagnose medical conditions, but rather our aim is to assist the therapist in making a physical therapy diagnosis regarding neuromusculoskeletal conditions.

Additionally, therapists often treat patients with true neuromusculoskeletal conditions who also have signs and symptoms associated with a known (or perhaps as yet undiagnosed) systemic disease. The purpose of the information within this textbook is to help to answer some of the therapist's questions with regard to such medical conditions and to provide a point of reference for determining when patients should be referred to a physician.

In each chapter in which visceral organs are discussed, a brief review of anatomy and physiology is provided. This review is meant only to acquaint the reader with the organs involved before discussing diseases that occur as a result of the pathophysiology of these organs. Because this is not a pathophysiology textbook, we do not attempt to provide an in-depth understanding of each disease entity. In the case of immunologic diseases, we have provided the reader with more information because of the broad and complex scope of this topic.

In the first chapter, we present a complete physical therapy interview that can be considered to be a basic or core interview. This interview can be used with all patients by modifying the extent and the detail of the questions, depending on the nature of the clinical setting (e.g., geriatrics, sports medicine, patient in the hospital, outpatient) and on the patient's chief complaint.

For example, in the case of a patient with an injury requiring knee rehabilitation, the therapist does not necessarily need a complete personal/family history or additional questions to determine the presence of signs and symptoms associated with systemic disease. However, when a patient presents with back or shoulder pain of unknown etiology, the therapist may require a more comprehensive review of the medical history and the interview to evaluate the need for further medical follow-up. In each subsequent chapter, we offer suggestions for Special Questions to Ask, which help to clarify the associated signs and symptoms.

A list of clinical signs and symptoms has been included for each disease, and this list is given at the beginning of each chapter to help readers to quickly and easily locate information. The Overview and Summary sections in each chapter serve as a review of the topics covered and as a quick reference source. Each chapter that describes systemic conditions also includes a list of signs and symptoms that require physician referral. This list, combined with Special Questions to Ask, should help the physical therapist to decide when it is necessary to refer a patient to a physician for further evaluation.

At the end of each chapter, one case study is provided to illustrate the material in the chapter. These case studies, which are based on actual experiences with patients in our practice, are presented in a way that should benefit the reader in a clinical setting. All case studies are directed toward using subjective evaluation skills of the physical therapy interview rather than focussing on how to evaluate patients objectively.

Because it is essential for the physical therapist to understand medical terminology in order to comprehend nurses' and physicians' notes and instructions and to be able to describe a patient's condition, a glossary has been provided at the end of the book.

Because *Differential Diagnosis in Physical Therapy: Musculoskeletal and Systemic Conditions* is the first textbook oriented toward independent practice, we would appreciate any constructive suggestions from students and therapists. We hope to eventually combine the pathophysiology of diseases with the information already presented here in order to provide a comprehensive medical textbook designed specifically for physical therapists.

CATHERINE CAVALLARO GOODMAN, M.B.A., P.T.

Acknowledgments

Differential Diagnosis in Physical Therapy: Musculoskeletal and Systemic Conditions is a direct result of experience in the military as an independent practitioner over a period of 7 years. In addition to the numerous men and women of the United States Army who have assisted in bringing this book to publication, special thanks go to:

Steven Stratton, Ph.D., for the introduction to knowledge of systemic origins of neuromusculoskeletal disorders.

Maureen Fleming, Ph.D., for advice and counsel from the start of this project.

Ray Murray, Ph.D., and Dorothy Patent, Ph.D., for their help and guidance in getting this book off the ground.

Cheryl McMullen, for her invaluable assistance with diction, grammar, spelling, and consistent use of language.

The physicians in our community, including Charles E. Bell, Thomas D. Bell, David W. Burgan, J.A. Cain, C. Paul Loehnen, C. Byron Olson, Dean E. Ross, Peggy Schlesinger, Stephen F. Speckart, John R. Stone, and Wesley W. Wilson.

Gene Mead, Ph.D., for keeping us up to date on the subject of acquired immunodeficiency syndrome (AIDS).

The staff of St. Patrick's Medical Library for the numerous times that they provided help and information at the last minute.

The many authors and publishers who have allowed us to publish some of their tables and drawings in order to help present the information in a quick reference format for both students and physical therapy clinicians.

William Bailey, P.T., for permission to reproduce the patient case study in Chapter 2.

Margaret Biblis, Shirley Kuhn, and the staff of W. B. Saunders Company for their suggestions in writing this textbook.

We would also like to express our appreciation to those experts who generously gave of their time to serve as reviewers. Their suggestions were invaluable in the development of this book:

Cara Adams, University of Alabama, Birmingham, Alabama

Jean Baldwin, Department of Physical Therapy, School of Pharmacology, University of Pacific, Stockton, California

Barbara Merrick Bourbon, P.T., Ph.D., Beaver College, Philadelphia College of Pharmacy and Science, Philadelphia, Pennsylvania

Linda D. Crane, M.MSc., P.T., C.C.S., Division of Physical Therapy, Department of Orthopedics and Rehabilitation, University of Miami, Miami, Florida
John Echternach, Ed.D., Old Dominion University, Program of Physical Therapy, Norfolk, Virginia
Sherrill H. Hayes, M.S., P.T., Director, Division of Physical Therapy, Department of Orthopaedics and Rehabilitation, School of Medicine, University of Miami, Coral Gables, Florida
Donna Keefe Marzouk, M.S., P.T., Physical Therapy Program, School of Medicine, Indiana University, Indianapolis, Indiana
James A. Martin, M.Ed., P.T., Hedrick Medical Center, Chillicothe, Missouri
Linda Woodruff, Department of Physical Therapy, Georgia State University, Atlanta, Georgia

To these people and to the many others who remain unnamed, we say thank you. Your support and encouragement have made *Differential Diagnosis in Physical Therapy: Musculoskeletal and Systemic Conditions* possible.

CATHERINE CAVALLARO GOODMAN
TERESA E. KELLY SNYDER

Contents

Chapter 1

Chapter 2

Chapter 3

Chapter 4

Chapter 7

Chapter 8

Chapter 9

Chapter 10

Chapter 11

Chapter 12

Chapter 1

Introduction to Differential Screening in Physical Therapy

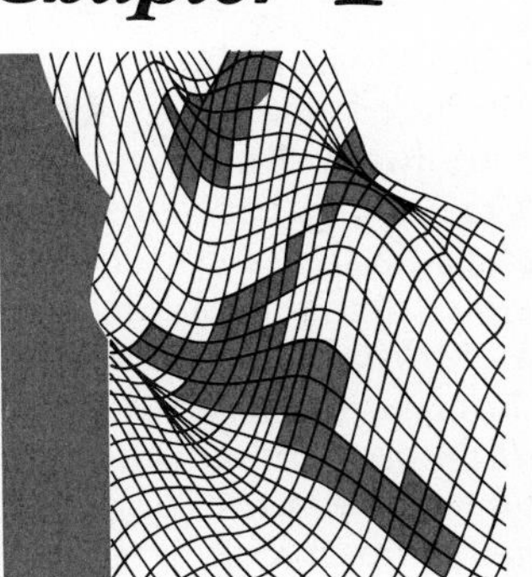

Following the model of independent practice under the increasingly prevalent Direct Access laws, physical therapists may have primary responsibility or become the first contact for some patients in the health care environment. It is important that physical therapists know when and how to refer patients to the appropriate health care practitioner. Such referral depends on the clinician's ability to quickly recognize problems that are beyond his or her expertise by being able to recognize major signs and symptoms of systemic illness.

This text provides both students and physical therapy clinicians alike with a step-by-step approach to patient evaluation, which follows the standards for competency established by the American Physical Therapy Association related to conducting a screening examination. By using the physical therapy interview as a foundation for subjectively evaluating each patient, each organ system is reviewed with regard to the most common disorders encountered, particularly those that may mimic primary musculoskeletal lesions.

To assist the physical therapist in making a treatment-versus-referral decision, specific pain patterns corresponding to systemic diseases are presented. Special follow-up questions are presented in the subjective examination to help the physical therapist to determine when these pain patterns are accompanied by associated signs and symptoms that indicate visceral involvement.

Throughout the text, guidelines for when and how to refer a patient to a physician (or other health care provider) for further evaluation or medical follow-up are provided. Each individual case must be reviewed carefully with regard to the patient's history, presenting pain patterns, and possible associated signs and symptoms and results from the objective evaluation when making a treatment-versus-referral decision.

PHYSICAL THERAPY DIAGNOSIS

Diagnosis is the recognition of disease. It is the determination of the cause and nature of pathologic conditions. Differential diagnosis is the comparison of symptoms of similar diseases so that a correct assessment of the patient's actual problem can be made. *Physical therapists do not make medical or differential diagnoses,* but like nurses who make *nursing diagnoses,* therapists are qualified to make a *physical therapy diagnosis* regarding primary neuromusculoskeletal conditions (American Physical Therapy Association, 1987; Sahrmann, 1988).

Physical therapists are required daily to make decisions regarding that which they are educated, trained, and licensed to provide—that is, physical therapy evaluation and treatment (American Physical Therapy Association, 1987). These decisions usually involve a determination of the location, severity, and treatment of a neuromusculoskeletal abnormality. According to the American Physical Therapy Association, physical therapy is directed toward the remedying of the symptoms or the sequelae of the injurious process and not toward developing a medical diagnosis or etiology (American Physical Therapy Association, 1987). Identification of causative factors or etiology by the physical therapist is limited primarily to those pathokinesiologic (study of movements related to a given disorder) problems associated with faulty biomechanical or neuromuscular action. Sahrmann (1988) noted that physical therapists' primary responsibility has been to understand anatomy and the components of kinesiology and kinesiopathology, or the study of disorders of movement, because this information is the basis of their practice. The practice of physical therapy includes performing and interpreting tests and measurements, planning initial and subsequent treatment programs, and administering treatment (American Physical Therapy Association, 1987).

Within this context, physical therapists communicate with physicians and other health care practitioners to request or recommend further medical evaluation. Additionally, whether in a private practice, home health, acute care hospital, or rehabilitation setting, the physical therapist may observe some important finding outside the realm of neuromusculoskeletal disorders requiring additional medical evaluation and treatment.

Direct Access

Physical therapists are working more and more in an environment that allows direct access to patients. The Physical Therapy Practice Act is being changed in many states to provide for the independent practice of physical therapists (Direct Access). Thus, a consumer (i.e., the patient) can be evaluated and treated by a physical therapist in those states with Direct Access without a physician or other practitioner first examining that patient and making a subsequent referral to a physical therapist.

Independent practice requires that the physical therapist should be able to knowledgeably evaluate a patient's complaint and determine whether the patient has signs and symptoms of a systemic disease or a medical condition that should be evaluated by a more appropriate health care provider. This text endeavors to provide the necessary information that will assist the physical therapist in making these decisions. The competencies for the physical therapy screening examination established by the American Physical Therapy Association in 1985 have been used to prepare this information.

The purpose and the scope of this text are not to teach physical therapists to be all-purpose diagnosticians, because the concern for physical therapists in relation to direct access to patients is in the differentiation of patients who need an appropriate referral. The purpose of this text is to provide a method for physical therapists to readily recognize (in a step-by-step problem-solving manner) areas that are beyond their expertise.

DECISION-MAKING PROCESS

This text is designed to help physical therapists (as the primary practitioner) to make appropriate decisions about treatment for the patient. To help physical therapists with those important decisions, this text includes:

- Diagnostic physical therapy interviewing
- Special features that include drawings of primary and referred pain patterns for quick reference
- Disease processes that mimic musculoskeletal pain
- Dual representation of signs and symptoms by the system and by the anatomic part

The text has an active participatory focus, with emphasis on interacting and on speaking with the patient and also on making treatment decisions. The following standards are within the competencies of the American Physical Therapy Association (1985) for conducting a screening examination:

> Describe the clinical manifestations of the more common disorders of organ systems other than neuromuscular system(s).
>
> Describe the etiology and clinical manifestations of disorders that mimic dysfunction of the neuromuscular system.
>
> Describe normal and abnormal reactions to common drugs; drugs that may affect the neuromusculoskeletal system(s); drug reactions that mimic disorders of these systems and drug interactions.
>
> Interpret information from the patient/client's history including a history that includes the patient/client's description and perception of the chief complaint, an accurate and comprehensive medical and family/social history, and a comprehensive and appropriately focused review of organ systems.
>
> Interpretation of the patient/client's history must be accurate, identify noncontributory information, identify chief and secondary problems, identify information that is inconsistent with the presenting complaint, generate a working hypothesis regarding possible causes of complaints and determine whether referral or consultation is indicated.

Case Studies

Case studies are provided with each chapter to provide the physical therapist with a working understanding of how to recognize the need for additional questions. In addition, information is given concerning the type of questions to ask and how to correlate the results with the objective findings. Whenever possible, information about when and how to refer a patient to the physician is given. Each case study is based on actual case histories to provide reasonable examples of what to expect when the physical therapist is functioning as an independent practitioner who assesses the patient as the primary care giver.

Clinical Signs and Symptoms

The major focus of this text is directed toward the recognition of signs and symptoms either reported by the patient subjectively or observed objectively by the physical therapist. *Signs* are observable findings detected by the physical therapist in an objective examination (e.g., unusual skin color, clubbing of the fingers [swelling of the terminal phalanges of the fingers or toes], hematoma [local collection of blood], effusion [fluid]). *Symptoms* are reported indications of disease that are perceived by the patient, but cannot be observed by the naked eye. Pain, discomfort, or other complaints, such as numbness, tingling, or "creeping" sensations, are symptoms that are difficult to quantify, but are most often reported as being the chief complaint.

Systemic signs and symptoms that are listed for each condition should serve as a warning to alert the informed physical therapist of the possible need for further questioning and medical referral. Because physical therapists spend a considerable amount of time investigating pain, it is easy to remain focused exclusively on this symptom when patients might otherwise bring to the forefront other important problems. Thus, the physical therapist is encouraged to become accustomed to using the word "symptoms" instead of "pain" when interviewing the patient. It is likewise prudent to refer to symptoms when talking to patients

Referral. A 32-year-old female university student was referred for physical therapy through the health service 2 weeks ago. The physician's referral reads: "Possible right oblique abdominus tear/possible right iliopsoas tear." This woman was screened initially by a faculty member, and the diagnosis was confirmed as being a right oblique abdominal strain.

History. Two months ago, while the patient was running her third mile, she felt "severe pain" in the right side of her stomach, which caused her to double over. She felt immediate nausea and had stomach distention. She couldn't change the position of her leg to relieve the pain at the time. Currently, she still cannot run without pain.

Presenting Symptoms. Pain increases during situps, walking fast, reaching, turning, and bending. Pain is eased by heat and is reduced by activity. Pain in the morning versus evening depends on body position. Once the pain starts, it is intermittent and aches. The patient describes the pain as being severe, depending on her body position. She is currently taking aspirin when necessary.

SAMPLE LETTER

Date

John Smith, M.D.
University of Montana Health Service
Eddy Street
Missoula, MT 59812

Re: Jane Doe

Dear Dr. Smith,
Your patient, Jane Doe was evaluated in our clinic on 5/2/88 with the following pertinent findings:

Subjective. The patient has severe pain in the right lower abdominal quadrant associated with nausea and abdominal distention. Although the patient notes that the onset of symptoms started while she was running, she denies any precipitating trauma. She describes the course of symptoms as having occurred 2 months ago with temporary resolution and now with exacerbation of earlier symptoms. Additionally, she has chronic fatigue and frequent night sweats.

Objective. Presenting pain is reproduced by resisted hip or trunk flexion with accompanying tenderness/tightness on palpation of the right iliopsoas muscle (compared with the left iliopsoas muscle). There are no implicating neurologic signs or symptoms.

Assessment. A musculoskeletal screening examination is consistent with your diagnosis of a possible iliopsoas or abdominal oblique tear. Jane appears to present with a combination of musculoskeletal and systemic symptoms, such as those outlined earlier. Of particular concern are the symptoms of fatigue, night sweats, abdominal distention, nausea, repeated episodes of exacerbation and remission, and severe quality of pain and location (right lower abdominal quadrant). These symptoms appear to be more of a systemic nature rather than caused by a musculoskeletal lesion.

Recommendations. I suggest that the patient should return to you for further medical follow-up to rule out any systemic involvement before the initiation of physical therapy services. I am concerned that my proposed treatment plan of ultrasound, soft-tissue mobilization, and stretching may aggravate an underlying disease process.

I will contact you directly by telephone by the end of the week to discuss these findings and to answer any questions that you may have. Thank you for this interesting referral.

Sincerely,

Catherine C. Goodman, M.B.A., P.T.

Figure 1–1.

Result. This patient returned to the physician who then ordered laboratory tests. After an acute recurrence of the symptoms described earlier, she had exploratory surgery. A diagnosis of a ruptured appendix and peritonitis was determined at surgery. In retrospect, the proposed treatment of ultrasound and soft-tissue mobilization would have been contraindicated in this situation.

Figure 1–1 *Continued* Sample letter of the physical therapist's findings given to the referring physician.

with chronic pain in order to move the focus away from pain.

Diagnostic Interviewing

The interview with the patient is very important because it helps the physical therapist to distinguish between problems that he or she can treat and problems that should be referred to a physician for diagnosis and treatment. This information establishes a solid basis for the physical therapy objective evaluation, assessment, and therefore treatment.

This material is intended to serve both as a reference guide for the skilled clinician and as a teaching text for use with physical therapy students. The student of physical therapy can use the book to develop necessary skills for clinical work, and the experienced clinician can refer to it as a guide for addressing specific clinical issues. For example, a student can use the detailed step-by-step breakdown of the interview with the patient to understand and practice each part of the process. The experienced clinician can refer to chapters on systemic problems and can have access to information about what specific questions to address to each patient depending on the presenting chief complaint. For example, the patient with chest pain should be asked specifically about both systemic and musculoskeletal origins of the present pain and symptoms.

An interviewing process is described which includes concrete and structured tools and techniques for conducting a thorough and informative interview. The use of follow-up questions is discussed because these questions help to structure the interview.

Reference Features

Pain Patterns

In each section, specific pain patterns characteristic of disease entities that can mimic musculoskeletal pain are discussed. Detailed information regarding the location, referral pattern, description, intensity, and duration of systemic pain is augmented by information about associated symptoms and relieving and aggravating factors. This information is compared with the presenting features of primary musculoskeletal lesions that have similar patterns of presentation.

Pain patterns of the chest, thoracic spine, shoulder, scapula, lumbar spine, groin, sacroiliac joint, and hip are included as being the most frequent sites of referred pain from a systemic disease process.

Disease Processes

Diseases are presented both by visceral (organ) system involved and by type of specialty. For example, organ systems that are discussed include heart, lungs, intestines, kidneys/bladder, and liver with specialty areas of study including cardiology, pulmonary medicine, hematology, gastroenterology, urology/nephrology, hepatic/biliary problems, endocrinology, oncology, and immunology.

Hematology, endocrinology, immunology, and oncology sections are included because the physical therapist may treat a patient with musculoskeletal problems who also has a disease involving one of these specialties. The information presented in these sections may assist the physical therapist in planning a treatment program that takes into consideration the patient's overall compromised health, especially when exercise may precipitate or aggravate one of these conditions.

With the continual expansion of physical therapy skills, physical therapy protocols are being developed for patients with diagnoses such as auto acquired immunodeficiency syndrome (AIDS), diabetes, allergies, asthma, and various cancers. The material in this text should provide the physical therapist with an overview of these disease entities.

PHYSICIAN REFERRAL

The hallmark of any health care professional is the ability to understand the limits of his or her professional knowledge. The physical therapist, either on reaching the limit of his or her knowledge or on reaching the limits prescribed by the patient's condition, should refer the patient to the physician (American Physical Therapy Association, 1987). Each physical therapist must work within the scope of his or her level of skill, knowledge, and practical experience.

Guidelines for appropriate referral to a physician (or other health care practitioner) have been outlined in the American Physical Therapy Code of Ethics, Guide for Professional Conduct and Standards for Physical Therapy Services and Physical Therapy Practitioners (American Physical Therapy Association, 1987):

If symptoms are present for which physical therapy is contraindicated or which are indicative of conditions for which treatment is outside the scope of his knowledge, the physical therapist must refer patients to a licensed practitioner of medicine.

In the event that a medical diagnosis is required and has not been established prior to treatment, then the physical therapist must refer to a licensed practitioner of medicine, dentistry, or podiatry.

Knowing how to refer the patient or how to notify the physician of important findings is not always clear. It is ultimately the patient's responsibility to act on the information provided by the physical therapist, whether this information is about a home program or involves a recommendation to seek additional medical care. In the case of a patient referred to physical therapy by a physician or dentist, a summary of findings is recommended, whether it is filed in the patient's chart in the hospital or sent in a letter to the outpatient's physician or dentist. (For a sample letter see Figure 1–1.)

When the patient has come to physical therapy without a medical referral (i.e., selfreferred) and the physical therapist recommends medical follow-up, the patient should be referred to the primary care physician. Occasionally, the patient indicates that he or she has not contacted a physician or was treated by a physician (whose name cannot be recalled) a long time ago, or that he or she has just moved to the area and does not have a physician. In these situations, the patient should be provided with a list of recommended physicians. It is not necessary to list every physician in the area, but the physical therapist should provide several appropriate choices. Whether or not the patient makes an appointment with a medical practitioner, the physical therapist is urged to carefully document subjective and objective findings and the recommendation made for medical follow-up. The patient should make these physical therapy records available to the consulting physician.

References

American Physical Therapy Association: Competencies in Physical Therapy—An Analysis of Practice. American Physical Therapy Association, March 1985.

American Physical Therapy Association: Direct Access to Physical Therapy: Information Packet. Division of Professional Relations, American Physical Therapy Association, June 1987.

Sahrmann, S.: Diagnosis by the physical therapist—a prerequisite for treatment. Phys. Ther., *68*:1705, 1988.

Chapter 2

Introduction to the Interviewing Process

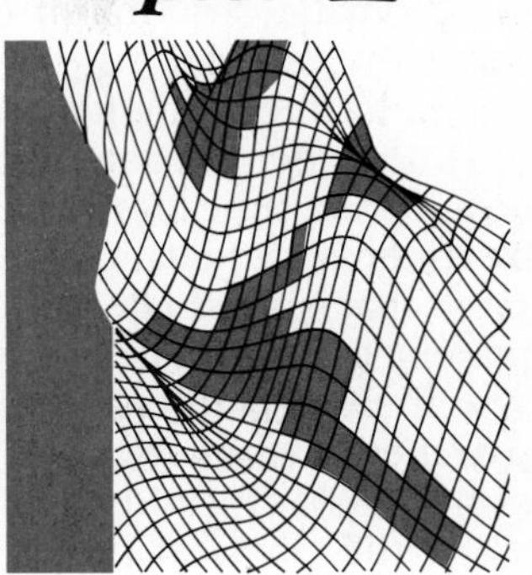

☐ ***Clinical Signs and Symptoms of:***
Conversion

You are interviewing a patient for the first time and she tells you, "The pain in my hip started 12 years ago when I was a corpsman in the navy standing on my feet 10 hours a day. It seems to bother me most when I am having premenstrual symptoms, such as food cravings or depression. My left leg is longer than my right leg, and my hip hurts when the scars from my bunionectomy ache. This pain occurs with any changes in the weather. I have a bleeding ulcer that bothers me, and the pain keeps me awake at night. I dislocated my shoulder 2 years ago, but I can lift weights now without any problems." She continues her dialogue, and you feel out of control and unsure of how to proceed. This scenario was taken directly from a clinical experience and represents what we term in the medical profession, "an organ recital." In this situation, the patient provides detailed information regarding all previously experienced illnesses and symptoms that may or may not be related to the current problem.

Interviewing is an important skill for the clinician to learn. It is generally agreed that 80% of the information needed to clarify the cause of symptoms is contained within the subjective assessment. This chapter is designed to provide the physical therapist with interviewing guidelines and important questions to ask the patient. The materials presented are not intended to teach the therapist how to interview a patient. Other more appropriate texts that emphasize interviewing for the health care professional are available (see the Bibliography).

Medical practitioners (including nurses, physicians, and therapists) begin the interview by determining the patient's chief complaint. The chief complaint is usually a symptomatic description by the patient (i.e., subjective sensations reported, such as fatigue, dizziness, night sweats, fever).

The subjective examination may also reveal any contraindications to physical therapy treatment or indications for the kind of treatment that is most likely to be effective (e.g., a patient examined by a physical therapist last year found that ultrasound was the most effective method for providing long-term relief of symptoms). Questioning the patient may also assist the physical therapist in determining whether an injury is in the acute, subacute, or chronic stage. This information guides the clinician in providing symptomatic relief for the acute injury, more aggressive treatment for the chronic problem, and a combination of both methods of treatment for the subacute lesion. The interviewing techniques, interviewing tools, core interview, and review of the inpatient hospital chart in this chapter will help the therapist to determine the location and potential significance of any symptom (including pain). The interview format provides detailed information regarding the frequency, duration, intensity, length, breadth, depth, and anatomic location as these relate to the patient's chief complaint. The physical therapist will later correlate this information with the objective findings of this examination to rule out possible systemic origin of symptoms. The information obtained from the interview guides the physical therapist in either referring the patient to a physician or in treating the patient in a clinic.

INTERVIEWING TECHNIQUES

An organized interview format assists the physical therapist in obtaining a complete and accurate data base. Using the same outline with each patient ensures that all pertinent information related to previous medical history and current medical problem(s) is included. This information is especially important when correlating the subjective data with objective findings from the physical examination.

Many interviewing techniques can be used by the skilled interviewer (Bernstein and Bernstein, 1985; Cash and Stewart, 1985). For the physical therapist, several techniques are essential building blocks that can be expanded on with experience. The most basic skills required for a physical therapy interview include:

- Open-ended questions
- Closed-ended questions
- Funnel sequence or technique
- Paraphrasing technique

Open-Ended and Closed-Ended Questions

Beginning an interview with an *open-ended question* (i.e., questions that elicit more than a one-word response) is advised even though this gives the patient opportunity to control and direct the interview. Initiating an interview with the open-ended directive, "Tell me why you are here" can potentially elicit more information in a relatively short (5 to 15 minute) period than a steady stream of *closed-ended questions* requiring a "yes" or "no" type of answer.

A patient who takes control of the interview by telling the therapist about every ache and pain of every friend and neighbor can be rechanneled effectively by interrupting the patient with a polite statement such as, "I'm beginning to get an idea of the nature of your problem. Now I would like to obtain some more specific information" (Kessler and Hertling, 1983). At this point, the interviewer may begin to use closed-ended questions (i.e., questions requiring the answer to be "yes" or "no") in order to characterize the symptoms more clearly. Moving from the open-ended line of questions to the closed-ended questions is referred to as the *funnel technique* or *funnel sequence.*

The following list highlights the differences between these two interview techniques.

OPEN-ENDED QUESTIONS	CLOSED-ENDED QUESTIONS
How does bedrest affect your back pain?	Do you have any pain after lying in bed all night?
Tell me how you cope with stress and what kinds of stressors you encounter on a daily basis.	Are you under any stress?
What makes the pain (better) worse?	Is the pain relieved by food?
How did you sleep last night?	Did you sleep well last night?

Each question format has advantages and limitations. The use of open-ended questions to initiate the interview may allow the patient to control the interview, but can also prevent a false-positive or false-negative response that would otherwise be elicited by starting with closed-ended (yes or no) questions. False responses elicited by closed-ended questions may develop from the patient's attempt to please the health care provider or to comply with what the patient believes is the correct response or expectation.

Closed-ended questions tend to be more impersonal and may set an impersonal tone for the relationship between the patient and the physical therapist. These questions are limited by the restrictive nature of the information received so that the patient may only respond to the category in question and may omit vital, but seemingly unrelated, information. Use of the funnel sequence to obtain as much information as possible through the open-ended format first (before moving on to the more restrictive but clarifying "yes" or "no" type of questions at the end) can establish an effective forum for trust between the patient and physical therapist.

Follow-up Questions

The *funnel sequence* is aided by the use of *f*ollow-*up* question*s* referred to as *FUPs* in the text. Beginning with one or two open-ended questions in each section, the interviewer may follow up with a series of closed-ended questions, which are listed in the core interview presented later in this chapter. For example: How does rest affect the pain or symptoms?

FUPs

- Are your symptoms aggravated or relieved by any activities?
  - If yes, what?
- How has this problem affected your daily life at work or at home?
- Your ability to care for yourself without assistance (e.g., dress, bathe, cook, drive)?

Paraphrasing Technique

A useful interviewing skill that can assist in synthesizing and integrating the information obtained during questioning is the paraphrasing technique. When using this technique, the interviewer repeats information presented by the patient. This technique can assist in fostering effective, accurate communication between the health care recipient and the health care provider. For example, once a patient has responded to the question, "What makes you feel better?," the physical therapist can paraphrase the reply by saying, "You've told me that the pain is relieved by such and such, is that right? What other activities or treatment brings you relief from your pain or symptoms?" If you cannot paraphrase what the patient has said, or you are unclear about the meaning of the patient's response, ask for clarification by requesting an example of what the patient is talking about.

INTERVIEWING TOOLS

With the changing requirements of hospital accreditation and third-party payment sources, physical therapists are required more and more to identify problems, to quantify symptoms (e.g., pain), and to demonstrate the effectiveness of treatment. The use of interviewing tools such as the *McGill Pain Questionnaire* (Melzack, 1975; Wolf, 1985) can also assist physical therapists in documenting a patient's progress and can assist in justifying services provided. This can be accomplished by utilizing information about the patient to establish objective and measurable goals against which progress can be measured.

There is no single instrument or method of pain measurement that can be considered to be the best under all circumstances (Jacox, 1977). However, for the clinician who is interested in quantifying pain as part of a goal-writing procedure and in order to measure improvement by using pain as a guide, some form of assessment is necessary. The McGill questionnaire is presented in this chapter in a form adapted for use by physical therapists. This particular questionnaire is included because it assesses overall pain experience and is not limited to a single disease, injury, or body part. Other forms of pain indices are available (Jacox, 1977) including assessment scales designed specifically for back pain and back disability (see the Bibliography).

McGill Pain Questionnaire

Classes of Word Descriptors

The McGill Pain Questionnaire, which was designed by Melzack (1975), consists of three major classes of word descriptors — sensory, affective, and evaluative — that are used by patients to describe subjective pain experience (Fig. 2-1). These three subgroups enable pain to be described by more than just a single scale of intensity (Table 2-1). *Sensory* words (Groups 1 to 10) describe pain in terms of time, space, pressure, heat, and other properties. *Affective* qualities (Groups 11 to 15) include aspects of tension, fear, and autonomic properties that are a part of the pain experience. *Evaluative* words (Group 16) describe the overall intensity of the pain phenomenon by using subjective labels (Jacox, 1977; Wolf, 1985).

The remaining groups (17 to 20) are considered to be a miscellaneous category. Each word selected in the miscellaneous category should be evaluated for possible etiology (e.g., radiating may be more neurogenic, whereas torturing is more descriptive of an affective quality). Words within each subgroup (1 to 20) were determined by Melzack and Torgerson (1971) to be ranked according to intensity of pain. For example, pounding pain is considered worse than pulsing pain, and stabbing implies more pain than boring which, in turn, represents more pain than pricking (Jacox, 1977).

Questionnaire Administration

The questionnaire was designed to provide quantitative measures of clinical pain that can be treated statistically. Proper questionnaire administration requires that the patient should select only one word from each category and the patient should describe only the present pain. The questionnaire should be administered by the physical therapist or by trained ancillary staff. The patient should be instructed to check only words listed that best describe the pain. Any categories that do not describe the patient's pain should remain blank.

The anatomic figure should be explained and presented at the same time. The physical therapist will note additional indicators between the two anatomical figures in the questionnaire (see Fig. 2-1) to outline areas of numbness, moderate or severe pain, or shooting pain. These descriptors were not part of the original questionnaire but have been added as a modification for use by physical therapists. These additional notations can be drawn in by the physical therapist while the patient is being interviewed regarding the description of pain sensation.

Questionnaire Scoring

The score is determined by adding the total number of checks in Groups 1 to 20. This total is then compared with the key provided (see Fig. 2-1). The results allow physical thera-

UNIVERSITY OF MONTANA
PHYSICAL THERAPY CLINIC

PATIENT'S NAME ____________________

DATE ____________________

DIRECTIONS: There are many words that describe pain. Some of these words are grouped below. IF YOU ARE EXPERIENCING ANY PAIN, check (√) any words that describe your pain.

1	Flickering ___, Quivering ___, Pulsing ___, Throbbing ___, Beating ___, Pounding ___
2	Jumping ___, Flashing ___, Shooting ___
3	Pricking ___, Boring ___, Drilling ___, Stabbing ___, Lancinating ___
4	Sharp ___, Cutting ___, Lacerating ___
5	Pinching ___, Pressing ___, Gnawing ___, Cramping ___, Crushing ___
6	Tugging ___, Pulling ___, Wrenching ___
7	Hot ___, Burning ___, Scalding ___, Searing ___
8	Tingling ___, Itchy ___, Smarting ___, Stinging ___
9	Dull ___, Sore ___, Hurting ___, Aching ___, Heavy ___
10	Tender ___, Taut ___, Rasping ___, Splitting ___
11	Tiring ___, Exhausting ___
12	Sickening ___, Suffocating ___
13	Fearful ___, Frightful ___, Terrifying ___
14	Punishing ___, Grueling ___, Cruel ___, Vicious ___, Killing ___
15	Wretched ___, Blinding ___
16	Annoying ___, Troublesome ___, Miserable ___, Intense ___, Unbearable ___
17	Spreading ___, Radiating ___, Penetrating ___, Piercing ___
18	Tight ___, Numb ___, Drawing ___, Squeezing ___, Tearing ___
19	Cool ___, Cold ___, Freezing ___
20	Nagging ___, Nauseating ___, Agonizing ___, Dreadful ___, Torturing ___

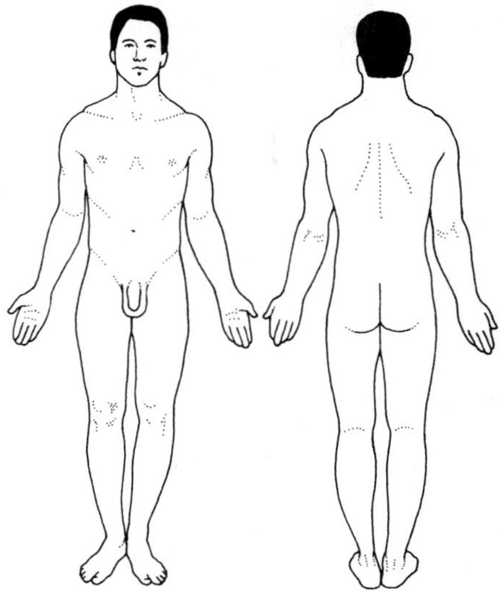

ACCOMPANYING SYMPTOMS:	SLEEP:	FOOD INTAKE:
Nausea ___	Good ___	Good ___
Headache ___	Fitful ___	Some ___
Dizziness ___	Can't sleep ___	Little ___
Drowsiness ___	COMMENTS:	None ___
Constipation ___		COMMENTS:
Diarrhea ___		
COMMENTS:	ACTIVITY:	COMMENTS:
	Good ___	
	Some ___	
	Little ___	
	None ___	

A form of the McGill Pain Questionnaire.

KEY:

Group 1	suggests vascular disorder
Groups 2-8	suggests neurogenic disorder
Group 9	suggests musculoskeletal disorder
Groups 10-20	suggests emotional lability

SCORING: Add up total number of checks. Patients who mark

4-8 = Within normal limits (WNL)
≥ 6 = may be getting a "little into pain"
≥ 10 = may be helped more by a clinical psychologist than by physical therapy
≥ 16 = unlikely to respond to therapy procedures

Figure 2–1. A form of the McGill pain questionnaire. The key and scoring information at the bottom are for the therapist's use only to determine the type of disorder and how to handle the disorder. (Adapted from Wolf, S.L.: Clinical decision making in physical therapy. *In* Paris, S.: Clinical Decision Making: Orthopedic Physical Therapy. Philadelphia, F.A. Davis, 1985)

Table 2–1. CLASSES AND SUBCLASSES OF PAIN DESCRIPTORS AS RATED BY PATIENTS*

Category	Descriptors
Sensory	
Temporal	Flickering Quivering Pulsing Throbbing Beating Pounding
Spatial	Jumping Flashing Spreading Radiating Shooting
Punctate pressure	Pricking Boring Drilling Stabbing Penetrating Piercing
Incisive pressure	Sharp Cutting Hurting Aching Drawing Heavy
Affective	
Autonomic	Nauseating Suffocating Choking
Sensory	Tender Taut Tearing
Tension	Nagging Fatiguing Tiring Exhausting
Punishment	Punishing Grueling Cruel Vicious
Constrictive pressure	Pinching Tight Squeezing Pressing Gnawing Cramping Gripping Crushing
Traction pressure	Tugging Pulling Wrenching
Thermal	Hot Burning Scalding Searing
Brightness	Tingling Itchy Smarting Stinging
Dullness	Dull Sore Numbing Killing Torturing
Evaluative	
	Annoying Troublesome Miserable Agonizing Intense Unbearable
Fear	Fearful Frightful Terrifying Dreadful Wretched Blinding

* Adapted from Melzack, R., and Torgerson, W.: On the language of pain. Anesthesiology, *34*:54, 1971.

pists to determine the degree of emotional involvement experienced by the patient. By reviewing the score and the categories selected by the patient to describe pain, the physical therapist may be able to recognize a potential need for psychologic counseling in place of, or as an adjunct to, physical therapy procedures (Melzack, 1975; Wolf, 1985).

Categories selected may also serve as a screen for symptoms of possible vascular, neurogenic (nervous system), or musculoskeletal involvement. For example, Group 1 suggests a vascular disorder, Groups 2 to 8 suggest a neurogenic disorder, and Group 9 suggests a musculoskeletal lesion. Accompanying (or associated) symptoms are more indicative of possible systemic involvement.

Physical therapists may choose to modify the standardized questionnaire procedure in order to assess previous and present pain patterns. This modification provides better understanding of the patient's history. If the test is not administered according to the standardization, then the scoring cannot be considered to be valid as described.

When used as intended, the McGill Pain Questionnaire should be administered after treatment to assess changes in pain. Although it was designed to be readministered after each treatment, individual physical therapists may determine a schedule of less frequent use depending on the type of facility, the type of patient, and time factors.* When the questionnaire is given after treatment, it is important to determine whether the patient tends to choose the same word descriptors on successive presentations of the questionnaire. Variations in the quality and intensity of pain, as well as changes in mood and other psychologic variables such as personality, would produce some variation in word choices on successive questionnaires. Patients who have a particular pain syndrome would be expected to show a considerable degree of consistency by choosing subclasses that characterize that pain syndrome (Melzack, 1975).

SUBJECTIVE EXAMINATION

The core interview is the primary substance of the subjective examination and is intended to provide a database that can be expanded to add information. Information obtained is extremely important in determining immediate treatment referral, and it must be conducted in a complete and organized manner. An example of a core interview follows. The subjective examination consists of several major components, each of which are discussed further in this chapter. These components include:

- Family/Personal History
    - Past medical history
    - Medical testing/previous surgery
    - General health
    - Special questions for women and men
    - Work environment
    - Vital signs
- Core Interview
    - History of present illness
    - Pain/symptom assessment
    - Medical treatment and medications
    - Current level of fitness
    - Sleep-related history
    - Stress

It is unnecessary and probably impossible to complete the entire subjective examination on the first day. Most clinics or health care facilities use what is called an initial intake form before the patient's first visit with the physical therapist. The *Family/Personal History* form is an example of an initial intake form.

For example, a patient who circles "Yes" on the Family/Personal History form indicating a history of ulcers or stomach problems now presents a chief complaint of back pain during the History of Present Illness. Obtaining further information at the first appointment with the patient by using "Special Questions to Ask" from Chapter 6 is necessary so that a decision regarding treatment or referral can be made immediately. This treatment-versus-referral decision is further clarified as the interview and other objective evaluation procedures continue. Thus, if further questioning fails to show any association of back pain with gastrointestinal symptoms and the objective findings from the back evaluation point to a true musculoskeletal lesion, medical referral is unnecessary and treatment with physical therapy can begin.

Each clinical situation requires slight adaptations or alterations to the interview. These modifications do, in turn, affect the depth and range of questioning. For example, a patient who has pain associated with an anterior shoulder dislocation and who has no history of other disease is unlikely to require in-depth questioning to rule out systemic origins of pain. Conversely, a woman with no history of trauma, previous history of breast cancer, self-referred to the physical therapist without a previous medical examination, and who complains of shoulder pain should be interviewed

* We have found that the *McGill Pain Questionnaire* is most useful in the case of patients with chronic pain or pain of unknown etiology. The major disadvantage of this tool is the use of uncommon words, such as lancinating, rasping, or lacerating.

more thoroughly. The simple question, "How will the answers to the questions I am asking permit me to help the patient?" can serve as a guide to you (Wolf, 1977).

Continued questioning may occur both during the objective examination and during treatment. In fact, the physical therapist is encouraged to carry on a continuous dialogue during the objective examination, both as an educational tool (i.e., for the patient's education) and as a method of reducing any apprehension on the part of the patient. This open communication may bring to light other important information (Swisher and Enelow, 1973).

The patient may wonder about the extensiveness of the interview, such as "Why is the therapist asking questions about bowel function when my primary concern relates to back pain?" The physical therapist may need to make a qualifying statement to the patient regarding the need for such detailed information. For example, questions about bowel function to rule out gallbladder involvement (which can refer pain to the back) may seem to be unrelated to the patient but make sense when the physical therapist explains the possible connection between back pain and systemic disease.

Throughout the questioning, record both positive and negative findings in the subjective and the objective reports in order to correlate information when making an initial assessment of the patient's problem. Efforts should be made to quantify all information by frequency, intensity, duration, and exact location (including length, breadth, depth, and anatomic location).

Family/Personal History

This component of the subjective examination can elicit valuable data regarding the patient's family history of disease and personal life style, including working environment and health habits. Once the patient has completed the *Family/Personal History* intake form, the clinician can then follow-up with appropriate questions based on any "Yes" selections made by the patient. This form may be set up in a variety of ways. One type is outlined in the sample on page 15. More detailed information and follow-up questions can be found in subsequent chapters under each system heading.

Physical therapists may modify the information required depending on individual differences in patient base and specialty areas served. For example, an orthopedic-based facility or a sports medicine center may want to include questions on the intake form concerning current level of fitness and orthopedic devices used, such as orthotics, splints, or braces. Physical therapists working with the geriatric population may want more information regarding levels of independence in activities of daily living.

Past Medical History

The initial Family/Personal History intake form also provides the physical therapist with some idea of the patient's previous medical history, medical testing, and current general health status. It is important to take time with these questions and to ensure that the patient understands what is being asked. As stated earlier, the interviewer may follow up on any "Yes" responses on the intake form. For example, a "Yes" response to questions on this form directed toward *allergies, asthma,* and *hayfever* should be followed up by asking the patient to list the allergies and to list the symptoms that may indicate a manifestation of allergies, asthma, or hay fever. The physical therapist can then be alert for any signs of respiratory distress or allergic reactions during exercise.

Likewise, patients may indicate the presence of *shortness of breath* with only mild exertion or without exertion, possibly even after waking at night. This condition of breathlessness can be associated with one of many conditions, including heart disease, bronchitis, asthma, obesity, emphysema, dietary deficiencies, pneumonia, and lung cancer. A "Yes" response to any question in this section would require further questioning, correlation to objective findings, and consideration of referral to the patient's physician.

FAMILY/PERSONAL HISTORY

DATE: ______________________________

PATIENT'S NAME __________________ DOB ______________________ AGE ______

DIAGNOSIS ________________________________ DATE OF ONSET __________

PHYSICIAN ____________ THERAPIST ____________ PRECAUTIONS __________

Past Medical History

Have you or any immediate family member ever been told you have:

Circle one:

(Do **NOT** complete) **For the therapist:**

Condition	Yes	No	Relation to Patient	Date of Onset	Current Status
• Cancer	Yes	No			
• Diabetes	Yes	No			
• Hypoglycemia	Yes	No			
• Hypertension or high blood pressure	Yes	No			
• Heart disease	Yes	No			
• Angina or chest pain	Yes	No			
• Shortness of breath	Yes	No			
• Stroke	Yes	No			
• Kidney disease/stones	Yes	No			
• Urinary tract infection	Yes	No			
• Allergies	Yes	No			
• Asthma, hay fever	Yes	No			
• Rheumatic/scarlet fever	Yes	No			
• Hepatitis/jaundice	Yes	No			
• Cirrhosis/liver disease	Yes	No			
• Polio	Yes	No			
• Chronic bronchitis	Yes	No			
• Pneumonia	Yes	No			
• Emphysema	Yes	No			
• Migraine headaches	Yes	No			
• Anemia	Yes	No			
• Ulcers/stomach problems	Yes	No			
• Arthritis/gout	Yes	No			
• Other	Yes	No			

Family/Personal History *(continued)*

Medical Testing

1. Are you taking any prescription or over-the-counter medications?

   Yes No

   If yes, please list:

2. Have you had any x-rays, sonograms, computed tomography (CT) scans, or magnetic resonance imaging (MRI) done recently?

   Yes No

   If yes, when? Where? Results?

3. Have you had any laboratory work done recently (urinalysis or blood tests)?

   Yes No

   If yes, when? Where? Results (if known)?

4. Please list any operations that you have ever had and the date(s) of surgery:

   Surgery Date

General Health

1. Have you had any recent illnesses within the last 3 weeks (e.g., colds, influenza, bladder or kidney infection)?

   Yes No

2. Have you noticed any lumps or thickening of skin or muscle anywhere on your body?

   Yes No

3. Do you have any sores that have not healed or any changes in size, shape, or color of a wart or mole?

   Yes No

4. Have you had any unexplained weight loss in the last month?

   Yes No

5. Do you smoke or chew tobacco?

   Yes No

   If yes, how many packs/day? ______________ For how many months or years? ______________

6. How much alcohol do you drink in the course of a week? ______________

7. How much caffeine do you consume daily (including soft drinks, coffee, tea, or chocolate)?

8. Are you on any special diet prescribed by a physician?

   Yes No

Special Questions for Women

1. Last pap smear:

Family/Personal History *(continued)*

2. Last breast examination
3. Do you perform a monthly self-breast examination?

Yes No

4. Do you take birth control pills or do you use an intrauterine device (IUD)?

Yes No

Special Questions for Men

1. Do you ever have difficulty with urination (e.g., difficulty in starting or continuing flow or a very slow flow of urine)?

Yes No

2. Do you ever have blood in your urine?

Yes No

3. Do you ever have pain on urination?

Yes No

Work Environment

1. Occupation:
2. Does your job involve:
   [ ] prolonged sitting (e.g., desk, computer, driving)
   [ ] prolonged standing (e.g., equipment operator, sales clerk)
   [ ] prolonged walking (e.g., mill worker, delivery service)
   [ ] use of large or small equipment (e.g., telephone, fork lift, typewriter, drill press, cash register)
   [ ] lifting, bending, twisting, climbing, turning
   [ ] exposure to chemicals or gases
   [ ] other: please describe
3. Do you use any special supports:
   [ ] back cushion, neck cushion
   [ ] back brace, corset
   [ ] other kind of brace or support for any body part

For the physical therapist:

Vital Signs

Resting pulse rate

Oral temperature

Blood pressure: 1st reading ________________ 2nd reading ________________

Position: Extremity:

Medical Testing

Tests contributing information to the physical therapy assessment may include radiography (x-rays, sonograms), CT scans, MRI, urinalysis, and blood tests. The patient's medical records may contain information regarding which tests have been performed and the results of the tests. It may be helpful to question the patient directly by asking:

- What medical test have you had for this condition?

After giving the patient time to respond, you may need to probe further by asking:

- Have you had any x-rays, sonograms, CT scans, or MRIs done in the last 2 years?
- Do you recall having any blood or urinalysis tests done?

If yes, the physical therapist will want to know when and where these tests were performed and the results (if known to the patient). Knowledge of where the tests took place provides the therapist with access to the results (with the patient's written permission for disclosure).

As often as possible, the physical therapist will want to examine the available test results either with a radiologist or with the patient's physician. Familiarity with the results of these tests, combined with an understanding of the patient's clinical presentation, can assist physical therapists in knowing what to look for clinically with patients in the future and to offer some guidelines for knowing when to suggest or recommend additional testing for patients who have not had a radiologic workup or other potentially appropriate medical testing.

For a current and informative comparison of each of these test procedures, including expected results, risk factors, advantages, and disadvantages, the reader and patient are referred to *The Patient's Guide to Medical Tests* (Pickney and Pickney, 1986). Laboratory values of interest to physical therapists are included in Chapter 3.

Previous Surgery

Previous surgery or surgery related to the patient's current symptoms may be indicated on the Family/Personal History intake form. Whenever treating a patient postoperatively, the physical therapist should try to read the surgical report and should look for any complications, blood transfusions, the position of the patient during the surgery, and the length of time in that position. Patients in an early postoperative stage (within 3 weeks of surgery) may have stiffness, aching, and musculoskeletal pain unrelated to the diagnosis, which may be attributed to position during the surgery. Specific follow-up questions differ from one patient to another depending on the type of surgery, age of patient, accompanying medical history, and so forth, but it is always helpful to assess how quickly the patient recovered from surgery in order to determine an appropriate pace for a therapy treatment program.

General Health

Recent Infections. Knowing that the patient has had a recent bladder or kidney infection or that the patient is likely to have such infections may help to explain back pain present in the absence of any musculoskeletal findings. The patient may confirm previous back pain associated with previous infections. If there is any doubt, a medical referral is recommended. Recent colds, influenza, or upper respiratory infections may be an extension of a chronic health pattern of systemic illness. Further questioning may reveal recurrent influenza-like symptoms associated with headaches and musculoskeletal complaints. These complaints could originate with medical problems, such as endocarditis (a bacterial infection of the heart) or pleuropulmonary disorders, which should be ruled out by a physician. On the other hand, patients with chest pain may have muscle exertion caused by repeated coughing after a recent upper respiratory infection.

Screening for Cancer. Any responses in the affirmative to early screening questions for cancer (General Health questions 2, 3, and 4) must be followed up by a physician. Changes in appetite and unexplained weight loss can be associated with cancer, onset of diabetes, depression, or pathologic anorexia (loss of appetite). Weight loss significant for neoplasm would be 10 to 15 lb in the same number of days separate from any intentional diet program or fasting.

Tobacco. The effects of tobacco use (whether in the form of chewing tobacco, pipe, or cigarette smoking) on the heart and lungs are well documented. For the patient with respiratory or cardiac problems, cigarette smoking stimulates the already compensated heart to beat faster, narrows the blood vessels, reduces the supply of oxygen to the heart, and increases the patient's chances of developing blood clots (Wong, 1981). These effects have a direct impact on the patient's ability to exercise and must be considered when planning a treatment program.

Alcohol. Alcohol has both vasodilatory (capable of opening blood vessels) and depressant effects that may produce fatigue and mental depression or alter the patient's perception of pain or symptoms. Additionally, alcohol may interact with prescribed medications to produce various effects, including death. Unless the patient has a dependency on alcohol, appropriate education may be sufficient for the patient experiencing negative effects of alcohol use during physical therapy treatment. For example, when interviewing the patient, you may want to inform the patient:

- Alcohol has an effect on your perception of pain and may mask or even increase other symptoms, that it is important that you think carefully about the amount of alcohol that you have consumed within the last 24 hours.

Patients who depend on alcohol require more in-depth medical treatment and follow-up. Because of the controversial nature of interviewing the alcohol- or drug-dependent patient, the following is only a suggested guideline of follow-up questions that may be considered:

- Do you ever drink alcoholic beverages (use drugs recreationally)?
- If yes, can you estimate how many drinks you consume on a weekly basis?

If the patient's answers seem to be questionable, pursue this information further by asking:

- How much alcohol would you estimate that you drink on an average day?
- When do you drink? Do you drink after work or lunch? Do you drink only with meals or before or after meals?

If the patient's breath smells of alcohol, you may want to ask more directly:

- I can smell alcohol on your breath today. How many drinks have you consumed?

Caffeine. Caffeine ingested in toxic (>250 mg/day or three cups of coffee) amounts has many effects, including nervousness, irritability, agitation, sensory disturbances, tachypnea (rapid breathing), heart palpitations (strong, fast, or irregular heartbeat), nausea, urinary frequency, diarrhea, and fatigue. Withdrawal from caffeine may produce headache, lethargy, poor concentration, and emotional instability (Blacklow, 1983). Caffeine may enhance the patient's perception of pain. Pain levels can be reduced dramatically by reducing the daily intake of caffeine.

Special Questions For Women

Gynecologic disorders can refer pain to the low back, hip, groin, or sacroiliac (SI) joint. In addition to the questions included in the Family/Personal History form, more specific questions for women who have pain in these areas are included in Chapter 12.

All women should be encouraged to have a pap smear done annually. Any woman over the age of 40 with a positive family history for cervical breast cancer should have a mammogram performed annually. Any woman with a positive family history for breast cancer who has chest or shoulder pain of unknown etiology should make an appointment with her physician. Any woman whose blood pressure is elevated and who is currently taking birth control pills should be monitored closely by her physician.

The hormone, relaxin, increases elongation of ligaments by placing ligaments at the end-range and, therefore, increasing the chances for injury. Relaxin is elevated in the woman's system during pregnancy and 7 to 10 days before menstruation begins. Women who have had multiple pregnancies or births may have SI or low back pain associated with poor abdominal tone and ligamentous laxity. The symptomatic SI problem may be aggravated by intercourse in the supine position.

Special questions directed toward women are included in the Family/Personal History intake form. Appropriate follow-up questions may include:

- When was your last menstrual cycle?
- At what point were you in your menstrual cycle when the symptoms or pain started?
- Do you have any discomfort associated with your menses?
    - If yes, elaborate and describe the intensity and duration of the discomfort.
- Do you have any premenstrual symptoms (e.g., water retention, mood changes [including depression], headaches, food cravings, painful or tender breasts)?
    - If yes, describe these symptoms.

Women who have a history of hip, SI, or low back pain without traumatic etiology should be referred for a gynecologic work-up if there is a history of fever or night sweats or an indication of correlation between menses and symptomatology.

Special Questions for Men

Men describing symptoms related to the groin, low back, or SI joint may have some urologic involvement. The screening questions presented on the intake form assess the need for further medical follow-up.

A positive response to any or all of these questions may be evaluated further following the format provided in Chapter 7. Additional "Special Questions to Ask" are listed in the urology section and may assist the physical therapist in making an appropriate referral for a possible urologic evaluation.

Work Environment

Questions related to the patient's daily work activities and work environment are included to assist the physical therapist in planning a program of patient education consistent with the objective findings and proposed treatment plan. For example, the physical therapist is alerted to the need for follow-up with a patient complaining of back pain who sits for prolonged periods without a back support or cushion. Likewise, a worker involved in bending and twisting complaining of lateral thoracic pain may be describing a muscular strain from repetitive overuse. These work-related questions may help the patient to report significant data contributing to symptoms that may otherwise have been undetected.

Vital Signs

Assessment of baseline vital signs including resting pulse, blood pressure, and temperature should be a part of the initial data collected so that correlations and comparisons with the baseline may be made available when necessary. Ancillary staff can be trained to perform these simple tests. Normal ranges of values for the vital signs are provided for your convenience. However, these ranges can be exceeded by a patient and still represent normalcy for that person. It is the unusual vital sign in combination with other signs and symptoms, medications, and medical status that gives clinical meaning to the pulse rate, blood pressure, and temperature.

Pulse Rate. A resting pulse rate (normal range: 60 to 100 beats/min), taken at the carotid artery or radial artery pulse point should be available for comparison with the pulse rate taken during treatment or after exercise. A pulse increase of over 20 beats/min, lasting for more than 3 minutes after rest or changing position, should be a warning to alert the physical therapist to the need for medical follow-up or intervention (Muthe, 1981). The resting pulse may be higher than normal with fever, anemia, infections, some medications, hyperthyroidism, or if the patient is in pain.

Blood Pressure. Blood pressure should also be obtained and correlated with any related diet or medication. The normal range varies slightly with age. These values range from 90/70 mm Hg to 140/90 mm Hg for young adults. The upper limit or normotensive values for elderly men are 160/100 mm Hg and for elderly women 170/90 mm Hg (Barnard and Evans, 1985). The blood pressure should be taken in the same arm and in the same position (supine or sitting) each time that blood pressure is measured, and this information should be recorded with the initial reading. Blood pressure depends on many factors including age, vessel size, blood viscosity, force of contraction, current medications, diet, and presence and perceived degree of pain. A change in blood pressure of 20 mm Hg (of either the diastolic or systolic reading) would require a change in position. A persistent fall or rise of blood pressure requires medical attention or intervention (Muthe, 1981).

Temperature. The temperature (normal range: 97 to 100.2°F) must be taken for any patient who has back, hip, SI, or groin pain. Temperature should also be assessed for any patient who has night sweats (gradual increase followed by a sudden drop in body temperature), pain, or symptoms of unknown etiology, and for patients who have not previously been medically screened by a physician. When measuring body temperature, the physical therapist should ask if the patient's normal temperature differs from 98.6°F.

Core Interview

History of Present Illness

The history of present illness (often referred to as the chief complaint) may best be obtained through the use of open-ended questions. This section of the interview attempts to elicit data described by the patient that is related specifically to the reason(s) for seeking clinical treatment.

Statements such as those following are appropriate to start an interview:

- Tell me why you are here today.
- Tell me about your injury.

An alternate form of these statements might be:

- What do you think is causing your problem or pain?

During this phase of the interview, allow the patient to carefully describe his or her current situation. FUPs and paraphrasing can now be used in conjunction with the primary, open-ended description. The core interview in its entirety with suggested follow-up questions is presented in the following chart on page 22.

Assessment of Pain and Symptoms

There are many possible reasons for pain and many types of pain. Physical therapists frequently see patients whose primary complaint is pain, which often leads to a loss of function. Usually, a careful assessment of pain behavior is invaluable in determining the nature and extent of the underlying pathology. Development of an appropriate treatment program and evaluation of progress may depend mainly on an assessment of pain (Kessler and Hertling, 1983). Therefore, this portion of the core interview regarding a patient's perception of pain is a critical factor in the evaluation of signs and symptoms.

The interviewing techniques and specific questions used foster a description of the patient that is clear, accurate, and comprehensive. Questions must be understood by the patient and should be presented in a nonjudgmental atmosphere. To elicit a more complete description of symptoms from the patient, the physical therapist may wish to use a term other than "pain." For example, referring to the patient's "symptoms" or using descriptors such as "hurt" or "sore" may be more helpful to some individuals (Jacox, 1977). If the patient has completed the McGill Pain Questionnaire, you may choose the most appropriate alternate word selected by the patient from the list to refer to the symptoms.

THE CORE INTERVIEW

History of Present Illness

Chief Complaint (Onset):

- Tell me why you are here today.
- Tell me about your injury.

Alternate question: What do you think is causing your problem/pain?

FUPs: How did this injury or illness begin?

Was your injury or illness associated with a fall, trauma, or repetitive activity (e.g., painting, cleaning, gardening, filing papers)?

When did the present problem arise and did it occur gradually or suddenly?

Systemic: gradual onset without known cause.

Have you ever had anything like this before? If yes, when did it occur? Describe the situation and the circumstances.

How many times has this illness occurred? Tell me about each occasion.

Is there any difference this time from the last episode?

How much time elapses between episodes?

Do these episodes occur more or less often?

Systemic disease may present in a gradual, progressive, cyclical onset: worse, better, worse.

Pain/Symptom Assessment

- Do you have any pain associated with your injury or illness? If yes, tell me about it.

Location

- Show me exactly where your pain is located.

FUPs: Do you have this same pain anywhere else?

Do you have any other pain or symptoms anywhere else?

If yes, what causes the pain or symptoms to occur in this other area?

Description

- What does it feel like?

FUPs: Has the pain changed in quality, intensity, frequency, or duration (how long it lasts) since it first began?

Pattern

- Tell me about the pattern of your pain or symptoms.
- Alternate question: How does your pain or symptoms change with time?

FUPs: Have you ever experienced anything like this before?

If yes, do these episodes occur more or less often?

When does your back/shoulder/(name body part) hurt?

Describe your pain/symptoms to me from first waking up in the morning to going to bed at night. (See the special questions regarding "sleep" that follow.)

Are your symptoms worse in the morning or in the evening?

The Core Interview *(continued)*

Frequency

- How often does the pain/symptoms occur?

FUPs: Is your pain constant or does it come and go (intermittent)?
Are you having this pain right now?
Did you notice these symptoms this morning immediately after awakening?

Duration

- How long does the pain/symptom(s) last?

Systemic disease: constant

Intensity

- On a scale from 0 to 10 with 0 being no pain and 10 being the worst pain you have experienced with this condition, what level of pain do you have right now?
- Alternate question: How strong is your pain (Melzack, 1975)?
  1 = mild
  2 = uncomfortable
  3 = distressing
  4 = horrible
  5 = excruciating

FUPs: Which word describes your pain right now? ____________
Which word describes the pain at its worst? ____________
Which word describes the least amount of pain? ____________

Systemic: tends to be intense

Associated Symptoms

- What other symptoms have you had that you can associate with this problem?

FUPs: Have you experienced any:

Burning	Hoarseness	Problems with vision
Difficulty in breathing	Nausea	Tingling
Difficulty in swallowing	Night sweats	Vomiting
Dizziness	Numbness	Weakness
Heart palpitations		

Systemic: presence of symptoms bilaterally (e.g., bilateral weakness, tingling, burning). Determine the frequency, duration, intensity, and pattern of symptoms. Blurred vision, double vision, scotomas (black spots before the eyes), or temporal blindness may indicate early symptoms of multiple sclerosis (MS), cerebral vascular accident (CVA), or other neurologic disorders.

Aggravating Factors

- What kinds of things affect the pain?

FUPs: What makes your pain/symptoms worse (e.g., eating, exercise, rest, specific positions, excitement, stress)?

Relieving Factors

- What makes it better?

The Core Interview *(continued)*

Systemic: unrelieved by change in position or by rest

- How does rest affect the pain/symptoms?

FUPs: Are your symptoms aggravated or relieved by any activities? If yes, what?
How has this problem affected your daily life at work or at home?
Your ability to care for yourself without assistance (e.g., dress, bathe, cook, drive)?

Medical Treatment and Medications

Treatment

- What medical treatment have you had for this condition?

FUPs: Have you been treated by a physical therapist for this condition before?
If yes, when?
Where?
How long?
What helped?
What didn't help?
Was there any treatment that made your symptoms worse? If yes, please elaborate.

Medications

- Are you taking any prescription or over-the-counter medications?

FUPs: If no, you may have to probe further regarding use of laxatives, aspirin, acetaminophen (Tylenol), and so forth.
If yes, what medication did you take?
How often?
What dose did you take?
What are you taking these medications for?
When was the last time that you took these medications? Have you taken these drugs today?
Do the medications relieve your pain or symptoms?
If yes, how soon after you take the medications do you notice an improvement?
If the drugs are on prescription, who prescribed them for you?
How long have you been taking these medications?
When did your physician last review these medications?

Current Level of Fitness

- What is your present exercise level?

FUPs: What type of exercise or sports do you participate in?
How many times do you participate each week (frequency)?
When did you start this exercise program (duration)?
How many minutes do you exercise during each session (intensity)?
Are there any activities that you cannot do now that you could do before your injury or illness? If yes, please describe.

Dyspnea: Do you ever experience any shortness of breath (SOB) or lack of air during any activities (e.g., walking, climbing stairs)?

The Core Interview *(continued)*

FUPs: Are you ever short of breath without exercising?
If yes, how often?
When does this occur?
Do you ever wake up at night and feel breathless?
If yes, how often?
When does this occur?

Sleep-Related

- Can you get to sleep at night? If no, try to determine if the reason is due to the sudden decrease in activity and quiet, which causes you to focus on the symptoms.
- Are you able to lie or sleep on that side?
  If yes, the condition may be considered to be chronic, and treatment would be more vigorous than if no, indicating a more acute condition requiring more conservative treatment.
- Do you ever wake up from a deep sleep by pain?

FUPs: If yes, do you awaken because you have rolled onto that side?
If yes, may indicate a subacute condition requiring a combination of treatment approaches depending on objective findings.

- Can you get back to sleep?

FUPs: If yes, what do you have to do (if anything) to get back to sleep?
(The answer may provide clues for treatment.)

- Have you had any unexplained fevers, night sweats, or unexplained perspiration?

Systemic: Fevers and night sweats are characteristic signs of systemic disease.

Stress

- What major life changes or stresses have you encountered that you would associate with your injury/illness?

Alternate questions: What situations in your life are "stressors" for you?

- On a scale from 0 to 10, with 0 being no stress and 10 being the most extreme stress you have ever experienced, in general, what number rating would you give to your stress at this time in your life?
- What number would you assign to your level of stress today?

Final Question

- Do you wish to tell me anything else about your injury, your health, or your present symptoms that we have not discussed yet?

The use of alternate words to describe a patient's symptoms may also aid in refocusing attention away from pain and more toward improvement of functional abilities.

Sources of Pain. When listening to the patient's description of pain there are four general sources of pain that must be considered:

Cutaneous (related to the skin). This source of pain includes superficial somatic structures located in the skin and subcutaneous tissue. The pain is well localized because the patient can point directly to the area that "hurts." Cutaneous (skin) tenderness may occur with both referred or deep somatic pain (Jacox, 1977).

Deep Somatic (related to the wall of the body cavity; parietal). This type of pain includes bone, nerve, muscle, tendon, ligaments, periosteum, cancellous (spongy) bone, arteries, and joints. Whereas the visceral pleura is insensitive to pain, the parietal pleura is well supplied with pain nerve endings. Deep somatic pain is poorly localized and may be referred to the body surface (cutaneous). This type of pain can be associated with an autonomic phenomenon, such as sweating, pallor, reduced blood pressure, and is commonly accompanied by a subjective feeling of nausea and faintness. Pain associated with deep somatic lesions follows patterns that relate to the embryologic development of the musculoskeletal system (Kessler and Hertling, 1983).

Visceral (related to internal organs). This type of pain includes all body organs located in the trunk or abdomen, such as the organs of the respiratory, digestive, urogenital, and endocrine systems, as well as the spleen, the heart, and the great vessels. The site of pain corresponds to dermatomes from which the diseased organ receives its innervation (see Fig. 6–1). Pain is not well localized because innervation of the viscera is multisegmental with few nerve endings. Additionally, although the viscera experience pain, the visceral pleura (membrane enveloping organs) is insensitive to pain. It is possible that a patient can have extensive disease without pain until the disease progresses enough to involve the parietal pleura (Bauwens and Paine, 1983; Travell and Simons, 1983; Way, 1983).

Referred (related to a remote origin). This source of pain includes all cutaneous, deep somatic, and visceral structures. It may occur in addition to or in the absence of deep somatic and true visceral pain. Referred pain is well localized (i.e., the patient can point directly to the area that hurts), but occurs in remote areas supplied by the same neurosegment as the diseased organ by way of shared central pathways for afferent neurons. Referred pain occurs usually when the painful stimulus is sufficiently intense or when the pain threshold of an organ has been lowered by disease (Blacklow, 1983). Referred pain can occur alone without accompanying visceral pain, but usually visceral pain precedes the development of referred pain when an organ is involved.

Characteristics of Pain. It is very important to be able to identify how the patient's description of pain as a symptom relates to these four sources. Many characteristics of pain can be elicited from the patient during the core interview to help to define the type of pain in question. These characteristics include:

- Location
- Description of sensation
- Pattern
- Frequency
- Intensity or duration

Other additional components are related to factors that aggravate the pain, factors that relieve the pain, and other symptoms that may occur that are associated with the pain. Specific questions are included for each descriptive component. Keep in mind that a gradual increase in frequency, intensity, or duration of symptoms over time can indicate systemic disease.

Location of Pain. Questions related to the location of pain focus the patient's description as precisely as possible. An opening statement might be:

- Show me exactly where your pain is located.

Follow-up questions may include:

- Do you have any other pain or symptoms anywhere else?
    - If yes, what causes the pain or symptoms to occur in this other area?

If the patient points to a small, localized area and pain does not spread, the cause is more likely to be a superficial lesion and is probably not severe. If the patient points to a small, localized area, but the pain does spread, this is more likely to be a diffuse, segmental referred pain that may originate in the viscera or deep somatic structure (Kessler and Hertling, 1983).

Description of the Sensation of Pain. To assist the physical therapist in obtaining a clear description of pain sensation, pose the question:

- What does it feel like?

Allow the patient some choices in potential descriptors. Some common words might include:

Knifelike	Dull
Boring	Burning
Throbbing	Prickly
Deep aching	Sharp

The use of an augmentary assessment tool such as the McGill Pain Questionnaire may assist in providing additional descriptors toward a more complete pain description. Follow-up questions may include:

- Has the pain changed in quality since it first began?
- Changed in intensity?
- Changed in frequency?
- Changed in duration (how long it lasts)?

When a patient describes the pain as knifelike, boring, or a deep aching feeling, this description should be a signal to the physical therapist to consider the possibility of a systemic origin of symptoms. Dull, somatic pain of an aching nature can be differentiated from the aching pain of a muscular lesion by squeezing or by pressing the muscle overlying the area of pain. Aching of muscular origin is reproduced by this method, whereas, aching of a deeper, somatic origin does not result in the reproduction of the symptoms.

Pattern of Pain. In determining the pattern of the pain, the patient should be asked to describe how the symptoms of pain change with time. Some choices may include (Melzack, 1975):

A	B	C
Continuous	Brief	Rhythmic
Steady	Momentary	Intermittent
Constant	Transient	Periodic

Follow-up questions may include:

- Have you ever had anything like this before?
- If yes, do these episodes occur more or less often?
- When does your back/shoulder (name the body part) hurt?
- Describe your pain/symptoms to me from when you wake up in the morning to when you go to bed at night. (See the following special questions regarding "Sleep.")

The pattern of pain associated with systemic disease is often a progressive pattern with a cyclical onset (i.e., the patient describes symptoms as being alternately worse, better, worse over a period of months). This pattern differs from the sudden sequestration of a discogenic lesion that presents with a pattern of increasingly worse symptoms followed by a sudden cessation of all symptoms. Such involvement of the disk occurs without the cyclical return of symptoms weeks or months later, which is more typical of a systemic disorder.

If the patient appears to be unsure of the pattern of symptoms or has "avoided paying any attention" to this component of pain description, it may be useful to keep a record at home assisting the patient to "live through" the symptoms for 24-hours. A chart such as the *McGill Home Recording Card* (Melzack, 1975) (Fig. 2–2) may help the patient to outline the existing pattern of the pain and can be used later in treatment to assist the therapist in detecting any change in symptoms.

A patient will frequently comment that the pain or symptoms have not changed despite 2 or 3 weeks of treatment with physical therapy. This information can be discouraging to both patient and therapist; however, when the symptoms are reviewed, there is in fact a de-

McGill Home Recording Card

NAME: ______________________ DATE STARTED: ______________

	Morning	Noon	Dinner	Bedtime
M				
Tu				
W				
Th				
F				
Sa				
Su				

Please record:

1. Pain intensity #:
   0 = no pain
   1 = mild
   2 = discomforting
   3 = distressing
   4 = horrible
   5 = excruciating
2. # analgesics taken
3. Note any unusual pain, symptoms or activities on back of card.
4. Record # hours slept in morning column.

Please note: If the patient previously rated the pain on a scale from 0–10, substitute the 0–10 scale in place of the 0-5 scale under Number 1 "Pain Intensity" above.

Figure 2–2. McGill home recording card. (From Melzack, R.: The McGill pain questionnaire: Major properties and scoring methods. Pain, *1*:298, 1975.)

crease in pain or other significant improvement in the pattern of symptoms. The improvement has been gradual and is best documented through the use of a baseline of pain activity established at an early stage in treatment by using a record such as the *Home Recording Card.*

Frequency and Duration. The frequency of occurrence is related closely to the pattern of the pain, and the patient should be asked about how often the symptoms occur and whether the pain is constant or intermittent. Duration of pain is a part of this description. How long do the symptoms last? For example, pain related to systemic disease has been shown to be a *constant* rather than an *intermittent* type of pain experience. Patients who indicate that the pain is constant should be asked:

- Do you have this pain right now?
- Did you notice these symptoms this morning immediately when you woke up?

Further responses may reveal that the pain is perceived as being constant but in fact is not actually present hourly.

Intensity. The level or intensity of the pain is an extremely important, but difficult, component to assess in the overall pain profile. Assist the patient with this evaluation by providing a rating scale. For example, the physical therapist might ask the patient to rate the pain on a scale from 0 (no pain) to 10 (worst pain experienced with this condition).

An alternative method provides a scale of one to 5 with word descriptions for each number (Melzack, 1975) and asks the question:

- How strong is your pain?
  1 = mild
  2 = discomforting
  3 = distressing
  4 = horrible
  5 = excruciating

As with the *Home Recording Card,* this scale for measuring the intensity of pain can be used to establish a baseline measure of pain for future reference. A patient who describes the pain as "excruciating" (or a 5 on the scale) during the initial interview may question the value of therapy when several weeks later there is no subjective report of improvement. A quick check of intensity by using this scale often reveals a decrease in the assigned number to pain levels. This can be compared with the initial rating, providing the patient with assurance and encouragement in the rehabilitation process.

Keep in mind that the description of intensity is highly subjective. What might be described as being "mild" for one person, could be "horrible" for another person. Careful assessment of the patient's nonverbal behavior (e.g., ease of movement, facial grimacing, guarding movements) and correlation of the patient's personality with his or her perception of the pain may help to clarify the description of the intensity of the pain. Pain of an intense, unrelenting (constant) nature is often associated with systemic disease.

Associated Symptoms. These symptoms may occur alone or in conjunction with the pain of systemic disease. The patient may or may not associate these additional symptoms with the chief complaint. The physical therapist may ask:

- What other symptoms have you had that you can associate with this problem?

If the patient denies any additional symptoms, follow up this question with a series of possibilities such as:

Burning
Difficulty in breathing
Difficulty in swallowing
Dizziness
Heart palpitations
Hoarseness
Nausea
Night sweats
Numbness
Problems with vision
Tingling
Vomiting

Any time the patient says "Yes" to such associated symptoms, check for the presence of these symptoms bilaterally. Additionally, bilateral weakness either proximally or distally should serve as an indicator of more than a musculoskeletal lesion.

Blurred vision, double vision, scotomas (black spots before the eyes), or temporary blindness may indicate early symptoms of MS or may possibly be warning signs of an impending CVA. The presence of any associated symptoms, such as those mentioned here, would require contact with the patient's physician to confirm the physician's knowledge of these symptoms.

Aggravating/Relieving Factors. Finally, a series of questions addressing aggravating and relieving factors must be included. The *McGill Pain Questionnaire* provides a chart like the one that follows that may be useful in determining the presence of relieving or aggravating factors (Melzack, 1975). A question related to aggravating factors could be:

- What kinds of things make your pain or symptoms worse (e.g., eating, exercise, rest, specific positions, excitement, stress)?

To assess relieving factors, ask the patient:

- What makes the pain better?

Follow-up questions include:

- How does rest affect the pain/symptoms?

	Indicate a + or a − opposite the appropriate factor*		
	Liquor		Sleep/rest
	Stimulants (e.g., caffeine)		Lying down
	Eating		Distraction (e.g., television)
	Heat		Urination/defecation
	Cold		Tension, stress
	Weather changes		Loud noises
	Massage		Going to work
	Pressure		Intercourse
	No movement		Mild exercise
	Movement		Fatigue
	Sitting		Standing

* From Melzack, R.: The McGill pain questionnaire: Major properties and scoring methods. Pain, *1*:277, 1975.

- Are your symptoms aggravated or relieved by any activities?
    - If yes, what?
- How has this problem affected your daily life at work or at home?
- How has this problem affected your ability to care for yourself without assistance (e.g., dress, bathe, cook, drive)?

Systemic pain tends to be relieved minimally, only relieved temporarily or unrelieved by change in position or by rest. However, musculoskeletal pain is *often* relieved both by a change of position and by rest.

In summary, careful, sensitive, and thorough questioning regarding the multifaceted experience of pain can elicit essential information necessary when making a decision regarding treatment or referral. The use of pain assessment tools may facilitate clear and accurate descriptions of this critical symptom.

Medical Treatment and Medications

Medical treatment includes any intervention performed by a physician (family practitioner or specialist), dentist, physician's assistant, nurse, nurse practitioner, physical therapist, or occupational therapist. The patient may also include chiropractic treatment when answering the question:

- What medical treatment have you had for this condition?

In addition to eliciting information regarding specific treatment performed by the medical community, follow-up questions key in on previous physical therapy treatment:

- Have you been treated by a physical therapist for this condition before?
    - If yes, when, where, and for how long?
- What helped and what didn't help?

- Was there any treatment that made your symptoms worse? If yes, please elaborate.

Knowing the patient's response to previous types of treatment techniques may assist the therapist in determining an appropriate treatment protocol for the current chief complaint. For example, previously successful treatment techniques described may provide a basis for initial treatment until the therapist can fully assess the objective data and consider all potential types of treatments.

Medications (either prescription or over-the-counter) may or may not be listed on the Family/Personal History intake form. Often, it is necessary to probe further regarding the use of aspirin, acetaminophen (Tylenol), laxatives, or other drugs that can alter the patient's symptoms. Knowing that medications can mask signs and symptoms or produce signs and symptoms that are seemingly unrelated to the patient's current medical problem, the therapist is advised to refer to a reference source (e.g., *Physician's Desk Reference [PDR], Nursing Drug Handbook 89,* or *United States Pharmacopeial Dispensing Information [USPDI],* usually available in hospital libraries or pharmacies) to check the potential side effects of all prescribed medications. For example, long-term use of steroids resulting in such side effects as proximal muscle weakness, tissue edema, and increased pain threshold may alter objective findings during the examination of the patient (Kessler and Hertling, 1983).

Appropriate FUPs include the following:

- Why are you taking these medications?
- When was the last time that you took these medications?
- Have you taken these drugs today?
- Do the medications relieve your pain or symptoms?
    - If yes, how soon after you take the medications do you notice an improvement?
- If prescription drugs, who prescribed this medication for you?
- How long have you been taking these medications?
- When did your physician last review these medications?

Many people who take prescribed medications cannot recall the name of the drug or tell you why they are taking it. If this is the case, the physician's office staff should be contacted to obtain information regarding the patient's prescribed medications. It is important to know whether the patient has taken the medication before the examination because the symptomatic relief obtained by the patient (or possible side effects) may alter the objective findings. Similarly, knowledge of the time when the patient obtains maximum relief from pain may point to the optimal treatment time for therapy.

In the case of hypertensive medications, it is important to ask if the patient has taken the medication today. The physical therapist often finds it necessary to re-educate the patient regarding the importance of taking medications as prescribed (on a daily or regular basis). It is not unusual to hear a patient report, "I take my blood pressure pills when I feel my heart start to pound." The same situation may occur with patients taking anti-inflammatory drugs, antibiotics, or any other medications that must be taken consistently for a specified period to be effective.

Current Level of Fitness

An assessment of current physical activity and level of fitness (or recent levels [i.e., just before the onset of the current problem]) can provide additional necessary information relating to the origin of the patient's symptomatology. The level of fitness can be a valuable indicator of potential response to treatment based on the patient's motivation (i.e., the patients who are more physically active and healthy seem to be more motivated to return to that level of fitness through disciplined self-rehabilitation).

It is important to know what type of exercise or sports activity the patient participates in, the number of times per week (frequency) that this activity is performed, the length (duration) of each exercise or sports session as well as how long the patient has been exercising (i.e., weeks, months, years), and the level of difficulty of each exercise session (intensity). It is very important to ask:

- Since the onset of symptoms, are there any activities that you can no longer accomplish?

The patient should give a detailed description concerning these activities including how physical activities have been affected by the symptoms.

Follow-up questions include:

- Do you ever experience SOB or lack of air during any activities (e.g., walking, climbing stairs)?
- Are you ever short of breath without exercising?
- Are you ever awakened at night breathless?
  - If yes, how often and when does this occur?

Sleep-Related History

Sleep patterns are valuable indicators of underlying physiologic and psychologic disease processes. The primary function of sleep is believed to be the restoration of body function. When the quality of this restorative sleep is decreased, the body and mind cannot perform at optimal levels. Physical problems that result in pain, increased urination, shortness of breath, changes in body temperature, perspiration, or side effects of medications are just a few causes of sleep disruption. Any factor precipitating sleep deprivation can contribute to an increase in the frequency, intensity, or duration of a patient's symptoms.

For example, fevers and night sweats are characteristic signs of systemic disease. Night sweats occur as a result of a gradual increase followed by a sudden drop in body temperature. This change in body temperature can be related to pathologic changes in immunologic, neurologic, and endocrine function. Certain neurologic lesions may produce local changes in sweating associated with nerve distribution. For example, a patient with a spinal cord tumor may report changes in skin temperature above and below the level of the tumor. Any patient presenting with a history of either night sweats or fevers should be referred to the primary physician. This is especially true for patients with back pain or multiple joint pain without traumatic origin.

Pain is usually perceived as being more intense during the night due to the lack of outside distraction when the patient lies quietly without activity. The sudden quiet surroundings and lack of external activity create an increased perception of pain that is a major disruptor of sleep. It is very important to ask the patient about pain during the night. Is the patient able to get to sleep? If not, the pain may be a primary focus and may become continuously intense so that falling asleep is a problem.

Does a change in body position affect the level of pain? If a change in position can increase or decrease the level of pain, it is more likely to be a musculoskeletal problem. If, however, the patient is awakened from a deep sleep by pain in any location, which is unrelated to physical trauma and is unaffected by a change in position, then it may be an ominous sign of serious systemic disease, particularly cancer. FUPs include:

- If you wake up because of pain, is it because you rolled onto that side?
- Can you get back to sleep?
  - If yes, what do you have to do (if anything) to get back to sleep? (This answer may provide clues for treatment.)

There are many other factors (primarily environmental and psychologic) associated with sleep disturbance, but a good, basic assessment of the main characteristics of physically related disturbances in sleep pattern can provide valuable information related to treatment or referral decisions.

Psychogenic Considerations

By using the interviewing tools and techniques described in this chapter, the physical therapist can communicate a willingness to consider all aspects of illness, whether biologic or psychologic. Patient self-disclosure is unlikely if there is no trust in the health professional, fear of a lack of confidentiality by the patient, or a sense of disinterest for the patient.

Stress. Most symptoms (pain included) are aggravated by unresolved emotional stress. Prolonged stress may lead gradually to physiologic changes. The effects of emotional stress may be increased by physiologic changes brought on by the use of medications or poor diet and health habits (e.g., cigarette smoking or ingestion of caffeine in any form). Finally, the patient's ability to remember secondary to the use of medications, age, depression, anxiety, or other factors may limit information given.

As part of the core interview, the physical therapist may assess the patient's subjective report of stress by asking:

- What major life changes or stresses have you encountered that you would associate with your injury/illness?

or

- What situations in your life are "stressors" for you?

It may be helpful to quantify the stress by asking the patient:

- On a scale from 0 to 10, with 0 being no stress and 10 being the most extreme stress you have ever experienced, what number rating would you give to your stress in general at this time in your life?

Emotions such as fear and anxiety are common reactions to illness and treatment and may increase the patient's awareness of pain and symptoms. These emotions may cause autonomic (branch of nervous system not subject to voluntary control) distress manifested in such symptoms as pallor, restlessness, muscular tension, perspiration, stomach pain, diarrhea or constipation, or headaches.

After the objective evaluation has been completed, the physical therapist can often provide immediate relief of emotionally based symptoms by explaining the cause of pain, by outlining a treatment plan, and by providing a realistic prognosis for improvement. This may not be possible if the patient demonstrates signs of hysterical symptoms or conversion symptoms.

Conversion Symptoms. Conversion symptoms are defined as a transformation of an emotion into a physical manifestation. These symptoms may present as hysterical pain, weakness, sensory changes, or paralysis. There is no etiology or disease that can explain the distribution of such symptoms. A conversion syndrome should be left up to the diagnosis and treatment management of a highly skilled specialist. However, the physical therapist should be able to recognize potential conversion symptoms in order to make an appropriate referral.

Clinical Signs of Conversion

These five clinical signs of conversion should be considered by the physical therapist during the core interview.

Bizarre Gait Pattern. The presenting feature is an unusual limp that cannot be explained by functional anatomy. Family members may be interviewed to assess whether there has been a change in the patient's gait and whether this is consistently present under the same aggravating factors. The physical therapist can look for a change in the wear pattern of the patient's shoes to decide whether this change in gait has been long-standing.

Muscle Strength. During manual muscle testing, true weakness results in smooth "giving way" of a muscle group; in hysterical weakness, the muscle "breaks" in a series of jerks.

Inconsistency. Extremity(ies) may appear to be flaccid during recumbency, yet the patient can walk on heels and toes when standing. A disparity occurs between manual muscle testing and functional performance that cannot be explained.

Movement Patterns. Various movements are performed slowly and extremely laboriously with facial grimaces. During functional tests, arms wave and the trunk oscillates with apparent tremendous effort.

Sensory Changes. Paresthesia or dysesthesia is a modification in sensation, usually with a sense of numbness or tingling, burning, or crawling. The sensation may be produced by slight pressure of clothes and may be described "as though worms are crawling over me" (Wolf, 1977). The physical therapist should carefully evaluate and document all sensory changes. Conversion symptoms are less likely to follow any dermatomal, myotomal, or sclerotomal patterns.

HOSPITAL INPATIENT INFORMATION

Medical Chart

The core interview presented in this chapter can provide the physical therapist with the basic information required for beginning to assess the patient's condition. Treatment of hospital or nursing home inpatients provides a slightly different interview (or information gathering) format. Reviewing the patient's chart thoroughly for information (see the following chart) will assist the physical therapist in developing a safe and effective treatment plan. It is important for the physical therapist to be aware of this vital information before beginning treatment. Important information to look for might include:

- Patient's age
- Diagnosis
- Surgery
- Physician's report
- Associated or additional problems relevant to physical therapy
- Medications
- Restrictions
- Laboratory results
- Vital signs

HOSPITAL INPATIENT INFORMATION

Medical Chart

- **Patient age**
- **Diagnosis**
- **Surgery:** Did the patient have surgery?
  - **FUPs:** See surgery on page 18 in this chapter.
- **Physician's Report**
  - **FUPs:** Check the physician's preoperative and postoperative orders (Was the patient treated preoperatively by a physical therapist for gait, strength, or range of motion evaluation?)
    - What are the short-term and long-term medical treatment plans?
    - Are there contraindications for treatment?
    - Are there weight-bearing limitations?
- **Associated or Additional Problems**

Such as diabetes, heart disease, peripheral vascular disease, respiratory involvement.

- **FUPs:** Are there complaints of any kind that may affect exercise?
  - If diabetic, what are the current blood/glucose levels (normal range: 70 to 120 mg/dl)?
  - When is insulin administered? (Use to determine the peak insulin levels in planning an exercise schedule).

- **Medications** (what, when received, what for, potential side effects).

FUPs: Is the patient receiving oxygen or receiving fluids/medications through an intravenous line?

- **Restrictions:** Are there any dietary or fluid restrictions?
  FUPs: If yes, check with the nursing staff to determine the patient's full limitation.
  Are ice chips or a wet washcloth permissible?
  How many ounces or cubic centimeters of fluid are allowed during therapy?
- **Laboratory Values:** Hematocrit/hemoglobin level (See Chapter 3 for normal values and significance of these tests.)
- **Vital signs:** Is the blood pressure stable?
  FUPs: If no, consider initiating standing with a tilt table or monitoring the blood pressure before, during, and after treatment.

Nursing Assessment

- **Medical Status:** What is the patient's current medical status?
- **Pain:** What is the nursing assessment of this patient's pain level and pain tolerance?
- **Physical Status:** Has the patient been up at all yet?
  FUPs: If yes, is the patient sitting, standing, or walking? What is the time frame and distance involved, and how much assistance is required?
- **Patient Orientation:** Is the patient oriented to time, place, and person?
  (i.e., does the patient know the date and the approximate time, where he or she is, and who he or she is?)
- **Discharge Plans:** Are there any known or suspected discharge plans?
  FUPs: If yes, what are these plans and when will the patient be discharged?
- **Final Question:** Is there anything else that I should know before exercising the patient?

An evaluation of the patient's medical status in conjunction with age and diagnosis can provide valuable guidelines for treatment. The neurophysiologic and behavioral implications of the aging process are well documented and should be considered on an individual basis (Jackson, 1987).

If the patient has had recent surgery, the physician's report should be scanned for preoperative and postoperative orders. For example, was the patient treated preoperatively with physical therapy for gait, strength, range of motion, or other objective assessments? Other valuable information that may be contained in the physician's report may include:

- What are the current short-term and long-term medical treatment plans?
- Are there any known or listed contraindications to physical therapy treatment?
- Does the patient have any weight-bearing limitations?

Associated or additional problems to the primary diagnosis may be found within the chart contents (e.g., diabetes, heart disease, peripheral vascular disease, or respiratory involvement). The physical therapist should look for any of these conditions in order to modify exercise accordingly and to look for any related signs and symptoms that might affect the exercise program.

- Are there complaints of any kind that may affect exercise (e.g., shortness of breath [dyspnea], heart palpitations, rapid heart rate (tachycardia), fatigue)?

If the patient is diabetic:

- What are the current blood-glucose levels?
- When is insulin administered?

The use of peak insulin levels in planning exercise schedules is discussed more completely in the Chapter 5. Other questions related to medications can follow the core interview outline with appropriate follow-up questions:

- Is the patient receiving oxygen or receiving fluids/medications through an intravenous line?
- Are there any dietary or fluid restrictions?
    - If so, check with the nursing staff to determine the patient's full limitations. For example:
- Are ice chips or wet washcloths permissible?
- How many ounces or milliliters of fluid are allowed during therapy?
- Where should this amount be recorded?

Laboratory values and vital signs should be reviewed. For example:

- Is the patient anemic?
- Is the patient's blood pressure stable?

Anemic patients may demonstrate an increased normal resting pulse rate that should be monitored during exercise. Patients with unstable blood pressure may require initial standing with a tilt table or monitoring of the blood pressure before, during, and after treatment. Check the nursing record for pulse rate at rest and blood pressure to use as a guide when taking vital signs in the clinic or at the patient's bedside.

Nursing Assessment

After reading the patient's chart, check with the nursing staff to determine the nursing assessment of the individual patient. The essential components of the nursing assessment that are of value to the physical therapist may include:

- Medical status
- Pain
- Physical status
- Patient orientation
- Discharge plans

The nursing staff are usually intimately aware of the patient's current medical and physical status. If pain is a factor:

- What is the nursing assessment of this patient's pain level and pain tolerance?

Pain tolerance is relative to the medications received by the patient; the number of days after surgery or after injury; fatigue; and the patient's personality.

To assess the patient's physical status, ask the nursing staff:

- Has the patient been up at all yet?
- If yes, how long has the patient been sitting, standing, or walking?
- How far has the patient walked?
- How much assistance does the patient require?

Ask about the patient's orientation.

- Is the patient oriented to time, place, and person?

In other words, does the patient know the date and the approximate time, where he or she is, and who he or she is? Treatment plans may be altered by the patient's awareness, for example, making a home program impossible without family compliance.

- Are there any known or expected discharge plans?
- If yes, what are these plans and when is the target date for discharge?

Cooperation between nurses and the physical therapist is an important part of the multidisciplinarian approach to planning the patient's treatment. The aforementioned questions to present and factors to consider provide the physical therapist with the basic hospital or nursing home-related information necessary to carry out an objective examination and to plan a treatment protocol. Each individual patient's situation may require that the physical therapist obtain additional information pertinent to each case.

PHYSICIAN REFERRAL

The physical therapist may be able to determine detailed and specific information regarding symptoms of possible systemic origin by using the questions presented in this chapter to interview the patient and then by correlating the patient's answers with family/personal history, vital signs, and objective findings from the physical examination. This information is not designed to be used to provide the patient with a medical diagnosis, but rather to accurately assess pain and systemic symptoms that may mimic or occur simultaneously with a musculoskeletal problem.

In each chapter, a list of possible signs or symptoms is provided for your consideration when making an evaluation and referral. The following list of systemic signs and symptoms were evaluated as part of the subjective examination. As always, correlate *history* with *patterns of pain* and any *unusual findings* that may indicate *systemic disease.*

Systemic Signs and Symptoms Requiring Physician Referral

Blood in urine
Constant pain
Cyclical pattern of symptoms
Difficulty swallowing
Difficulty with urination
Dizziness
Dyspnea (shortness of breath)
Faintness
Fever
Heart palpitations
Nausea
Night pain
Night sweats
Pain description
  Boring
  Knifelike
  Deep ache
Pain on urination
Problems with vision
Symptoms present bilaterally
Temporary relief or no relief with rest or change of position
Unexplained excessive perspiration
Unusual menstrual history
Vomiting
Weight loss

SUMMARY

Careful questioning during the subjective assessment can save time and can provide direction in planning the objective examination. All information (either positive or negative) from the interview must be correlated with objective findings before an accurate assessment of the patient's condition can be determined. In turn, the assessment is the basis for establishing goals and for determining the treatment plan.

Briefly, the areas addressed within this chapter have included:

- Interviewing techniques
- Interviewing tools
- Subjective examination
    - Family/personal history
    - Core interview
- Hospital inpatient medical chart and nursing assessment
- Psychogenic considerations

The information presented in this chapter is based on the assumption that the reader has taken a course or has completed some extra reading about interviewing techniques. The guidelines presented here provide information that should supplement previous knowledge of these techniques and tools. Any clinician who decides to use the interview tools presented here is advised to read the original articles describing the research and intentions for use of these pain scales.

Finally, the following list of **dos** and **don'ts** is a summary of the preceding text and is by no means an exhaustive record of interviewing skills.

LIST OF THINGS TO DO AND NOT TO DO

DOs

Do use a sequence of questions that begins with open-ended questions.

Do leave closed-ended questions for the end as clarifying questions.

Do select a private location where confidentiality can be maintained.

Do listen attentively and show it both in your body language and by occasionally making reassuring verbal prompts, such as "I see" or "Go on."

Do ask one question at a time and allow the patient to answer the question completely before continuing with the next question.

Do encourage the patient to ask questions throughout the interview.

Do listen with the intention of assessing the patient's current level of understanding and knowledge of this person's current medical condition.

Do eliminate unnecessary information and speak to the patient at his or her level of understanding.

Do correlate signs and symptoms with medical history and objective findings to rule out systemic disease.

Do provide several choices or selections to questions that require a descriptive response.

DON'Ts

Don't jump to premature conclusions based on the answers to one or two questions. Correlate all subjective and objective information and consult with a physician.

Don't interrupt or takeover the conversation when the patient is speaking.

Don't destroy helpful open-ended questions with closed-ended follow-up questions before the patient has a chance to respond (e.g., How do you feel this morning? Has your pain gone?).

Don't use professional or medical jargon when it is possible to use common language (e.g., using the term myocardial infarct versus heart attack).

Don't overact to information presented. Common overeactions include raised eyebrows, puzzled facial expressions, gasps, or other verbal exclamations such as "Oh, really?" or "Wow!" Less dramatic reactions may include facial expressions or gestures that indicate approval or disapproval, surprise or sudden interest. These responses may influence what the patient does or does not tell you.

Don't use leading questions. Pain is difficult to describe, and it may be easier for the patient to agree with a partially correct statement than to attempt to clarify points of discrepancy between your statement and his or her pain experience (Jacox, 1977).

Leading Questions	Better Presentation of the Same Question
Where is your pain?	Do you have any pain associated with your injury? If yes, tell me about it.
Does it hurt when you first get out of bed?	When does your back hurt?
Does the pain radiate down your leg?	Do you have this pain anywhere else?
Do you have pain in your lower back?	Point to the exact location of your pain.

CASE STUDY*

Referral

Your latest referral is a 28-year-old, white man who has had a diagnosed progressive idiopathic Raynaud syndrome of the bilateral upper extremities for the last 4 years. The patient has been examined by numerous physicians and by an orthopedist. He has complete numbness and cyanosis of the right second, third, fourth, and fifth digits upon contact with even a mild decrease in temperature. He says that his symptoms have progressed to the extent that they appear within seconds if he picks up a glass of cold water.

He works almost entirely outside, often in cold weather, and uses saws and other power equipment. The numbness has created a very unsafe job situation.

The patient received a gunshot wound in a hunting accident 6 years ago. The bullet entered the posterior left thoracic region, lateral to the lateral border of the scapula, and came out through the anterior, lateral, superior chest wall. He says that he feels as if his shoulders are constantly rolled forward. He reports no cervical, shoulder, or elbow pain or injury.

Physical Therapy Interview

Please note that not all of these questions would necessarily be presented to the patient, because his answers may determine the next question and may eliminate some questions.

Tell me why you are here today (open-ended question)?

Pain

Do you have any pain associated with your past gunshot wound?
If yes, describe your pain.
FUPs: Give the patient a chance to answer and prompt only if necessary

---

*This case study was adapted and used with permission from the primary physical therapist.

CASE STUDY

with suggested adjectives such as, "Is your pain sharp, dull, boring, or burning?" or "Show me on your body where you have pain."

To pursue this line of questioning, if appropriate:

FUPs: What makes your pain better or worse?

What is your pain like when you first get up in the morning, during the day, and in the evening?

Is your pain constant or does it come and go?

On a scale from 0 to 10 with zero being no pain and ten being the worst pain you have ever experienced with this problem, what level of pain would you say that you have ***right now***?

Do you have any other pain or symptoms that are not related to your old injury?

If yes, pursue as above to find out about the onset of pain, etc.

You indicated that you have numbness in your right hand. How long does this last?

FUPs: Besides, picking up a glass of cold water, what else brings it on?

How long have you had this problem?

You indicated that this numbness has progressed over time. How quickly has this progression occurred?

Do you ever have similar symptoms in your left hand?

Associated Symptoms

Even though this patient has been seen by numerous physicians, it is important to ask appropriate questions to rule out systemic origin of current symptoms, especially if there has been a recent change in the symptoms or presentation of symptoms bilaterally. For example:

What other symptoms have you had that you can associate with this problem?

In addition to the numbness, have you had any:

- Tingling
- Burning
- Weakness
- Vomiting
- Hoarseness
- Difficulty with breathing
- Nausea
- Dizziness
- Difficulty with swallowing
- Heart palpitations or fluttering
- Unexplained sweating or night sweats
- Problems with your vision

How well do you sleep at night? (Open-ended question)

Do you have trouble sleeping at night? (Closed-ended question)

Does the pain awaken you out of a sound sleep? Can you sleep on either side comfortably?

Medications

Are you taking any medications?

If yes, and the patient doesn't volunteer the information, probe further:

What medications?

What are you taking this medication for?

When did you take the medications last?

CASE STUDY

Do you think the medication is easing the symptoms or helping in any way?

Have you noticed any side effects? If yes, what are these effects?

Previous Medical Treatment

Have you had any recent x-rays?

If yes, find out where the x-rays were taken and also when and what parts of the body were x-rayed.

Tell me about your gunshot wound: Were you treated immediately?

Did you have any surgery at that time or since then?

If yes, pursue details with regard to what type of surgery, and where and when it occurred.

Did you have physical therapy treatment at any time after your accident?

If yes, relate when, for how long, with whom, what was done, did it help?

Functional Capacity

Are you right handed?

How do your symptoms affect your ability to do your job or work around the house?

In caring for yourself (showering, shaving, other activities of daily living such as eating or writing)?

Final Question

Is there anything else you feel that I should know about concerning your injury, such as your health or your present symptoms, that I have not asked about?

Note: If this patient had been a woman, the interview would have included questions about breast pain, the date when she was last screened for cancer with a physician (cervical and breast), and whether she does monthly self-screening examinations of her breasts.

References

Barnard, C., and Evans, P.: Your Healthy Heart. New York, McGraw-Hill, 1985.

Bauwens, D.B., and Paine, R.: Thoracic pain. *In* Blacklow, R.S. (ed): MacBryde's Signs and Symptoms, 6th ed. Philadelphia, J.B. Lippincott, 1983, pp. 139–164.

Bernstein, L., and Bernstein, R.: Interviewing: A Guide for Health Professionals. Norwalk, Appleton-Century-Crofts, 1985.

Blacklow, R.S. (ed): MacBryde's Signs and Symptoms, 6th ed. Philadelphia, J.B. Lippincott, 1983.

Cash, W.B., Jr., and Stewart, C.J.: Interviewing: Principles and Practices. Dubuque, W.C. Brown, 1985.

Jackson, O.L. (ed): Therapeutic Considerations for the Elderly. New York, Churchill-Livingstone, 1987.

Jacox, A.: Pain: A Source Book for Nurses and Other Health Professionals. Boston, Little, Brown, 1977.

Kessler, R.M., and Hertling, D.: Management of Common Musculoskeletal Disorders. Philadelphia, J.B. Lippincott, 1983.

Melzack, R.: The McGill pain questionnaire: Major properties and scoring methods. Pain, *1*:277, 1975.

Melzack, R., and Torgerson, W.S.: On the language of pain. Anesthesiology, *34*:50, 1971.

Muthe, N.C.: Endocrinology: A Nursing Approach. Boston, Little, Brown, 1981.

Pickney, C., and Pickney, E.R.: The Patient's Guide to Medical Tests, 3rd ed. New York, Facts on File, 1986.

Swisher, S.N., and Enelow, A.J.: Interviewing and Patient Care. London, Oxford University Press, 1973.

Travell, J.G., and Simons, D.G.: Myofascial Pain and Dysfunction: The Trigger Point Manual. Baltimore, Williams & Wilkins, 1983.

Way, L.W.: Abdominal pain. *In* Sleisenger, M.H., and Fortran, J.S. (eds): Gastrointestinal Disease, 2nd ed. Philadelphia, W.B. Saunders Company, 1983, pp. 207–221.

Wolf, G.A., Jr.: Collecting Data from Patients. Baltimore, University Park Press, 1977.

Wolf, S.L.: Clinical decision making in physical therapy. *In* Paris, S.: Clinical Decision Making: Orthopedic Physical Therapy. Philadelphia, F.A. Davis, 1985.

Wong, C.: Learning to Live with Angina. New York, MIPI Publications, 1981.

Bibliography

Advice for the patient, Vol. 2, 7th ed. United States Pharmacopeial Dispensing Information (USPDI), Rockville, 1987.

Barnhart, E.R. (ed): Physicians' Desk Reference, 43rd ed. Oradell, NJ, Medical Economics Co., Inc., 1989.

Bergner, M., Bobbitt, R.A., and Kressel, S.: The sickness impact profile: Conceptual formulation and methodology for the development of a health status measure. Int. J. Health Serv., *6*:393, 1976.

Fairbanks, J.C.T., Couper, J. Davies, J.B., and O'Brien, J.P.: The Oswestry low back pain disability questionnaire. Physiotherapy, *66*:271, 1980.

McKenzie, R.A.: The Lumbar Spine: Mechanical Diagnosis and Therapy. New Zealand, Spinal Publications, 1981.

Million, R., Hall, W., and Haavik, R.D.: Assessment of the progress of the back-pain patient. Spine, *7*:204, 1982.

Nursing 89 Drug Handbook. Springhouse, PA, Springhouse Corporation, 1989.

Roland, M., and Morris, R.: A study of the natural history of back pain. Part I: Development of a reliable and sensitive measure of disability in low-back pain. Spine, *2*:141, 1983.

Rose, S.J., Shulman, A.D., and Strube, M.J.: Functional assessment of patients with low back syndrome. Top. Geriatric Rehabilitation, *1*:9, 1986.

Shealy, N.C.: Electrical stimulation: The primary method of choice: Compr. Ther., *1*:41, 1975.

Waddell, G., and Main, C.J.: Assessment of severity of low-back disorders. Spine, *9*:204, 1984.

Chapter 3

Overview of Cardiovascular Signs and Symptoms

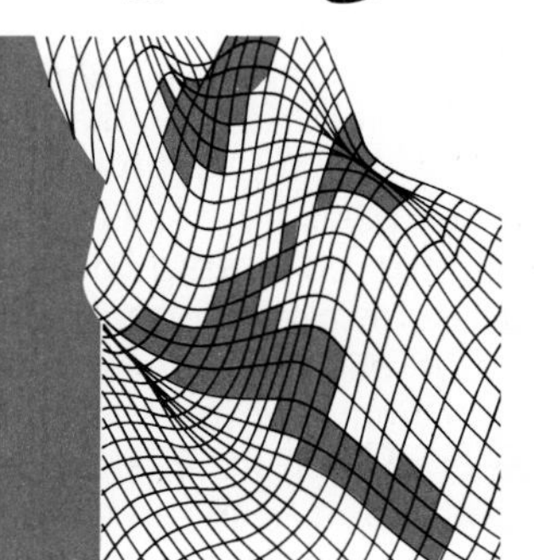

☐ ***Clinical Signs and Symptoms of:***

- Myocardial Ischemia
- Angina Pectoris
- Myocardial Infarct
- Pericarditis
- Left-Sided Heart Failure
- Right-Sided Heart Failure
- Aneurysm
- Cardiac Valvular Disease
- Rheumatic Fever
- Rheumatic Heart Disease
- Endocarditis
- Fibrillation
- Tachycardia
- Bradycardia
- Herpes Zoster (Shingles)
- Dorsal Nerve Root Irritation
- Thoracic Outlet Syndrome
- Gastrointestinal Disorders
- Breast Pathology
- Anxiety-Producing Chest Pain
- Arterial Disease
- Diabetic Coronary Atherosclerosis
- Arteriosclerosis Obliterans
- Buerger's Disease
- Venous Disorders
- Lymphedema
- Hypertension
- Transient Ischemic Attacks
- Orthostatic Hypotension

Heart disease today is the leading cause of death in industrialized nations. In the United States alone, cardiovascular disease (CVD) is responsible for approximately one million fatalities every year. Fortunately, during the last two decades, cardiovascular research has greatly increased our understanding of the structure and function of the cardiovascular system in health and disease; and despite the formidable statistics regarding the prevalence of CVD, during the last 15 years, a steady decline in mortality from cardiovascular disorders has been witnessed. Effective application of the increased knowledge regarding CVD and its risk factors will assist health care professionals to educate clients in achieving and maintaining cardiovascular health (Kavanagh, 1987).

CARDIAC PHYSIOLOGY

(Kavanagh, 1987)

Heart

The heart is a relatively small organ located in the middle of the mediastinum, where the lungs partially overlap it. This pulsatile four-chambered pump beats approximately 72 times/min and pumps more than 5 liters of blood each minute or about 2,000 gal/day. It continually propels oxygenated blood into the arterial system and receives poorly oxygenated blood from the venous system. The heart muscle rests on the diaphragm and is tilted forward and to the left so that the apex of the heart is rotated anteriorly.

The heart is enclosed by the pericardium, which consists of two layers (Fig. 3–1):

- Visceral pericardium (the inner layer)
- Parietal pericardium (the outer layer)

The two pericardial surfaces are separated by a pericardial space that normally contains approximately 10 to 20 ml of thin, clear pericardial fluid. This lubricating fluid moistens the contacting surfaces of the pericardial layers and serves to reduce the friction produced by the pumping action of the heart. The visceral pericardium actually encases the heart

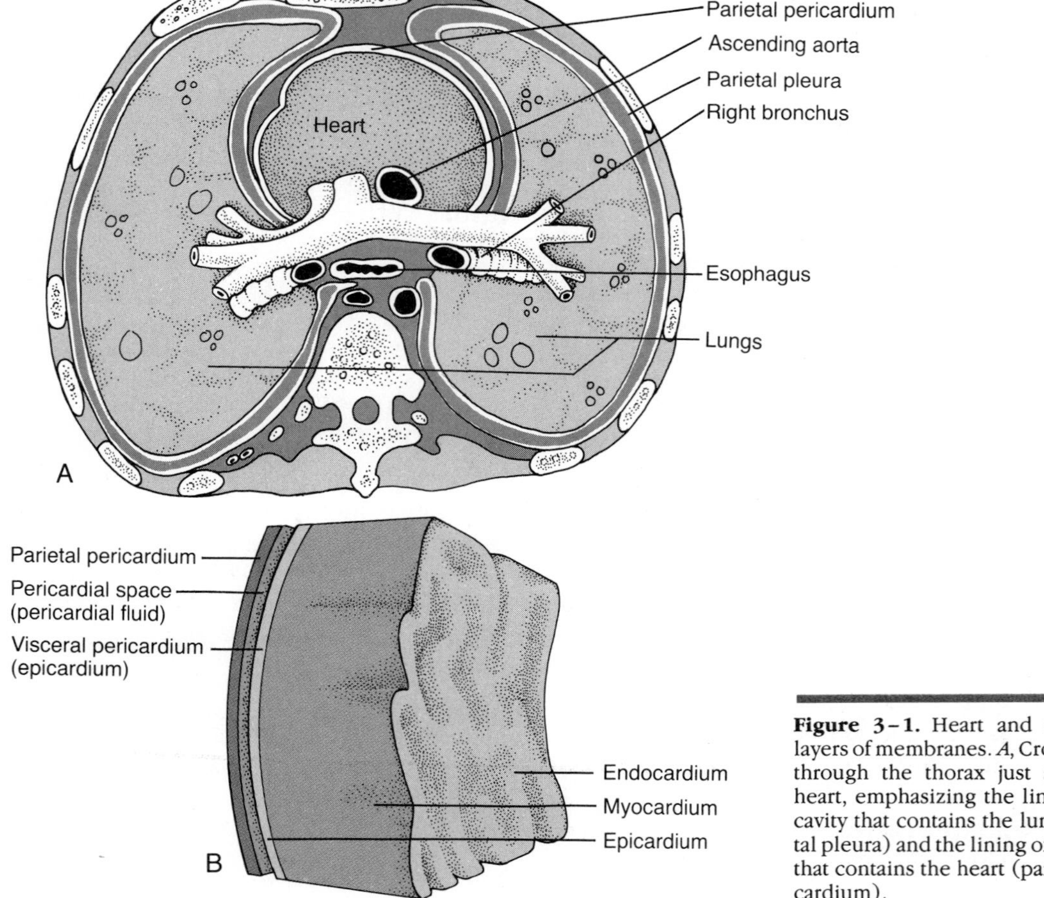

Figure 3–1. Heart and associated layers of membranes. *A*, Cross section through the thorax just above the heart, emphasizing the lining of the cavity that contains the lungs (parietal pleura) and the lining of the cavity that contains the heart (parietal pericardium).

and extends several centimeters onto each of the great vessels. The parietal pericardium is attached anteriorly to the manubrium and xiphoid process of the sternum, posteriorly to the vertebral column, and inferiorly to the diaphragm.

There are three layers of cardiac tissue:

- Epicardium (outer layer of the heart, which has the same structure as the visceral pericardium)
- Myocardium (middle layer of the heart, composed of striated muscle fibers)
- Endocardium (inner layer, consisting of endothelial tissue that lines the inside of the heart's chambers and covers the heart valves)

Coronary Arteries

The coronary arteries arise from the aorta (just behind the cusps of the aortic valve) in an area known as the sinuses of Valsalva. The function of the coronary artery system is to provide an adequate blood supply to the myocardium. Despite scientific advances in the field of cardiology, coronary artery disease and its complications are still the leading cause of death in the United States.

Two main coronary arteries supply blood to the myocardium. This supply occurs almost exclusively during diastole (heart relaxed between contractions), when coronary vascular resistance is diminished. During systole (heart contraction), coronary vascular resistance increases because of the increased ventricular wall tension produced by ventricular contraction.

Valves

The four cardiac valves are flaplike structures that function to maintain unidirectional (forward) blood flow through the heart chambers. These valves open and close in response to changes in pressure and volume within the heart chambers. The cardiac valves can be classified into two types: the atrioventricular (AV) valves, which separate the atria from the ventricles; and the semilunar valves, which separate the pulmonary artery and the aorta from their respective ventricles.

Atrioventricular

The AV valves include the:

- Tricuspid valve (located between the right atrium and the right ventricle)
- Bicuspid (mitral) valve (located between the left atrium and left ventricle)

The tricuspid valve contains three leaflets held in place by fibrous cords called the chordae tendineae. The mitral valve on the left side of the heart is a bicuspid valve with two valve cusps or leaflets. It is also attached by the chordae tendineae, which are extremely important because of the support they give to the AV valves during ventricular systole to prevent valvular prolapse (falling downward) into the atrium. There is also a degree of leaflet overlapping during closure of the AV valves, which helps to prevent the backward flow of blood.

Semilunar

The semilunar valves include the:

- Aortic valves
- Pulmonic valves

The structural design of the semilunar valves consists of three cuplike cusps. The valves lie between each ventricle and the great vessel into which it empties. These valves are open during ventricular systole (contraction) to permit blood flow into the aorta and pulmonary artery. They are closed during diastole (relaxation) to prevent retrograde (backward) flow from the aorta and pulmonary artery back into the ventricle when it is relaxed.

Cardiac Nervous System

The pacemaking center of the normal heart is the sinoatrial (SA) or "sinus" node, which is located in the right atrium near the root of the superior vena cava. This node consists of two types of specialized cells within a network of dense fibers. P cells in the center of the node initiate impulses at a rate of 60 to 100/min under normal conditions. T cells on the circumference transmit these impulses to surrounding atrial muscle.

Purkinje's fibers (modified cardiac muscle fibers) lie as a network on the endocardial surface and penetrate the myocardium of both ventricles. They transmit the impulse to both ventricular walls. Cells outside the conduction system also play a role in the conduction of an impulse, but further discussion of this mechanism is beyond the scope of this text.

Depolarization (rapid reversal of the resting membrane potential to generate an electrical current) is initiated by an impulse from the SA node. The impulse first spreads through the right atrium and then activates the left atrium. Shortly after the impulse reaches the left atrium, it also activates the region at the junction, and subsequently, the AV node. The impulse continues to activate the ventricular muscle from the apex toward the base of the heart to complete the process.

The heart rate is controlled primarily by the autonomic nervous system, but other factors such as body temperature, medication, hormones, and electrolyte concentrations can affect the heart rate. The control of the autonomic nervous system on the heart is mediated by neurotransmitters, but impulses from the cerebral cortex can have a significant effect on the heart rate. For example, pain, fear, anger, and excitement can all cause a substantial increase in the heart rate.

CARDIAC PATHOPHYSIOLOGY

Three components of cardiac disease are discussed:

Diseases affecting the heart muscle

Diseases affecting heart valves

Defects of the cardiac nervous system

Within these categories, there are diseases that are not mentioned, either because these diseases are rare or because they do not mimic musculoskeletal symptoms.

Diseases affecting the *heart muscle* include:

- Arterial diseases, such as coronary artery disease (CAD)
- Myocardial infarction
- Infections, such as pericarditis*
- Congestive heart failure (CHF; the heart's inability to pump adequately enough to circulate blood)
- Aneurysms (sac formed by the dilatation of the wall of an artery, a vein, or the heart)

Diseases affecting the *heart valves* include:

- Rheumatic fever
- Endocarditis (inflammation of the lining covering the heart and valves)
- Congenital deformities

Defects of the *cardiac nervous system* include:

- Arrhythmias (irregularity of the heartbeat), such as fibrillations (twitching of the heart muscle fibrils, but not the cardiac muscle as a whole)
- Tachycardia (rapid beating of the heart)
- Bradycardia (slowness of the heart beat)

Diseases Affecting the Heart Muscle

Coronary Artery Disease

CAD may also be referred to as arterial disease or coronary heart disease (CHD). In 1948, the United States government decided to investigate the etiology, incidence, and pathology of CAD by studying a typical small town in the United States called Framingham, Massachusetts. Over a period of 10, 20, and 30 years, the participants in the study began to die and when possible, postmortem examinations were conducted to ascertain the causes of death (Barnard and Evans, 1985). The research revealed important modifiable and

* The numerous terms to describe cardiac diseases and anatomy can be confusing. The reader is advised to refer to the glossary for a more complete definition of this term and others.

nonmodifiable risk factors associated with death caused by CHD.

Modifiable risk factors include smoking, hypertension, diabetes mellitus, gout, elevated serum (blood) cholesterol levels, sedentary life style, obesity, and the controversial type "A" personality (characterized by hostility anger, irritability, impatience, insecurity, and competitive drive). Nonmodifiable risk factors are sex (men are at greater risk), family history of heart disease, and age (Dawber et al, 1951).

CAD includes atheroma, which involves the slow deterioration of arteries in which fatty deposits or lipids such as triglycerides and cholesterol are laid down in the inner lining of

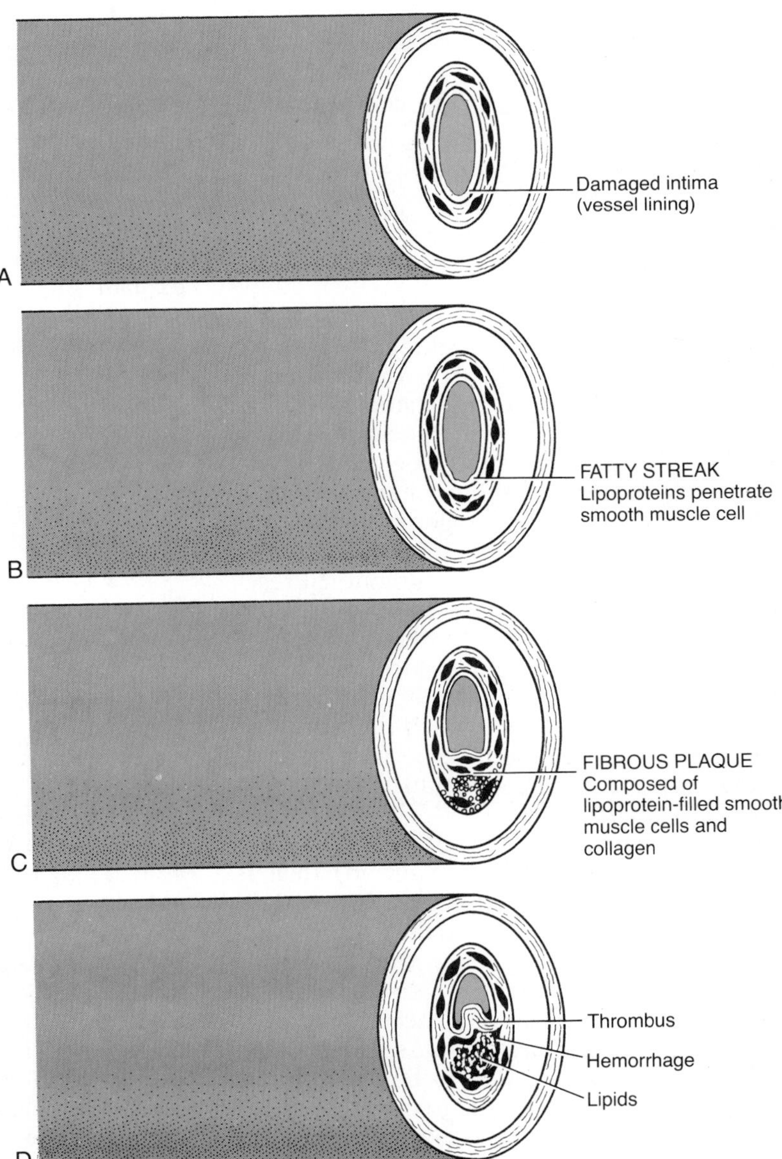

Figure 3-2. Hardening of the arteries. *A*, Atherosclerosis begins with an injury to the endothelial lining of the artery (intimal layer) that makes the vessel permeable to circulating lipoproteins. *B*, Penetration of lipoproteins into the smooth muscle cells of the intima produce "fatty streaks." *C*, A fibrous plaque large enough to decrease blood flow through the artery develops. *D*, Calcification with rupture or hemorrhage of the fibrous plaque is the final advanced stage. Thrombosis may occur to further occlude the lumen of the blood vessel.

the arterial walls, and arteriosclerosis, which is the thickening and hardening of the usually supple arterial walls (Fig. 3–2) (Barnard and Evans, 1985). The resultant plaque formation, a mixture of fat, cholesterol, blood cells, and fibrous tissue progressively narrows the arteries that carry blood rich in oxygen to the myocardium (the middle layer of the heart consisting of the heart muscle) and leads eventually to ischemia (inadequate circulation of blood) and to necrosis (death of tissue) of the heart muscle.

CLINICAL SYMPTOMS OF MYOCARDIAL ISCHEMIA

- Angina pectoris (chest pain)
- Eventual myocardial infarct (MI, i.e., necrosis or death of the heart muscle)

Angina Pectoris (Hindle and Wallace, 1987; Nursing 84). One of the most common and typical symptomatic indicators of CAD is pain in the chest or angina pectoris. Angina occurs when the cardiac workload and oxygen demands exceed the ability of affected coronary arteries to supply oxygen to myocardial tissue. In its chronic form, angina is activated usually by physical exertion, emotional reactions, a heavy meal, or exposure to the cold (Barnard and Evans, 1985). Although angina is a symptom of obstructed or decreased blood supply to the heart muscle, it is a transient symptom that is relieved when the workload of the heart is decreased. No permanent damage to myocardial tissue results when the patient has angina.

When the heart is required to supply greater blood flow (e.g., physical exertion) than is possible through clogged, constricted, or rigid arteries, ischemia occurs and the patient experiences the chest pain referred to as angina. The present theory of heart pain suggests that pain occurs as a result of an accumulation of metabolites within an ischemic segment of the myocardium. The transient ischemia of angina or the prolonged, necrotic ischemic of an MI sets off pain impulses secondary to rapid accumulation of metabolites in the heart muscle.

Angina is often confused with indigestion. The patient may indicate the location of the symptoms by placing a clenched fist against the sternum. Angina radiates most commonly to the left shoulder and down the inside of the arm to the fingers; but it can also refer pain to the neck, jaw, teeth, upper back, possibly down the right arm, and occasionally to the abdomen (see Fig. 3–6).

Pain associated with angina and myocardial infarction occurring along the inner aspect of the arm and corresponding to the ulnar nerve distribution, results from common connections between the cardiac and brachial plexus. Cardiac pain referred to the jaw occurs through internuncial (neurons connecting other neurons) fibers from cervical spinal cord posterior horns to the spinal nucleus of the trigeminal nerve. Abdominal pain produced by referred cardiac pain is more difficult to explain and may be due to the overflow of segmental levels to which visceral afferent nerve pathways flow (see Fig. 6–1). This overflow increases the chances that final common pain pathways between the chest and the abdomen may occur.

CLINICAL SYMPTOMS OF ANGINA PECTORIS

- Gripping, vicelike feeling of pain or pressure behind the breast bone
- Pain may radiate to the neck, jaw, back, shoulder, or arms (most often the left arm)
- Toothache
- Burning indigestion
- Dyspnea (shortness of breath)
- Nausea
- Belching

Types of Anginal Pain. Anginal pain as a direct result of myocardial ischemia typically lasts from 1 to 3 minutes, but usually lasts no more than 5 minutes. It is relieved by rest or nitroglycerin (a coronary artery vasodilator). There are a number of types of anginal pain, including the chronic stable angina (also referred to as "walk-through" angina), resting angina or angina decubitus, unstable angina, nocturnal angina, atypical angina, new-onset angina, and Prinzmetal's or "variant" angina.

Chronic stable angina occurs at a predictable level of physical or emotional stress and responds promptly to rest or to nitroglycerin. No pain occurs at rest, and the location, duration, intensity, and frequently of chest pain is consistent over time. *Resting angina or angina decubitus* is chest pain that occurs when the patient is at rest in the supine position and frequently occurs at the same time every day. The pain is neither brought on by exercise nor relieved by rest. *Unstable angina* is an abrupt change in the intensity and frequency of symptoms or decreased threshold of stimulus, such as the onset of chest pain while at rest. The duration of these attacks is longer than the usual 1 to 5 minutes and may last for up 20 to 30 minutes. Such changes in the pattern of angina require immediate medical follow-up by the patient's physician.

Nocturnal angina may awaken a patient from sleep with the same sensation experienced during exertion. During sleep, this exertion is usually caused by dreams. This type of angina may be associated with underlying CHF. *Atypical angina* refers to unusual symptoms (e.g., toothache or earache) related to physical or emotional exertion. These symptoms subside with rest or nitroglycerin. *New-onset angina* describes angina that has developed for the first time within the last 60 days. *Prinzmetal's or "variant" angina* produces symptoms similar to typical angina, but is caused by coronary artery spasm. This form of angina occurs at rest and can be difficult to induce by exercise. It is cyclic and frequently occurs at the same time each day.

Myocardial Infarct

Coronary blood flow is affected by the tonus (tone) of the coronary arteries. Arteries "clogged" by plaque formation become rigid, and resultant spasm may be provoked by cold and by exercise, which can explain the adverse effect of both factors on patients with angina (Bauwens and Paine, 1983). However, if the requirements for blood are not eased (e.g., by decreased activity), the heart attempts to continue meeting the increased demands for oxygen with an inadequate blood supply, which leads to an MI.

Many health care professionals do not like the term "heart attack," which is used most often by patients to describe the sudden blockage of a coronary artery known as "coronary thrombosis." The effects of arterial diseases may be to block the blood flow partially or completely, to form thromboses (blood clots), to weaken the artery wall causing hemorrhage, to reduce the arterial elasticity ("hardening of the arteries"), or to cause spasm of the circular muscle surrounding the artery resulting in a loss of blood flow. This spasm may be a causative factor in the development of an MI. A coronary embolus secondary to rheumatic heart disease, endocarditis, or aortic stenosis may also be indicated (Berkow, 1987).

The onset of an infarct may be characterized by severe fatigue for several days before the attack. People who have MIs may not experience any pain and may be unaware that damage is occurring to the heart muscle as a result of prolonged ischemia. They may have severe unrelenting anginal pain (lasting 30 minutes or more), which is not alleviated by rest or by nitroglycerin (see Fig. 3–7). These people may interpret the pain of MI as indigestion, and a medical evaluation may be difficult because many patients have coexisting hiatus hernia, peptic ulcer, or gallbladder disease (Berkow, 1987).

CLINICAL SYMPTOMS OF MYOCARDIAL INFARCT

- Severe substernal chest pain or squeezing pressure
- Pain possibly radiating down both arms
- Feeling of indigestion
- Angina lasting for 30 minutes or more
- Angina unrelieved by rest or nitroglycerin
- Pain of infarct unrelieved by a change in position
- Nausea

- Pallor
- Diaphoresis (heavy perspiration)
- Shortness of breath
- Weakness and feelings of faintness
- Painful shoulder-hand syndrome perhaps occurring 1 to 3 months after infarction (shoulder pain; hand is swollen, shiny, stiff, and discolored)

Hurst (1986) noted that the shoulder-hand syndrome was a common complication of myocardial infarction when patients were treated with strict, prolonged bed rest and immobilization. The change from prolonged bed rest to early ambulation has almost eliminated this problem.

An MI can lead to more serious complications such as sudden death or myocardial dysfunction that results in impaired pump performance, decreased cardiac output, and CHF.

Pericarditis

Pericarditis is an inflammation of the epicardium (visceral surface) and parietal pericardium (fluidlike membrane between the [fibrous] pericardium and the epicardium of the heart) may present the patient with no external signs or symptoms (see Fig. 3–1). However, over time, the inflammatory process may result in an accumulation of fluid in the pericardial sac, preventing the heart from expanding fully and from reducing cardiac output. The subsequent pain of pericarditis (see Figure 3–8) closely mimics that of an MI, but can be differentiated by the pattern of relieving and aggravating factors. For example, the pain of an MI is unaffected by position, breathing, or movement, whereas the pain associated with pericarditis may be relieved in various ways.

CLINICAL SYMPTOMS OF PERICARDITIS

- Substernal pain that may radiate to the neck, upper back, upper trapezius, left supraclavicular area, down the left arm to the costal margins
- Difficulty in swallowing
- Relieved by leaning forward or by sitting upright
- Aggravated by movement associated with deep breathing (laughing, coughing, deep inspiration)
- Aggravated by trunk movements (side bending or rotation)
- History of fever, chills, weakness, or heart disease. A recent MI accompanying the pattern of symptoms may alert the physical therapist to the need for medical referral to rule out cardiac involvement.

Congestive Heart Failure or Heart Failure

CHF can be defined most simply as the heart's inability to pump enough blood for the body to function well. In CHF, the heart muscles gradually fail to contract vigorously enough to adequately cycle the total volume of circulating blood. This condition develops when the muscle fibers of the left ventricle, weakened by a poor blood supply from thickened coronary arteries of CAD and scarred by earlier infarcts, begin to pump poorly. When the heart fails to propel blood forward normally, congestion occurs in the pulmonary circulation as blood accumulates in the lungs.

The right ventricle, which is rarely affected by CHD, continues to pump more blood into the lungs. The immediate result is shortness of breath, and, if the process continues, actual flooding of the air spaces of the lungs with fluid seeping from the distended blood vessels. This last phenomenon is called pulmonary congestion or pulmonary edema (Friedman and Rosenman, 1974). Because a properly functioning heart depends on both ventricles, failure of one ventricle almost always leads to failure of the other ventricle. Right-sided ventricular failure (right-sided heart failure) causes congestion of the peripheral tissues and viscera (Nursing 84, 1984). The liver may enlarge, the ankles swell, and the patient develops ascites (fluid accumulates in the abdomen).

CLINICAL SIGNS AND SYMPTOMS OF LEFT-SIDED HEART FAILURE

- Fatigue and dyspnea (subjective sensation of breathlessness) after mild physical exertion or exercise
- Persistent spasmodic cough, especially when lying down, while fluid moves from the extremities to the lungs
- Paroxysmal nocturnal dyspnea (occurring suddenly at night)
- Orthopnea (person must be in the upright position to breathe)
- Tachycardia
- Muscle weakness
- Edema and weight gain
- Irritability/restlessness
- Decreased renal function or frequent urination at night

CLINICAL SIGNS AND SYMPTOMS OF RIGHT-SIDED HEART FAILURE

- Signs of right-sided heart failure vary according to the presence and extent of left-sided heart failure, but typically include:
- Increased fatigue
- Dependent edema (usually beginning in the ankles)
- Pitting edema (after 5 to 10 lb of edema accumulates)
- Edema in the sacral area or the back of the thighs (often developing in patients who are bedridden)

Aneurysm

An aneurysm is an abnormal dilatation (commonly a saclike formation) in the weakened and diseased arterial wall. Aneurysms occur when the vessel wall becomes weakened from trauma, congenital vascular disease, infection, and atherosclerosis (Kavanagh, 1987). Thoracic aneurysms usually involve the ascending, transverse, or descending portion of the aorta; abdominal aneurysms generally involve the aorta between the renal arteries and iliac branches; peripheral arterial aneurysms affect the femoral and popliteal arteries. A dissecting aneurysm (most often a thoracic aneurysm) splits and penetrates the arterial wall, creating a false vessel. Most patients with dissecting aneurysms have had preexisting arterial hypertension. Marked elevation of blood pressure may facilitate rapid disruption and final rupture of the aortic wall when a small tear in the intima has occurred (Bauwens and Paine, 1983).

Abdominal Aortic Aneurysm. Recognition of a dissecting or ruptured aneurysm is critical for lifesaving, but is often difficult to achieve. Most abdominal aneurysms are asymptomatic until rupture is imminent. Thoracic aortic aneurysms occur most frequently in hypertensive men between the ages of 40 and 70. These aneurysms can develop in the ascending, transverse, or descending aorta and are the most likely aneurysms to dissect. Many of the symptoms mentioned are related to pressure from the sac of the aneurysm pressing against internal structures (Kavanagh, 1987).

CLINICAL SIGNS AND SYMPTOMS OF ANEURYSM

- Palpable, pulsating abdominal mass
- Abdominal "heart-beat" felt by the patient when lying down
- Dull ache in the midabdominal left flank or low back that may indicate an impending rupture

Thoracic aneurysms may cause various clinical effects according to the size and location of the aneurysm, but the most common symptoms are:

- Sudden chest pain occurs with a tearing sensation (see Fig. 3–9)
- Chest pain occurs when the person is supine
- Pain may extend to the neck, shoulders, lower back, or abdomen, but rarely to the joints and arms (which distinguishes it from MI) (Nursing 84, 1984)

- Extreme pain may be felt at the base of the neck and along the back, particularly in the interscapular area, while dissection proceeds over the aortic arch and into the descending aorta (Bauwens and Paine, 1983)
- Cough
- Dyspnea
- Hoarseness
- Dysphagia

Diseases Affecting the Heart Valves

The second category of heart problems occurs secondary to impairment of the valves caused by disease (e.g., rheumatic fever or coronary thrombosis), congenital deformity, or infection such as endocarditis. Three types of valve deformities may affect aortic, mitral, tricuspid, or pulmonic valves: stenosis, insufficiency, or prolapse. Stenosis is a narrowing or constriction that prevents the valve from opening fully and may be caused by growths, scars, or abnormal deposits on the leaflets. Insufficiency (also referred to as regurgitation) occurs when the valve does not close properly and causes blood to flow back into the heart chamber. Prolapse affects only the mitral valve and occurs when enlarged valve leaflets bulge backward into the left atrium.

These valve conditions increase the workload of the heart and require the heart to pump harder to force blood through a stenosed valve or to maintain adequate flow if blood is seeping back. A further complication for people with a malfunctioning valve may occur secondary to a bacterial infection of the valves (endocarditis).

Patients affected by diseases of the heart valves may be asymptomatic and require extensive auscultation with a stethoscope and diagnostic study to differentiate one condition from another. In early symptomatic stages, cardiac valvular disease causes easy fatigue. As stenosis or insufficiency progresses, the main symptom of heart failure (breathlessness or dyspnea) appears (Gasner and McCleary, 1984).

CLINICAL SIGNS AND SYMPTOMS OF CARDIAC VALVULAR DISEASE

- Easy fatigue
- Dyspnea
- Palpitation (subjective sensation of throbbing, skipping, rapid, or forcible pulsation of the heart)
- Chest pain
- Pitting edema
- Orthopnea or paroxysmal dyspnea
- Dizziness and syncope (episodes of fainting or loss of consciousness)

Rheumatic Fever

Rheumatic fever is an infection caused by streptococcal bacteria that can be fatal or may lead to rheumatic heart disease, a chronic condition due to scarring and deformity of the heart valves (Fig. 3–3). It is called rheumatic fever because two of the cost common symptoms are fever and joint pain (Miller and Keane, 1987). These bacteria stimulate an immunologic reaction by the body. The infection generally starts with strep throat in children between the ages of 5 and 15 and damages the heart in approximately 50% of the cases. In the last two or three decades, the aggressive use of specific antibiotics in the treatment of strep throat has effectively removed rheumatic fever from first place as the primary cause of valvular damage in the United States (Nursing 84, 1984).

The membranes around the joints (usually the ankles, knees, elbows, or wrists; however, the shoulders, hips, and small joints of the hands and feet may also be involved and all layers of the heart (epicardium, endocardium, myocardium, and pericardium) may be involved, and the heart valves are affected by this inflammatory reaction. The most characteristic and potentially dangerous anatomic lesion of rheumatic inflammation is the gross effect on cardiac valves, most commonly, the mitral and aortic valves. These valves, if left damaged and scarred, may become narrow or may leak later in life.

Arthritis is the most common clinical mani-

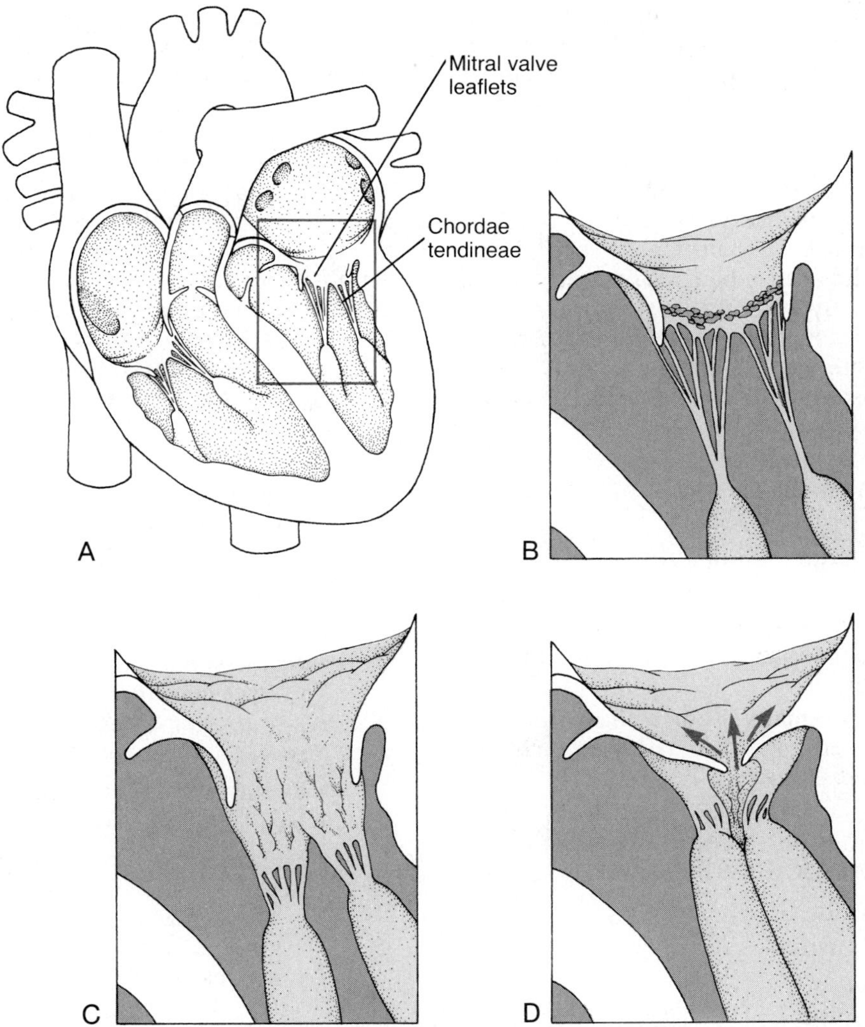

Figure 3–3. Cardiac valvular disease caused by rheumatic fever. *A*, Inflammation of the membrane over the mitral (and aortic) valves may cause edema and accumulation of fibrin and platelets on the chordae tendineae. *B*, This accumulation of inflammatory materials produces rheumatic vegetations that affect the support provided by the chordae tendineae to the AV valves. *C*, In this view, the mitral valve leaflets have become thickened with scar tissue so that the valves fail to close properly (mitral stenosis). *D*, Regurgitation or back flow of blood into the atrium develops when the scarred valve fails to close tightly. Prolonged, severe stenosis with mitral regurgitation leads to symptoms of congestive heart failure.

festation of rheumatic fever and gives the disease its name. The joints become painful and tender and may also become red, hot, and swollen, sometimes with effusion. The involved joints are usually ankles, knees, elbows, or wrists. The shoulders, hips, and small joints of the hands and feet may be involved, but almost never alone (Berkow, 1987). Rheumatic chorea (also called chorea or St. Vitus' dance) may occur 1 to 3 months after the strep infection and always occurs after polyarthritis. The patient develops rapid, purposeless, nonrepetitive movements that may involve all muscles except the eyes. This chorea may last for 1 week or for several months or may persist for several years without permanent impairment of the central nervous system (Berkow, 1987; Stollerman, 1986).

Rheumatic Heart Disease. Adults with rheumatic heart disease (especially the more common mitral valve prolapse) secondary to rheumatic fever may be asymptomatic or may present with symptoms that are poorly related to exertion and do not subside with rest or nitroglycerin. The chest pain is rarely severe: It may last for hours and is unlike angina in quality or duration.

CLINICAL SIGNS AND SYMPTOMS OF RHEUMATIC FEVER

- Migratory joint pain
- Subcutaneous nodules on the exterior surface of joints
- Fever secondary to streptococcal infection
- Occasionally, skin lesions characterized by a flat, painless rash of short duration

CLINICAL SIGNS AND SYMPTOMS OF RHEUMATIC HEART DISEASE

- Nonanginal chest pain
- Palpitations
- Fatigue
- Dyspnea

Endocarditis

Bacterial endocarditis, another common heart infection, causes inflammation of the cardiac endothelium (layer of cells lining the cavities of the heart) and damages the tricuspid, aortic, or mitral valve. This infection may be caused by bacteria or may occur as a result of abnormal growths on the closure lines of previously damaged valves. These growths consist of collagen fibers and may separate from the valve, embolize, and cause infarction in the myocardium, kidney, brain, spleen, abdomen, or extremities (Nursing 84, 1984). This infection is often a consequence of receiving dental treatment due to the increased opportunities for normal oral microorganisms to gain entrance to the circulatory system by way of the highly vascularized oral structures. Patients who are susceptible may take antibiotics as a precaution (Bernard and Evans, 1985). In addition to patients with previous valvular damage, intravenous drug users and postcardiac surgical patients are at high risk for developing endocarditis.

CLINICAL SIGNS AND SYMPTOMS OF ENDOCARDITIS

- Fever
- Night sweats
- Petechiae (pinpoint sized hemorrhagic spots) of the skin and mucus of eyes and mouth
- Splinter hemorrhages in the nail beds
- Recurrent influenza-like illness
- Headaches
- Musculoskeletal complaints including:
    - Myalgias (muscular pain)
    - Arthralgias (joint pain)
    - Back pains

Congenital Valvular Defects

Congenital malformations of the heart occur in approximately 1 of every 100 babies born in the United States (Barnard and Evans, 1985). The most common defects include ventricular or atrial septal defect (hole between the ventricles or atria), tetralogy of Fallot (combination of four defects), patent ductus arteriosus (shunt caused by an opening between the aorta and the pulmonary artery), or congenital

Figure 3–4. Congenital malformations of the heart. *A*, Ventricular septal defect. *B*, Atrial septal defect. *C*, Patent ductus arteriosus. *D*, Coarctation of the aorta. *E*, Tetralogy of Fallot: (1) Stenosis of the pulmonary valve; (2) ventricular septal

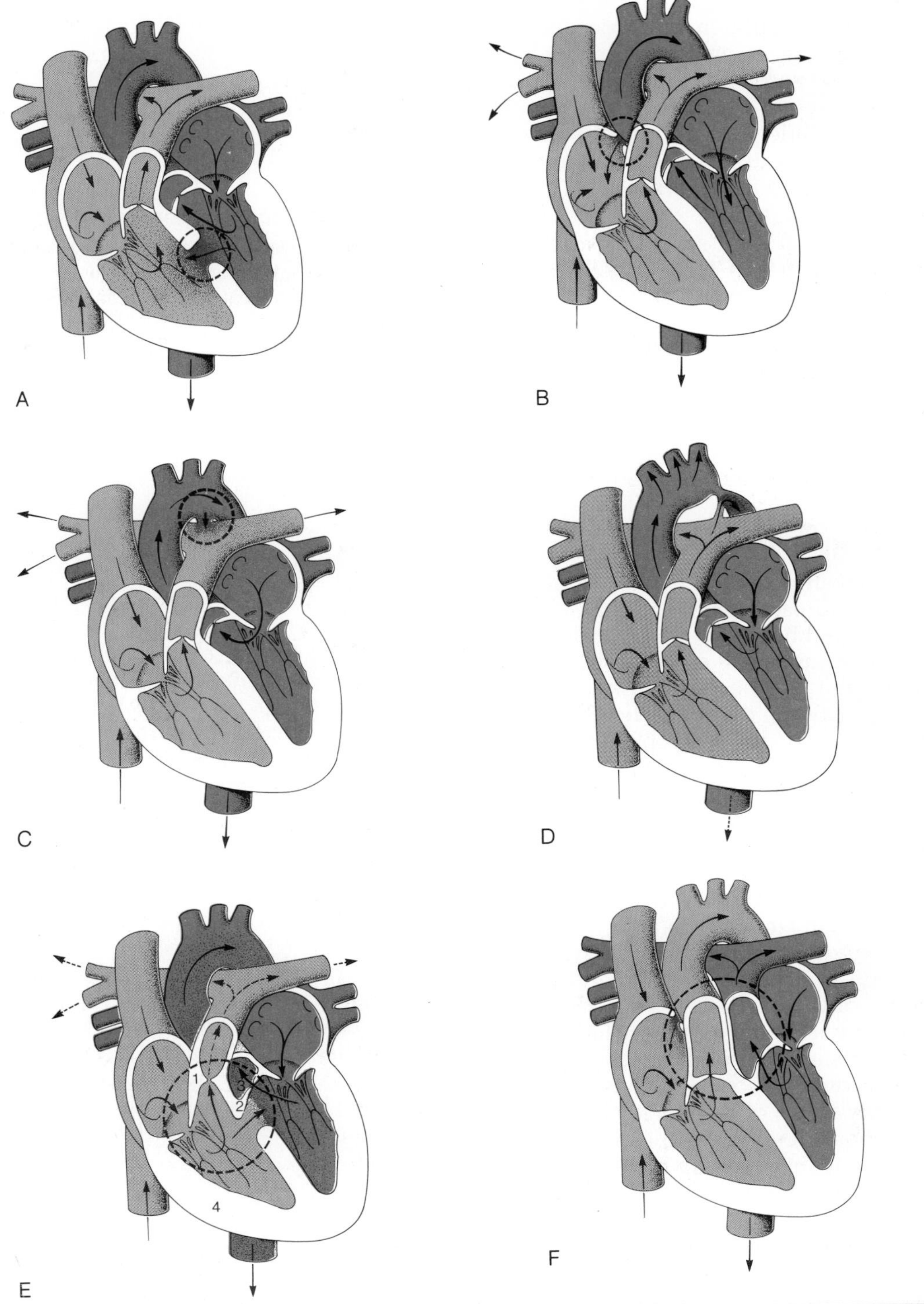

defect; (3) aorta has communication with both ventricles; (4) enlargement of the right ventricle wall. *F*, Transposition of the great arteries.

stenosis of the pulmonary, aortic, and tricuspid valves (Fig. 3–4). These congenital defects require surgical correction and may be part of the patient's *past medical history*. They are not conditions that are likely to mimic musculoskeletal lesions and are therefore not covered in detail in this text.

Defects of the Cardiac Nervous System

The third type of problem is caused by failure of the heart's nervous system to conduct normal electrical impulses. Arrhythmias (disorders of rhythm) may cause the heart to beat too quickly (tachycardia), too slowly (bradycardia), or with extra beats and fibrillations.

Fibrillation

The sinoatrial node (or cardiac pacemaker) initiates and paces the heart beat. During an MI, damaged heart muscle cells, deprived of oxygen, release small electrical impulses that may disrupt the heart's normal conduction pathway between the ventricles. The heart attack may suddenly develop into ventricular fibrillation that can result in sudden death. Similarly, a heart damaged by CAD (with or without previous infarcts), can go into fibrillation.

Atrial fibrillation is characterized by a total disorganization of atrial activity without effective atrial contraction. This arrhythmia is seen commonly in patients who have rheumatic mitral stenosis, hypertensive heart disease, pericarditis, or CHD (Zipes and Maloy, 1987).

Symptoms of fibrillation vary depending on the functional state of the heart, and fibrillation may exist without symptoms. The patient is usually aware of the irregular heart action and reports feeling "palpitations." Careful questioning may be required to pinpoint the exact description of sensations reported by the patient.

Palpitation often results from emotional or psychic disturbance and does not necessarily imply an organic cardiac condition (Massie and Kleiger, 1983). Separate from disturbances of cardiac rhythm, palpitations may result from effort, excitement, tobacco, caffeine, alcohol, or infection.

CLINICAL SIGNS AND SYMPTOMS OF FIBRILLATION

- Subjective report of palpitations
- Sensations of fluttering, skipping, irregular beating or pounding, heaving action
- Dyspnea
- Chest pain
- Anxiety
- Pallor
- Nervousness
- Cyanosis

Tachycardia (Zipes and Maloy, 1987)

The conduction pathway in sinus tachycardia is the same as that found in normal sinus rhythm; however, because of enhanced discharge at the sinus node, the sinus rate is between 100 and 180 beats/min and may be higher in the case of extreme exertion and in infants.

Sinus tachycardia is the normal reaction to various physiologic stresses, such as fever, hypotension, anemia, anxiety, exertion, pulmonary emboli, myocardial ischemia, CHF, or shock. Inflammation such as pericarditis may produce tachycardia. Tachycardia usually has no physiologic significance; however, in patients with organic myocardial disease, reduced cardiac output, CHF, or arrhythmias may result in association with tachycardia. Because heart rate is a major determinant of oxygen requirements, angina, or perhaps an increase in the size of an infarction may accompany persistent tachycardia in patients with CAD.

CLINICAL SYMPTOMS OF TACHYCARDIA

The symptoms of tachycardia vary from one person to another and may range from an increased pulse rate to a group of symptoms that would restrict the normal activity of the patient. This group of symptoms include:

- Palpitation (most common symptom)
- Restlessness
- Chest discomfort or pain
- Agitation
- Anxiety and apprehension, the latter depending on the pain threshold and emotional reaction of the patient (Massie and Kleiger, 1983)

Bradycardia

In sinus bradycardia, impulses travel down the same pathway as in a normal sinus rhythm, but the sinus node discharges at a rate less than 60 beats/min. Bradycardia may be normal in athletes or young adults and is therefore asymptomatic. Eye surgery, meningitis, intracranial tumors, cervical and mediastinal tumors, myocardial infarction, and obstructive jaundice may produce sinus bradycardia (Zipes and Maloy, 1987).

CLINICAL SIGNS AND SYMPTOMS OF BRADYCARDIA

- Reduced pulse rate
- Syncope (may be preceded by sudden onset of weakness, sweating, nausea, pallor, vomiting, and distortion or dimming of vision)
- Signs and symptoms remit promptly when the patient is placed in the horizontal position (Berkow, 1987)

CHEST PAIN

The four types of pain discussed in Chapter 2 including cutaneous, deep somatic (or parietal), visceral, and referred pain also apply to chest pain. The pathways and referral of pain in the thorax are not well understood. It is clear that within the chest cavity, parietal pleura (the cavity linings) have sensory nerve fibers that respond to chemical and mechanical forces exerted on this pleura. However, there are few nerve endings (if any) in the visceral pleura (linings of the various organs), such as the heart or lungs. The exception to this statement is in the area of the pericardium (sac enclosed around the entire heart), which is adjacent to the diaphragm (see Fig. 3–1).

Experiments by Capps and Coleman (1932) have shown that pain fibers do exist in the lower parietal pericardium, adjacent to the diaphragm. Stimulation of this portion of the parietal membrane results in sharp pain along the superior border of the trapezius muscle. This referral pattern is identical to the pattern that occurs as a result of stimulation of the central diaphragm and is postulated to be carried by the phrenic nerves that innervate the diaphragm (Fig. 3–5). Extensive disease may occur within the body cavities without the occurrence of pain until the process extends to the parietal pleura (lining of the chest or abdominal cavity wall). Neuritis (constant irritation of nerve endings) in the parietal pleura then produces pain (Bauwens and Paine, 1983).

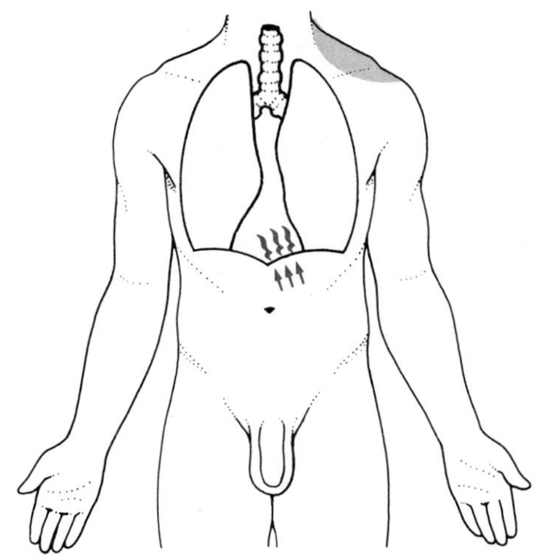

Figure 3–5. Irritation of the peritoneal (outside) or pleural (inside) surface of the central area of the diaphragm refers pain to the upper trapezius muscle, neck, and supraclavicular fossa. The pain pattern is ipsilateral to the area of irritation.

Pain fibers, originating in the parietal pleura, are conveyed through the chest wall as fine twigs of the intercostal nerves. Irritation of these nerve fibers results in pain in the chest wall that is usually described by the patient as knifelike and is sharply localized, occurring cutaneously (in the skin). This pain may be aggravated by any respiratory movement involving the diaphragm, such as sighing, deep breathing, coughing, sneezing, laughing, or the hiccups and may be referred along the costal margins or into the upper abdominal quadrants. Chest pain can occur as a result of cervical spine disorders because nerves originating as high as C34 can extend as far as the nipple line. For example, pectoral, suprascapular, dorsal scapular, and long thoracic nerves originating in lower cervical levels can cause pain in the chest, midscapular regions, and postscapular regions when irritated (Bauwens and Paine, 1983).

There are many causes of chest pain, both cardiac and noncardiac in origin. As discussed, cardiac-related pain may arise secondary to angina, myocardial infarction, pericarditis, or dissecting aortic aneurysm. Cardiac-related chest pain can also occur when there is normal coronary circulation, such as in the case of patients with pernicious anemia (chronic, progressive reduction of red blood cells, and subsequent loss of oxygen). These patients may have angina on physical exertion because of the lack of nutrition to the myocardium.

Coronary disease may go unnoticed because the patient has had no anginal or infarct pain associated with ischemia. This situation occurs when a collateral circulation is established to counteract an obstruction of the blood flow to the heart muscle. Gradual occlusion of principal coronary vessels may be accompanied by anastomoses (connecting channels) between the branches of the right and left coronary arteries eliminating the patient's perception of pain.

Noncardiac Causes

- Pleuropulmonary disorders
  - Pulmonary embolism
  - Cor pulmonale
  - Pulmonary hypertension
  - Pleurisy with pneumonia
  - Spontaneous pneumothorax
- Musculoskeletal disorders
  - Myalgia
  - Fractured ribs
  - Myofascial trigger points
  - Costochondritis
- Neurologic disorders
  - Intercostal neuritis
  - Dorsal nerve root radiculitis
  - Thoracic outlet syndrome
- Gastrointestinal disorders
- Breast pain
- Anxiety states

Pleuropulmonary Disorders

Pulmonary chest pain results usually from obstruction, restriction, dilation, or distention of the large airways or large pulmonary artery walls (Forshee, 1987). Pleuropulmonary disorders are discussed in detail in Chapter 4.

Musculoskeletal Disorders

Musculoskeletal disorders such as myalgia associated with muscle exertion, myofascial trigger points, costochondritis, or xyphoiditis can produce pain in the chest and arms. Compared with angina pectoris, the pain associated with these conditions may last for seconds or hours, and prompt relief does not occur with the ingestion of nitroglycerin (Andreoli et al, 1979).

Muscle exertion secondary to prolonged or repeated movement may create a condition of *myalgia* or muscular pain. Myalgia of chest muscles caused by repeated coughing may be associated with a recent upper respiratory infection. This information is brought to the examiner's attention when reviewing the *Family/Personal History* form. Patients who have chest pain should be asked during the physical therapy interview about recent activities of a repetitive nature that could cause sore muscles (e.g., painting or washing walls; calisthenics, including pushups or recent repetitive lifting of heavy boxes or weights).

Fractured ribs can cause sharp, localized pain at the level of the fracture with an increase in symptoms associated with respiratory movements such as deep inspiration, laughing, sneezing, or coughing.

Myofascial trigger points (Travell and Simons, 1983), which are defined as hypersensitive spots in the skeletal musculature involving the serratus anterior, pectoralis, sternalis, or upper rectus abdominus muscles, may produce precordial (the region over the heart and lower part of the thorax) pain (see Fig. 3–10*A* to *D*). Abdominal muscles have multiple referred pain patterns that may reach up into the chest or midback and produce heartburn or deep epigastric (upper middle region of the abdomen, lower sternum) pain. The patient may present with a history of prolonged, vigorous activity that requires forceful abdominal breathing, such as bending and lifting.

Chest pain from serratus anterior trigger points may present at rest in severe cases. Patients with this myofascial syndrome may report that they are "short of breath" or that they are in pain when they take a deep breath. Serratus anterior trigger points on the left side of the chest can contribute to the pain associated with myocardial infarction. This pain is rarely aggravated by the usual tests for range of motion at the shoulder, but may result from a strong effort to protract the scapula. Palpation reveals tender points that increase the patient's symptoms, and there is usually a palpable taut band present within the involved muscles.

There may be a history of muscle strain from lifting weights overhead, pushups, prolonged running, or severe coughing. When active trigger points occur in the left pectoralis major muscle, the referred pain (anterior chest, to the precordium and down the inner aspect of the left arm) is easily confused with that due to coronary insufficiency. Chest pain that persists long after an acute myocardial infarction is often due to myofascial trigger points. As with all myofascial syndromes, inactivation of the trigger points eliminates the patient's symptoms of chest pain.

Costochondritis or *xyphoiditis* involves local swelling and pain of the associated costochondral, chondrosternal, or xiphisternal joints. The second costocartilage on either side is the most common area of involvement, but any costochondral articulations can be involved. Pain and tenderness may be reproduced by palpation of the local areas. The condition may persist for months without fever or systemic symptoms (Hurst, 1986). The details of clinical signs and symptoms of this disorder are reviewed in detail in Chapter 12.

Neurologic Disorders

Herpes Zoster

Neurologic disorders such as intercostal neuritis and dorsal nerve root radiculitis or a neurovascular disorder such as thoracic outlet syndrome can cause chest pain. The most commonly recognized neuritis is *herpes zoster (shingles),* which usually occurs in older people.

Shingles is produced by infection of the dorsal nerve root by a virus. This neuritis is identified by the appearance of a vesicular rash in the area of discomfort. Neuritic chest wall conditions are usually dermatomal in distribution; pain and skin rash are confined to the somatic distribution of one of the spinal nerves. The pattern of the pain differs from coronary pain because the neuritis is unrelated to effort and lasts for prolonged periods (Andreoli et al, 1979).

CLINICAL SIGNS AND SYMPTOMS OF HERPES ZOSTER (SHINGLES)

- Chills
- Fever
- Headache and malaise
- Skin eruptions appear 4 or 5 days after the other symptoms

Dorsal Nerve Root Irritation

Other conditions of neuritis involve the dorsal nerve roots of the thoracic spine and can refer pain to the lateral and anterior chest wall. This somatic pain can be localized to the point of irritation or is referred to any point along the peripheral nerve. Pain may be described as sharp or dull and aching, with referral possibly to one or both arms through branches of the brachial plexus.

Pain associated with dorsal nerve root irritation is accompanied commonly by a history of back pain, pain more superficial than cardiac pain, which is usually aggravated by exertion of just the upper body and is accompanied by other neurologic signs (e.g., numbness, tingling, and muscle atrophy). Lesions producing dorsal nerve root pain may be infectious (e.g., *radiculitis,* which is an inflammation within or beneath the dura mater [intradural] of the spinal nerve root). However, the pain is more likely to be the result of mechanical irritation of the root due to spinal disease or deformity (e.g., bony spurs secondary to osteoarthritis, or to the presence of cervical ribs placing pressure on the brachial plexus) (Bauwens and Paine, 1983).

CLINICAL SIGNS AND SYMPTOMS OF DORSAL NERVE ROOT IRRITATION

- Lateral or anterior chest wall pain
- History of back pain
- Pain is aggravated by exertion of only the upper body
- May be accompanied by neurologic signs
  - Numbness
  - Tingling
  - Muscle atrophy

Thoracic Outlet Syndrome

Thoracic outlet syndrome refers to compression of the neural and vascular structures that leave, or pass over, the superior rim of the thoracic cage. Various names have been given to the condition, including first thoracic rib, cervical rib, scalenus anticus, costoclavicular, and hyperabduction syndrome.

The pain associated with thoracic outlet syndrome may occur mainly in the anterior chest wall and suggests CHD, but the pain resulting from somatic nerve compression usually affects the upper extremity in the distribution of the ulnar nerve. Pain may radiate into the neck, shoulder, scapula, or axilla with associated paresthesias (burning, pricking sensation) and hypoesthesias (abnormal decreases in sensitivity to stimulation).

Palpation of the supraclavicular space may elicit tenderness or may define a prominence indicative of a cervical rib. The effect on pulse of Adson's maneuver (deep inspiration with the neck fully extended and the head rotated toward the side of symptoms), the hyperabduction test (arm extended overhead), and the costoclavicular test (exaggerated military attention posture) should be compared in both arms (Smith, 1986).

CLINICAL SIGNS AND SYMPTOMS OF THORACIC OUTLET SYNDROME

- Paresthesia of fingers
- Weakness and atrophy of small muscles of the hand
- Positive Adson's sign
- Positive result from a hyperabduction test
- Positive result from a costoclavicular test
- Pain in the anterior chest wall

Gastrointestinal Disorders

Gastrointestinal disorders may cause chest pain with radiation of pain to the shoulders and back (see Fig. 3–11). Cholecystitis (inflammation of the gallbladder) can be mistaken for angina pectoris and myocardial infarction. Acute pancreatitis is more likely to be confused with acute myocardial infarction and the hypotension that may occur with pancreatitis can produce a reduction of coronary blood flow with the production of angina pectoris.

Gastric duodenal peptic ulcer may occasionally cause pain in the lower chest rather than in the upper abdomen. Pain in the lower substernal area may arise as a result of reflux esophagitis. It may be gripping, squeezing, or burning and may sometimes be accompanied by regurgitation. Like that of angina pectoris, the discomfort of reflux esophagitis may be precipitated by recumbency or by meals; however, unlike angina, it is not precipitated by exercise (Andreoli et al, 1979).

For a more thorough description of these conditions, refer to Chapter 6 in this text.

SYMPTOMS ASSOCIATED WITH GASTROINTESTINAL DISORDERS

- Nausea
- Vomiting
- Blood in stools
- Pain on swallowing or associated with meals

Breast Pain

Breast pain (see Fig. 3–12) is caused most commonly by benign and malignant tumors, inflammatory breast disease such as mastitis (inflammation of the breast), or mastodynia (mammary neuralgia). Mastodynia is a unilateral breast pain caused by irritation of the upper dorsal intercostal nerves and is associated almost always with ovulatory cycles. This association between symptoms and menses may be discovered during the physical therapy interview when the patient responds to *Special Questions for Women.* The pain occurs initially at the premenstrual period, and later it may become persistent.

Breast cancer and cysts develop more frequently in individuals who have a family history of the disease (Berkow, 1987). Any indication of such a family history on the *Family/Personal History* form in association with breast pain requires medical follow-up. The patient's subjective report of family history of breast disease or report of palpable breast nodules or lumps and previous history of chronic mastitis is very important.

The patient who presents with a painful or tender breast may have trigger points in the lateral margin of the pectoralis major muscle. These "trigger points" or hypersensitive spots in the skeletal musculature can refer pain to the chest in a manner that confusingly simulates the pain of coronary insufficiency in persons with no history or evidence of cardiac disease. Although these patterns strongly mimic cardiac pain, myofascial trigger-point pain shows a much wider variation in its response to daily activity than does the more consistent limit imposed by angina pectoris (Travell and Simons, 1983).

This breast pain pattern may be differentiated from the aching pain arising from the pectoral muscles by a history of upper extremity overuse usually associated with pectoral myalgia. Resistance to isometric movement of the upper extremities reproduces the symptoms of a pectoral myalgia, but does not usually aggravate pain associated with breast tissue.

Travell notes that in acute myocardial infarction, pain is commonly referred from the heart to the midregion of the pectoralis major and minor muscles. The injury to the heart muscle initiates a viscerosomatic process that activates trigger points in the pectoral muscles. After recovery from the acute infarction, these selfperpetuating trigger points tend to persist in the chest wall, unless they are inactivated.

The skin surface over a tumor may be red, warm, edematous, firm, and painful. There may be skin dimpling over the lesion with attachment of the mass to surrounding tissues preventing normal mobilization of skin, fascia, and muscle. Jarring or movement of the breasts and movement of the arms may aggravate the pain with radiation of pain to the inner aspects of the arm(s).

CLINICAL SIGNS AND SYMPTOMS OF BREAST PATHOLOGY

- Family history of breast disease
- Palpable breast nodules or lumps

and previous history of chronic mastitis

- Breast pain with possible radiation to inner aspect of arm(s)
- Skin surface over a tumor may be red, warm, edematous, firm, and painful
- Firm, painful site under the skin surface
- Skin dimpling over the lesion with attachment of the mass to surrounding tissues, preventing normal mobilization of skin, fascia, and muscle
- Pain aggravated by jarring or by movement of the breasts
- Pain that is not aggravated by resistance to isometric movement of the upper extremities

Anxiety State

An anxiety state producing chest pain is the most common noncardiovascular cause of chest pain. Psychogenic chest pain may be manifested in the form of cardiac or respiratory symptoms mimicking myocardial infarction. Clues to the patient's underlying state of anxiety may be observed during the physical therapy interview. For example, the patient may indicate that the symptoms of chest pain are aggravated by crowded places (claustrophobia), or the patient may manifest sighing respirations (hyperventilation). The pain rarely radiates to other locations and is not aggravated by breathing, but it is associated with hyperventilation.

CLINICAL SIGNS AND SYMPTOMS OF ANXIETY-PRODUCING CHEST PAIN

- Dull, aching discomfort in the substernal region and in the anterior chest
- Sinus tachycardia
- Fatigue
- Fear of closed-in places

CARDIOVASCULAR DISORDERS

Peripheral Vascular Disorders

Impaired circulation may be caused by a number of acute or chronic medical conditions known as peripheral vascular diseases (PVD). PVDs can affect the arterial venous, or lymphatic circulatory systems (Kisner and Colby, 1985). Vascular disorders secondary to occlusive arterial disease have an underlying atherosclerotic process that causes disturbances of circulation to the extremities and can result in significant loss of function of either the upper or lower extremities.

Arterial Disease

Arterial diseases include acute arterial occlusion caused by:

Thrombus, embolism, or trauma to an artery

Arteriosclerosis obliterans (occlusive disease of the aorta and its branches to the extremities as a result of atherosclerosis) (Young, 1986)

Thromboangitis obliterans or Buerger's disease (an intense inflammatory reaction of the veins and arteries to tobacco in smokers)

Raynaud's disease (vasospasm of digital arteries with blanching and numbness of fingers)

The pain associated with arterial disease is generally felt as a dull, aching tightness deep in the muscle, but it may be described as a boring, stabbing, squeezing, pulling, or even burning sensation. Although the pain is sometimes referred to as cramp, there is no actual spasm in the painful muscles. The location of the pain is determined by the site of the major arterial occlusion. The most frequent lesion, which is present in about two thirds of the patients, is occlusion of the superficial femoral artery between the groin and the knee, producing pain in the calf that sometimes radiates to the popliteal region and to the lower thigh. Aortoiliac occlusive disease induces pain in the gluteal and quadriceps muscles, whereas occlusion of the popliteal or more distal arteries causes pain in the foot (Layzer, 1985).

In the typical case of superficial femoral artery occlusion, there is a good femoral pulse at the groin, but arterial pulses are absent at the knee and foot, although resting circulation appears to be good in the foot. After exercise, the patient may have numbness in the foot as well as pain in the calf. The foot may be cold and pale, which is an indication that the circulation has been diverted to the arteriolar bed of the leg muscles (Layzer, 1985).

CLINICAL SIGNS AND SYMPTOMS OF ARTERIAL DISEASE

- Intermittent claudication (limping due to pain, ache, or cramp in the muscles of the lower extremities caused by ischemia or insufficient blood flow)
- Reduced or absent pulses distal to the obstruction
- Burning, ischemic pain at rest
- Rest pain may be aggravated by elevating the extremity and relieved by hanging the foot over the side of the bed or chair
- Ischemic extremities are characterized by decreased skin temperature, dry and scaly or shiny skin, poor nail and hair growth, and possible ulcerations on weight-bearing surfaces (e.g., toes or heel)

Diabetes mellitus increases the susceptibility to CHD, but the specific mechanism by which this happens is poorly understood (Wenger and Schlant, 1986). PVD has been estimated to occur 11 times more frequently and to develop about 10 years earlier in diabetics than in nondiabetics. Gangrene is about 50 times more frequent in diabetic men than in nondiabetic men over the age of 40 and is 70 times more frequent in women in this age group (Berkow, 1987).

CLINICAL SIGNS AND SYMPTOMS OF DIABETIC CORONARY ATHEROSCLEROSIS

- Fatigue on exertion
- Changes in vision
- In later stages—hypertension, edema, hematuria (blood in the urine)

Arteriosclerosis Obliterans (Young, 1986). Arteriosclerosis obliterans is also known as atherosclerotic occlusive disease, chronic occlusive arterial disease, obliterative arteriosclerosis, and peripheral arterial disease. It is the most common occlusive arterial disease that causes chronic ischemia of the lower extremities and accounts for about 95% of the cases (Juergens et al, 1980). This disease is most often seen in elderly patients and is commonly associated with diabetes mellitus (Kisner and Colby, 1985).

Other risk factors in arteriosclerosis obliterans are smoking, hypertension, obesity, and atherosclerosis in the coronary arteries. As with atherosclerosis elsewhere, arteriosclerosis obliterans develops slowly and insidiously over a period of years. Initially, the patient is asymptomatic as collateral circulation develops. Over time, the collateral vessels may become occluded, causing more ischemia.

CLINICAL SIGNS AND SYMPTOMS OF ARTERIOSCLEROSIS OBLITERANS

- Intermittent claudication (limping due to pain, ache, or cramp in the muscles of the lower extremities caused by ischemia or insufficient blood flow)
- Pain at rest
- Ulceration and gangrene

Buerger's Disease. This disease (Berkow, 1987) occurs predominantly in men aged 20 to 40 who smoke cigarettes. The exact etiology is unknown, but the relationship of smoking to the occurrence and progression of the disease is apparent. The incidence of this disease has decreased in recent years and, although relatively rare, it is second to arteriosclerosis obliterans as a cause of chronic, occlusive arterial disease of the extremities (Young, 1986). The onset is gradual, starting in the most distal small-sized and medium-sized arteries and resulting in the development of distal gangrene.

CLINICAL SIGNS AND SYMPTOMS OF BUERGER'S DISEASE

- Intermittent claudication
- Raynaud's phenomenon
- Coldness, numbness, tingling, or burning of the affected hand or foot

Raynaud's Phenomenon and Disease. The spasm of arteries in the fingers results in a condition characterized by the blanched, cyanotic, shiny appearance of the fingers referred to as Raynaud's phenomenon. This phenomenon may be idiopathic (Raynaud's disease) or secondary to other conditions such as:

- Connective tissue disorders
    - Scleroderma
    - Rheumatoid arthritis
    - Systemic lupus erythematosus
    - Polymyositis/dermatomyositis
    - Mixed connective tissue disease
- Neurogenic lesions
    - Thoracic outlet syndrome
- Pulmonary hypertension
- Trauma

During an attack of Raynaud's phenomenon, the blood vessels in the fingers or toes become narrow, preventing normal blood flow. The affected digits may change color from white (lack of blood) to blue (blood remains in veins without flowing) and red or purple as blood flow returns to normal. The affected areas may hurt and feel numb and cold when blood flow is compromised and then begin to swell, tingle, ache, and feel warm as the blood flow returns to normal. Precipitating factors for idiopathic Raynaud's phenomenon may include exposure to cold, emotional disturbance (e.g., anxiety, excitement), and the use of vibrating equipment such as jackhammers (Arthritis Foundation, 1985).

Idiopathic Raynaud's disease is differentiated from secondary Raynaud's phenomenon by a history of symptoms for at least 2 years with no progression of the symptoms and no evidence of an underlying cause (Berkow, 1987).

Venous Disorders

The major venous disorders are varicose veins (dilated or distended veins) and thrombophlebitis (inflammation of a vein accompanied by thrombus or blood clot formation). Varicose veins result from valve incompetence or dilatation of the affected vessel commonly associated with a history of pregnancy, obesity, prolonged standing, abdominal tumors, or ascites. These factors increase pressure in the veins, causing venous distention and eventually causing incompetence of the valves.

Superficial and deep-vein thrombophlebitis result from inflammation or occlusion of the affected vessel (Nursing 84, 1984). Thrombophlebitis is an acute disease with symptoms lasting during a period of hours to several days. The actual disease process is usually self-limiting and lasts for 1 to 2 weeks. However, phlebitis (inflammation of a vein) of one of the deep veins can result in a pulmonary embolism and is life-threatening (Fell and Strandness, 1982). Symptoms are usually relieved with elevation, rest, ice, and elastic support for the lower extremities.

CLINICAL SIGNS AND SYMPTOMS OF VENOUS DISORDERS

- Swelling
- Warmth and blue discoloration of the extremity
- Pain
- Dependent edema
- Prominence of superficial veins
- Skin ulcerations and tenderness

- Deep calf tenderness can be elicited and is often difficult to differentiate from the muscle pain of gastric/soleus muscles when using Homans' sign (slight pain at the back of the knee or calf when the ankle is forcibly dorsiflexed, indicative of thrombus in the veins of the leg)

In the case of deep-vein thrombosis, the patient may be asymptomatic or some of the following signs and symptoms may appear:

- Fever
- Chills
- Malaise
- Cyanosis of the affected extremity

Lymphedema

The third type of peripheral vascular disorder, lymphedema (an excessive accumulation of fluid in tissue spaces), typically occurs secondary to an obstruction of the lymphatic system from trauma, infection, radiation, or surgery (Kisner and Colby, 1985).

CLINICAL SIGNS AND SYMPTOMS OF LYMPHEDEMA

- Usually unilateral
- Worse after prolonged dependency
- Edema of the dorsum of the foot or hand
- No discomfort or skin changes

Hypertension

Hypertension is defined as a consistent diastolic pressure of more than 90 mm Hg and a consistent systolic pressure of more than 140 mm Hg, measured on at least two occasions — in other words, a *sustained* elevation of blood pressure (Nursing 84, 1984; Walsh and Woloszyn, 1987). Hypertension can be classified in two ways: by type and severity.

Primary (or *essential*) hypertension is the first type, and the etiology is unknown. It exists in approximately 90 to 95% of all hypertensive patients. The second type of hypertension is *secondary* hypertension associated with other factors such as renal disease, use of oral contraceptives, Cushing's syndrome, or hyperthyroidism. People with intermittently elevated blood pressure are considered to have *labile* hypertension. Hypertension is *resistant* when it does not respond to medical treatment.

The severity of hypertension is classified by degrees as follows:

Class I (mild)	90 – 104 mm Hg
Class II (moderate)	105 – 114 mm Hg
Class III (severe)	115 mm Hg or greater

Hypertension is often considered in conjunction with peripheral vascular disorders for several reasons. Both are disorders of the circulation; the courses of both diseases are affected by similar factors; and hypertension is a major risk factor in atherosclerosis, the largest single cause of PVD. Hypertension is a major cause of heart failure, stroke, and kidney failure. Aneurysm formation and CHF are also associated with hypertension (Walsh and Woloszyn, 1987).

CLINICAL SIGNS AND SYMPTOMS OF HYPERTENSION

Hypertensive patients are asymptomatic in early stages, but when symptoms do occur, they include:

- Headache (usually occipital and present in the early morning)
- Vertigo (dizziness)
- Flushed face
- Spontaneous epistaxis (nosebleed)
- Blurred vision or nocturnal urinary frequency

Persistent, elevated diastolic pressure damages the intimal layer of the small vessels, which causes an accumulation of fibrin, local edema, and, possibly, intravascular clotting. Eventually, these damaging changes diminish blood flow to vital organs, such as the heart, kidneys, and brain, resulting in complications such as heart failure, renal failure, and cerebrovascular accidents or stroke.

Many people have brief episodes of transient ischemic attacks before they have an actual stroke. The attacks occur when the blood supply to part of the brain has been temporarily disrupted. These ischemic episodes last from 5 to 20 minutes, although they may last for as long as 24 hours. Transient ischemic attacks are important warning signals that an obstruction exists in an artery leading to the brain.

CLINICAL SIGNS AND SYMPTOMS OF TRANSIENT ISCHEMIC ATTACKS

- Slurred speech or sudden difficulty with speech
- Temporary blindness or other dramatic visual problems
- Paralysis or extreme weakness, usually affecting one side of the body

Orthostatic Hypotension

Orthostatic hypotension, an excessive fall in blood pressure of 20 mm Hg or more on assuming the erect position, is not a disease, but a manifestation of abnormalities in normal blood pressure regulation. This condition may occur secondary to the effects of drugs such as hypertensives, diuretics and antidepressants, venous pooling (e.g., pregnancy, prolonged bed rest, or standing), or neurogenic origins. The latter includes diseases affecting the autonomic nervous system such as Guillain-Barré syndrome, diabetes mellitus, or multiple sclerosis.

CLINICAL SIGNS AND SYMPTOMS OF ORTHOSTATIC HYPOTENSION

- Lightheadedness
- Syncope
- Mental or visual blurring
- Sense of weakness or "rubbery" legs

These postural symptoms are often accentuated in the morning and are aggravated by heat, humidity, heavy meals, and exercise.

OVERVIEW OF CARDIAC PAIN PATTERNS (Andreoli, 1986, 1987; Nursing 82; Nursing 84)

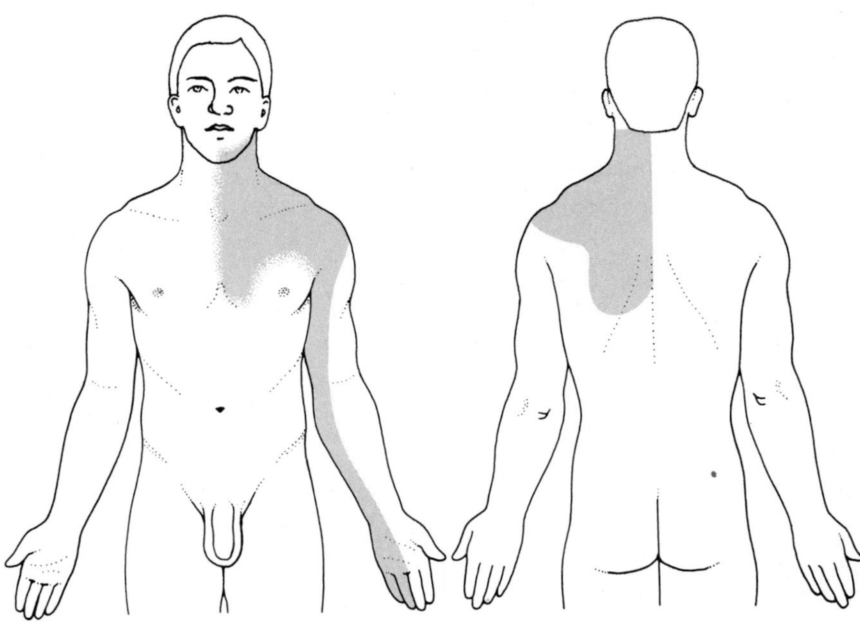

Figure 3–6. Pain patterns associated with angina. *A*, Area of substernal discomfort projected to the left shoulder and arm over the distribution of the ulnar nerve. Referred pain may be present only in the left shoulder or in the shoulder and along the arm only to the elbow. *B*, Occasionally, anginal pain may be referred to the back in the area of the left scapula or the interscapular region.

Angina

Location:	Substernal/retrosternal (beneath the sternum)
Referral (Fig. 3–6):	Neck, jaw, back, shoulder, or arms (most commonly the left arm)
	May only have a toothache
	Occasionally to the abdomen
Description:	Vicelike pressure, squeezing, heaviness, burning indigestion
Intensity*:	Mild to moderate
	Builds up gradually or may be sudden
Duration:	Usually less than 10 minutes
	Never more than 30 minutes
	Average: 3–5 minutes

* For each pattern reviewed throughout this text, intensity is related directly to the degree of noxious stimuli.

Associated Signs and Symptoms:	Shortness of breath (dyspnea)
	Nausea
	Diaphoresis (heavy perspiration)
	Anxiety or apprehension
	Belching (eructation)
Relieving Factors:	Rest or nitroglycerin
Aggravating Factors:	Exercise or physical exertion
	Cold weather or wind
	Heavy meals
	Emotional stress

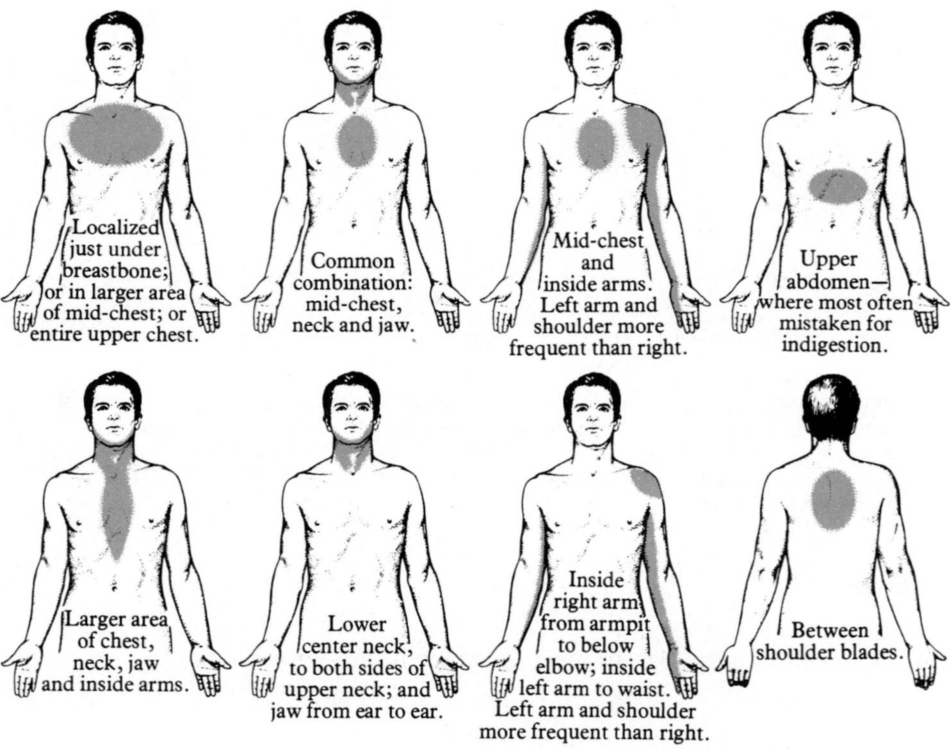

Figure 3–7. Early warning signs of a heart attack.

Myocardial Infarction

Location:	Substernal, anterior chest
Referral (Fig. 3–7):	May radiate like angina, frequently down both arms

Description:	Burning, stabbing, vicelike pressure, squeezing, heaviness
Intensity:	Severe
Duration:	Usually at least 30 minutes; may last 1 to 2 hours Residual soreness 1 to 3 days
Associated Signs and Symptoms:	Dizziness, feeling faint Nausea, vomiting Pallor Diaphoresis (heavy perspiration) Apprehension, severe anxiety Fatigue, sudden weakness Dyspnea May be followed by painful shoulder-hand syndrome (see text)
Relieving Factors:	None, unrelieved by rest or nitroglycerin taken every 5 minutes for 20 minutes
Aggravating Factors:	Not necessarily anything; may occur at rest or follow emotional stress or physical exertion

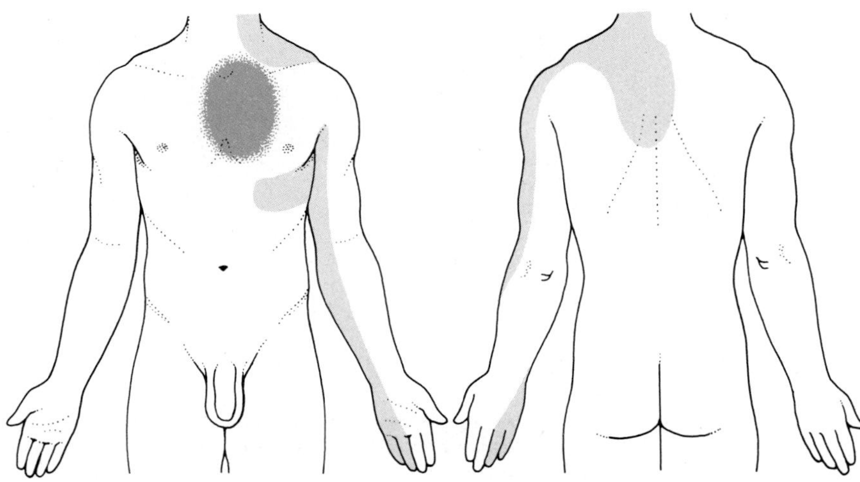

Figure 3–8. Substernal pain associated with pericarditis (***dark red***) may radiate anteriorly (*light red*) to the costal margins, neck, upper back, upper trapezius, left supraclavicular area, or down the left arm.

Pericarditis

Location (Fig. 3–8):	Substernal or over the sternum, sometimes to the left of midline toward the cardiac apex
Referral:	Neck, upper back, upper trapezius, left supraclavicular area, down the left arm, costal margins

Description: More localized than pain of myocardial infarction

Sharp, stabbing, knifelike

Intensity: Moderate to severe

Duration: Continuous, may last hours or days with residual soreness following

Associated Signs and Symptoms: Usually medically determined associated symptoms (e.g., by chest auscultation using a stethoscope)

Relieving Factors: Sitting upright or leaning forward

Aggravating Factors: Muscle movement associated with deep breathing (e.g., laughter, inspiration, coughing)

Left lateral (side) bending of the upper trunk

Trunk rotation (either to the right or to the left)

Supine position

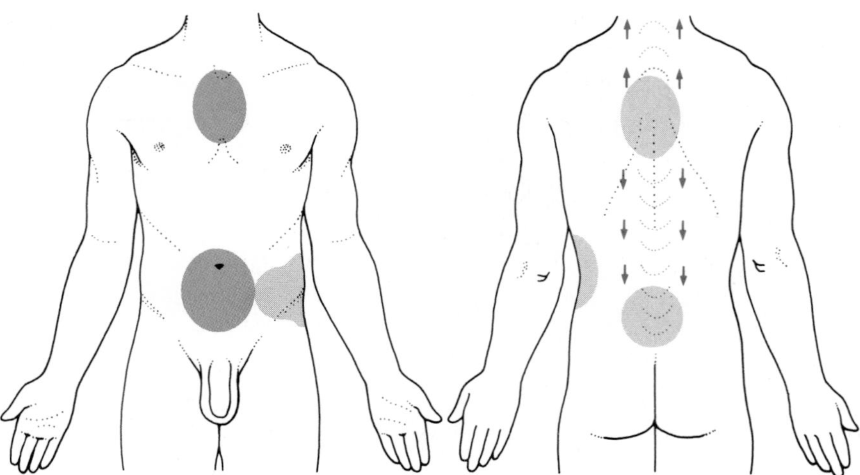

Figure 3–9. Chest pain (*dark red*) associated with thoracic aneurysms may radiate (*light red*) to the neck, interscapular area, shoulders, lower back, or abdomen. Early warning signs of an impending rupture may include an abdominal heartbeat when lying down (not shown) or a dull ache in the midabdominal left flank or lower back (*light red*).

Dissecting Aortic Aneurysm

Location: Anterior chest (thoracic aneurysm)

Abdomen (abdominal aneurysm)

Referral (Fig. 3–9): Thoracic area of back

Pain may move in the chest as dissection progresses

Pain may extend to the neck, shoulders, interscapular area, or lower back

Description:	Knifelike, tearing (thoracic aneurysm)
	Dull ache in the lower back or midabdominal left flank (abdominal aneurysm)
Intensity:	Severe, excruciating
Duration:	Hours
Associated Signs and Symptoms:	Pulses absent
	Patient senses "heartbeat" when lying down
	Palpable, pulsating abdominal mass
	Lower blood pressure in one arm
	Other medically determined symptoms
Relieving Factors:	None
Aggravating Factors:	None

OVERVIEW OF NONCARDIAC CHEST PAIN PATTERNS (Andreoli et al, 1979, 1986; Nursing 82)

Musculoskeletal Disorders

Location (Fig. 3–10):	Variable
	Costochondritis (inflammation of the costal cartilage) may occur at the sternum or rib margins
	Upper rectus abdominis trigger points on the left side; pectoralis, serratus anterior or sternalis muscles may produce precordial pain
Referral:	Variable depending on the structure involved
	Abdominal oblique trigger points have multiple referred pain patterns that may reach up into the chest (Travell and Simons, 1983)
	Pectoralis trigger points refer pain down the inner aspect of the arms along the ulnar distribution to the fourth and fifth digits
Description:	Aching or soreness
Intensity:	Mild to severe; may depend on patient's anxiety level—if fearful of a "serious" condition, the pain level may be accentuated and often decreases with medical reassurance that the condition is not an early sign of heart disease
Duration:	Seconds or hours
	Days to weeks, may become chronic over months if continually aggravated

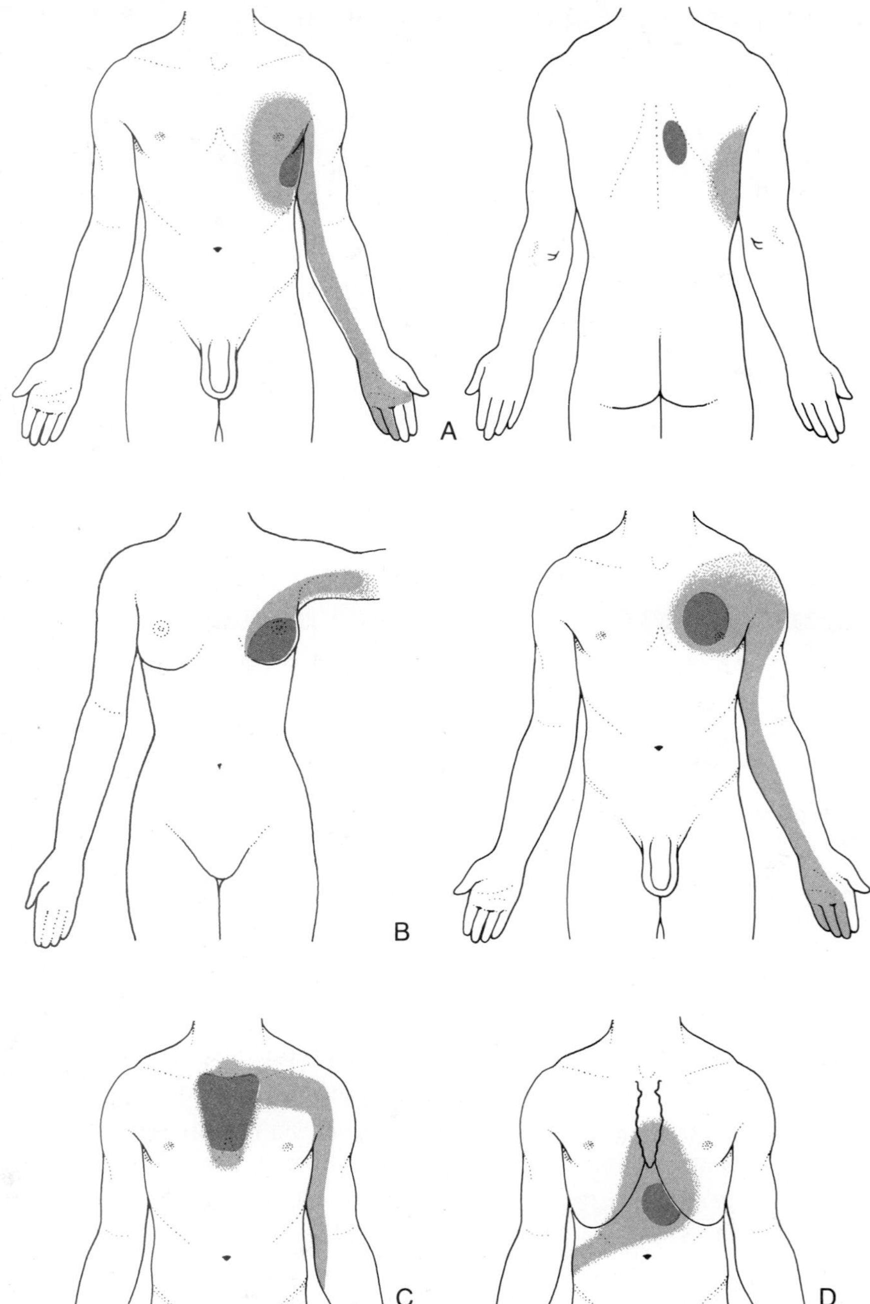

Figure 3–10. *A*, Referred pain pattern from the left serratus anterior muscle. *B*, Left pectoralis major muscle: Referred pain pattern in the woman and man. *C*, Referred pain pattern from the left sternalis muscle. *D*, Referred pain from the external oblique abdominal muscle can cause "heartburn" in the anterior chest wall. (*A, C,* and *D,* From Travell, J. G., and Simons, D. G.: Myofascial Pain and Dysfunction: The Trigger Point Manual. Baltimore, Williams & Wilkins, 1983. *B,* Adapted from Travell, J. G., and Simons, D. G.: Myofascial Pain and Dysfunction: The Trigger Point Manual. Baltimore, Williams & Wilkins, 1983.)

Associated Signs and Symptoms:	Usually none
	History of muscle exertion often associated with prolonged or repeated coughing secondary to upper respiratory infection
	Myofascial syndrome causing restricted chest expansion may be associated with shortness of breath, difficulty in taking a deep breath or in finishing a single sentence without stopping to breathe (Travell and Simons, 1983)
Relieving Factors:	Heat, immobilization during acute phase, medication relief does *not* occur with ingestion of nitroglycerin
Aggravating Factors:	Chest wall movement such as coughing, deep inspiration
	Tender to palpatory pressure; muscles involve ache when palpated or squeezed firmly
	Myofascial syndrome may be aggravated by a strong effort to protract the scapula (Travell and Simons, 1983)

Neurologic Disorders

Location:	May be localized around the precordium (upper central region of the abdomen, the diaphragm)
Referral:	May be localized along the course of the inflamed nerve at the sternum, in the axillary lines, or on either side of the vertebrae
	May be referred to the lateral and anterior chest wall
	Referral occasionally to one or both arms through branches of the brachial plexus; described as aching
Description:	Burning, stabbing, knifelike, exquisite tenderness to pressure
Intensity:	Usually intense
Duration:	Days to weeks, condition usually persists if untreated
Associated Signs and Symptoms:	Vesicular (blister) rash accompanies herpes zoster or "shingles," a distinctive form of dorsal nerve root irritation
	Hyperesthesia (increased sensitivity to touch or other sensory stimuli) may occur with herpes zoster
	Chills, fever, headache, malaise with neuritis of the chest wall
	Positive result on Adson's test, hyperabduction, or costoclavicular tests with thoracic outlet syndrome
	Neurologic signs associated with dorsal nerve root irritation (e.g., numbness, tingling, muscle atrophy)
Relieving Factors:	Heat, medication
Aggravating Factors:	Cold, palpatory pressure, exertion of the upper body

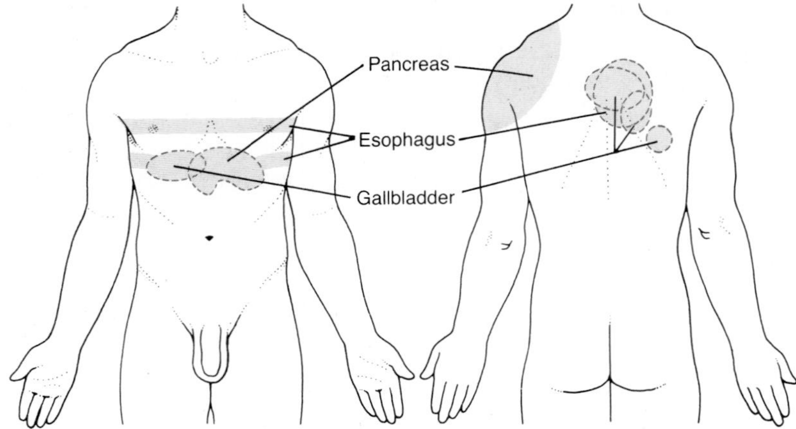

Figure 3–11. Chest pain caused by gastrointestinal disease with referred pain to the shoulder and back.

Gastrointestinal Disorders (patterns described in greater detail in Chapter 6)

Location:	Substernal, epigastric area of upper abdominal quadrants
Referral (Fig. 3–11):	May radiate around chest to shoulders, upper back
Description:	Burning, knotlike pain, "heartburn"
Intensity:	Mild to severe
Duration:	Minutes to hours
Associated Signs and Symptoms:	Nausea, jaundice, vomiting, blood in stool (melena), pain on swallowing associated with esophageal disorders
Relieving Factors:	Belching, antacids, upright position
Aggravating Factors:	Supine position, meals

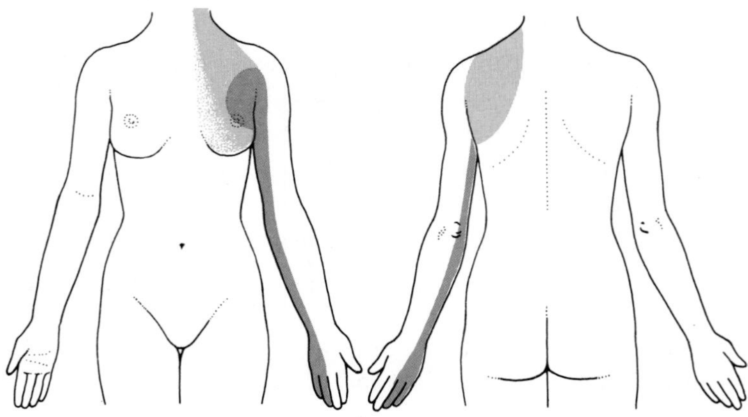

Figure 3–12. Pain arising from the breast showing (*A*) mammary pain referred into the axilla along the medial aspect of the arm; (*B*) referral pattern to the supraclavicular level and into the neck; (*C*) breast pain may diffuse around the thorax through the intercostal nerves. Pain may be referred to the back and to the posterior shoulder (not shown).

Breast Pain

Location (Fig. 3–12):	Specifically within the breast tissue
	May be localized in pectoral and supraclavicular areas
Referral:	Around the chest into the axilla, to the back at the level of the breast, occasionally into the neck and posterior aspect of the shoulder girdle
	Along the medial aspects of the arm(s) to fourth and fifth digits
Description:	Sharp, cutting, sharp aching
Intensity:	Mild to severe
Duration:	Intermittent to constant (may coincide with menstrual cycle)
Associated Signs and Symptoms:	May have no other symptoms
	May report change in breasts (e.g., discharge or bleeding from breasts, lumps, retracted nipple, distorted nipple or breast contour)
	Enlarged or tender lymph nodes
	Edematous and red, warm skin over the area of involvement
	Hypersensitivity of the nipple with intolerance to clothing
	Trigger points in the chest wall musculature associated with muscle exertion and resultant myalgia
	Previous history of MI with resultant pectoral trigger points
Relieving Factors:	Temporary relief may be obtained from rest, heat, or ice
Aggravating Factors:	Jarring or bouncing movement of the breasts
	Movement of the upper extremities
	Resistance to isometric movement of the upper extremities (pectoral myalgia)

Anxiety States

Location:	Variable but commonly in the substernal region and anterior chest
	Usually localized to a point
Referral:	Does not radiate
Description:	Sharp, stabbing, vague discomfort, pressure, burning, crushing
Intensity:	Mild to severe
Duration:	Usually brief, may last from minutes to hours
Associated Signs and Symptoms:	Dyspnea
	Fatigue

	Sighing respirations (hyperventilation)
	Chest wall tenderness
	Tachycardia
Relieving Factors:	Relaxation techniques, medications, rest
Aggravating Factors:	Intense emotion (e.g., anger, fear worry)
	Crowded places
	Not aggravated by deep inspiration

LABORATORY VALUES

The results of diagnostic tests can provide the therapist with information to assist in patient education. The patient often reports test results to the therapist and asks for information regarding the significance of those results. *The Patient's Guide to Medical Tests* (Pinckney and Pinckney, 1986) answers both patient's and therapist's specific questions. The information presented discusses potential causes for abnormal text values and includes comprehensive coverage of all available test procedures.

A basic understanding of laboratory tests used specifically in the diagnosis and monitoring of cardiovascular problems can provide the therapist with additional information regarding the patient's status. Some of the tests commonly used in the management and diagnosis of cardiovascular problems include cholesterol (including low-density lipoprotein [LDL]/high-density lipoprotein [HDL]) and triglyceride levels.

Other laboratory measurements of importance in the overall evaluation of the patient with CVD include red blood cell values (e.g., red blood cell count, hemoglobin, and hematocrit). Those values (see Chapter 5) provide valuable information regarding the oxygen-carrying capability of the blood and the subsequent oxygenation of body tissues such as the heart muscle.

Cholesterol

Cholesterol is a waxy substance and is a normal constituent of bile. High levels of serum cholesterol have been associated with the development of atherosclerosis, the formation of fatty plaques within the surface of blood vessel walls. A build-up of such deposits can occlude blood circulation to the heart muscle and can result in death of the heart muscle (myocardial infarction).

Excessive dietary intake of cholesterol and saturated fats increases the total blood cholesterol levels. There also seems to be an inherited tendency toward increased cholesterol levels. The following cholesterol values presented here can serve as a reference guide for the therapist. Cholesterol values vary according to age and may be elevated at the time of testing due to external circumstances (e.g., pregnancy, secondary to medications, position, ingestion of vitamins).

In the last few years, there has been disagreement among physicians with regard to the "normal" value of cholesterol. Some researchers and physicians suggest that the normal values listed should be considered abnormal and that much lower values should be applied as normal. At this time, the lower values suggested reflect more of an opinion than scientific fact (Pinckney and Pinckney, 1986).

The list of cholesterol values provided in Table 3-1 accounts for variance according to

Table 3-1. BLOOD CHOLESTEROL LEVELS

Age (Yrs)	Values (mg/dl)
<25	125-200
25-40	140-250
40-50	160-260
50-65	170-265
>65	175-280

age, which is a common method of categorization of cholesterol values. Blood cholesterol levels of greater than 250 mg/dl place the patient at "high risk" for the development of cardiovascular disease (Cella and Watson, 1989).

Triglycerides

Triglycerides are fats circulating in the bloodstream that are used in the body to provide energy for various metabolic activities. Excessive amounts of triglyceride are stored in adipose tissue. Triglyceride levels increase rapidly in response to foods high in calories, sugar, and fat. Triglyceride levels decrease with exercise. High levels of triglycerides are associated with increased risk of CVD. Triglyceride levels tend to increase with age and are slightly different for men and women. The values listed in Table 3-2 are guidelines for reference and may vary according to the same variables described for serum cholesterol. Levels greater than 250 mg/dl are believed to carry a greater risk of heart disease (Cella and Watson, 1989).

Low-Density Lipoprotein/ High-Density Lipoprotein

LDL and HDL are the two major types of cholesterol circulating in the blood serum. HDLs are thought to be formed in the liver and are the source of "good" or readily transportable cholesterol. Research has suggested that high levels of HDL and low levels of LDL are associated with decreased risk of CVD. HDL levels have been found to increase with exercise. Low levels of HDL and high levels of LDL are considered to be risk factors for the development of atherosclerotic heart disease (Cella and Watson, 1989).

Table 3-2. TRIGLYCERIDE LEVELS

Age (Yrs)	Value (mg/dl)
Infant	5-40
2-20	10-140
20-40	10-140 (women)
	10-150 (men)
40-60	10-180 (women)
	10-190 (men)

SUMMARY

When a patient mentions signs and symptoms, these may be clues to systemic disease processes that mimic musculoskeletal pain and dysfunction. Patients often confide in physical therapists and describe symptoms of a more serious nature. Cardiac symptoms unknown to the physician may be mentioned to the therapist during the opening interview or in subsequent visits.

The materials presented in this chapter help to prepare the therapist for making referral decisions. An understanding of the nature of thoracic pain provides a knowledge base for recognizing cardiac and noncardiac chest pain patterns and the systemic signs and symptoms associated with these patterns.

In addition to the systemic symptoms shown in Chapter 2 the therapist should review the signs and symptoms listed here for consideration when making a medical referral. The findings of the objective assessment in correlation with the medical history and presentation of any of these symptoms will help to clarify the referral decision.

Systemic Signs and Symptoms that Require Physician Referral

- Absent pulses
- Anxiety or apprehension
- Bradycardia
- Breast lumps or nodules
- Chest pain caused by exertion
- Chest pressure
- Claudication
- Cold sweat
- Diaphoresis
- Difficulty in swallowing
- Distortion of vision or speech
- Dyspnea
- Edema and weight gain
- Eructation
- Fever

"Heartbeat" in the back or abdomen
Heart fibrillation
Heart palpitations
Hemoptysis
Irritability
Migratory joint pain
Nausea/vomiting
Night sweats
Orthopnea
Nocturnal dyspnea
Painful shoulder-hand syndrome
Pallor
Persistent cough
Positive Homans' sign
Restlessness
Severe fatigue
Skin rashes or petechiae
Skipped heart beats
Sudden incoordination
Sudden weakness
Syncope
Tachycardia
Transient paralysis

SUBJECTIVE EXAMINATION

Special Questions to Ask

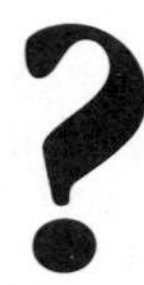

Past Medical History

- □ Has a doctor ever said that you have heart trouble?
- □ Have you ever had a heart attack?

  If yes, when? Please describe.
- □ Do you associate your current symptoms with your heart problems?
- □ Have you ever had rheumatic fever, growing pains, twitching of the limbs called St. Vitus' dance, or rheumatic heart disease?
- □ Have you ever had an abnormal electrocardiogram (ECG)?
- □ Have you ever had an ECG taken while you were exercising (e.g., climbing up and down steps or walking on a treadmill) which was not normal?
- □ Do you have a pacemaker, artificial heart, or any other device to assist your heart?

Angina/Myocardial Infarct

- □ Do you have angina (pectoris)?

  If yes, please describe the symptoms and tell me when it occurs.

  If no, pursue further with the following questions.
- □ Do you ever have discomfort or tightness in your chest?
- □ Have you ever had a crushing sensation in your chest with or without pain down your left arm?
- □ Do you have pain in your jaw either alone or in combination with chest pain?

Subjective Exam

Special Questions to Ask

□ If you climb a few flights of stairs fairly rapidly, do you have tightness or pressing pain in your chest?

□ Do you get pressure or pain or tightness in the chest if you walk in the cold wind or face a cold blast of air?

□ Have you ever had pain or pressure or a squeezing feeling in the chest that occurred during exercise, walking, or any other physical or sexual activity?

Associated Symptoms

□ Do you ever have bouts of rapid heart action, irregular heart beats, or palpitations of your heart?

□ Have you ever felt a heartbeat in your abdomen when you lie down?

If yes, is this associated with low back pain or left flank pain? **(Abdominal aneurysm)**

□ Do you ever notice sweating, nausea, or chest pain when your current symptoms (e.g., back pain, shoulder pain) occur?

□ Do you have frequent attacks of heartburn or do you take antacids to relieve heartburn or acid indigestion? **(Noncardiac cause of chest pain, abdominal muscle trigger point, gastrointestinal disorder)**

□ Do you get very short of breath during activities that do not make other people short of breath? **(Dyspnea)**

□ Do you ever wake up at night gasping for a air or short breath? **(Paroxysmal nocturnal dyspnea)**

□ Do you ever need to sleep on more than one pillow to breathe comfortably? **(Orthopnea)**

□ Do you ever get cramps in your legs if you walk for several blocks? **(Intermittent claudication)**

□ Do you ever have swollen feet or ankles?

If yes, are they swollen when you get up in the morning? **(Edema/CHF)**

□ Have you gained unexpected weight during a fairly short period of time (i.e., less than 1 week)? **(Edema, CHF)**

□ Do you ever feel dizzy or have fainting spells? **(Valvular insufficiency, bradycardia, pulmonary hypertension, orthostatic hypotension)**

□ Have you had any significant changes in your urine (e.g., increased amount, concentrated urine, frequency at night or decreased amount)? **(CHF, diabetes, hypertension)**

□ Do you ever have sudden difficulty with speech, temporary blindness, or other changes in your vision? **(Transient ischemic attacks)**

□ Have you ever had sudden weakness or paralysis down one side of your body or just in an arm or a leg? **(Transient ischemic attacks)**

Subjective Exam

Special Questions to Ask

Medications

□ Have you ever taken digitalis, nitroglycerin, or any other drug for your heart?

□ Have you been on a diet or taken medications to lower your blood cholesterol?

(For patients taking nitroglycerin)

□ Do you ever have headaches, dizziness, or a flushed sensation after taking nitroglycerin? (Most common side effects)

□ How quickly does your nitroglycerin reduce or eliminate your chest pain? (Use as a guideline in the clinic when the patient has angina during exercise; refer to a physician if angina is consistently unrelieved with nitroglycerin or rest after the usual period of time)

For Patients with Breast Pain

□ Do you have any discharge from your breasts or nipples?

□ Have you examined yourself for any lumps or nodules?

□ Have you been involved in any activities of a repetitive nature that could cause sore muscles (e.g., painting, washing walls, pushups, or other calisthenics, heavy lifting or pushing, overhead movements, prolonged running or fast walking)?

□ Have you recently been coughing excessively?

For Patients with Joint Pain

□ Have you had any skin rashes or dotlike hemorrhages under the skin? **(Rheumatic fever, endocarditis)**

If yes, did this occur after a visit to the dentist? **(Endocarditis)**

PHYSICIAN REFERRAL

The description and location of chest pain associated with pericarditis, myocardial infarction, angina, breast pain, gastrointestinal disorders, and anxiety are often similar. The physician is able to distinguish among these conditions through a careful history, medical examination, and medical testing.

For example, the severe substernal pain of pericarditis closely mimics the pain of acute myocardial infarction, but the two disorders differ in aggravating and relieving factors. Pain associated with gastrointestinal disorders involving the esophagus may create pain like that of angina pectoris, with discomfort precipitated by recumbency or by meals. However, the esophageal pain is not aggravated by exercise, whereas true angina is caused by exercise or by physical exertion and is relieved by rest (Andreoli et al, 1979). In both these examples, chest auscultation and an ECG provide the physician with valuable diagnostic information.

It is not the physical therapist's responsibility to differentiate diagnostically among the various causes of chest pain, but rather to recognize the systemic origin of signs and symptoms that may mimic musculoskeletal disorders. For example, compared with angina, the pain of true musculoskeletal disorders may last for seconds or for hours, is not relieved by nitroglycerin, and may be aggravated by exertion of just the upper body. The physical therapy interview presented in Chapter 2 is the primary mechanism used to begin exploring a patient's symptoms and is accomplished by carefully questioning the patient to determine the location, duration, intensity, frequency, associated symptoms, and relieving or aggravating factors related to pain or symptoms.

When to Refer Patient to Physician

Referral by the therapist to the physician is recommended when the patient presents with any combination of systemic signs or symptoms discussed throughout this chapter. These signs and symptoms should always be correlated with the patient's history to rule out systemic involvement or to identify musculoskeletal or neurologic disorders that would be appropriate for physical therapy treatment.

GUIDELINES FOR PHYSICIAN REFERRAL

- When a patient presents with any combination of systemic signs or symptoms
- Women with chest or breast pain who have a positive family history of breast cancer should always be referred to a physician for a follow-up examination
- Cardiac patients should be sent back to their physician under the following conditions:
    - Nitroglycerin tablets do not relieve anginal pain
    - Pattern of angina changes
    - Patient has abnormally severe chest pain
    - Anginal pain radiates to the jaw or to the left arm
    - Anginal pain is not relieved by rest
    - Upper back feels abnormally cool, sweaty, or moist to touch
    - Patient has any doubt about his or her present condition

IMMEDIATE MEDICAL ATTENTION

In the clinic setting, the onset of an anginal attack requires immediate cessation of exercise and rest. If the patient is currently taking nitroglycerin, self-administration of medication is recommended. Relief from pain should occur within 1 to 2 minutes. The dose may be repeated according to the prescribed direction. If anginal pain is not relieved in 20 minutes or if the patient has nausea, vomiting, or profuse sweating, immediate medical intervention may be indicated.

Changes in the pattern of angina, such as increased intensity, decreased threshold of stimulus, or longer duration of pain require immediate intervention by the physician. Patients in treatment under these circumstances should either be returned to the care of the nursing staff or, in the case of an outpatient, should be encouraged to contact their physician by telephone for further instructions before leaving the physical therapy department. The patient should be advised not to leave unaccompanied.

GUIDELINES FOR IMMEDIATE MEDICAL ATTENTION

- If anginal pain is not relieved in 20 minutes
- If the patient has nausea, vomiting, or profuse sweating

CASE STUDY

Referral

A 30-year-old woman with five children comes to you for an evaluation on the recommendation of her friend who received physical therapy from you last year. She has not been to a physician since her last child was delivered by her obstetrician 4 years ago. Her chief complaint is pain in the left shoulder and left upper trapezius with pain radiating into the chest and referred pain down the medial aspect of the arm to the thumb and first two fingers. When the medical history is being taken, she mentions that she was told 5 years ago that she had a mitral valve prolapse secondary to rheumatic fever, which she had when she was 12 years old.

There is no reported injury or trauma to the neck or shoulder, and the symptoms subside with rest. Physical exertion, such as carrying groceries up the stairs or laundry outside, aggravates the symptoms, but she is uncertain whether just using her upper body has the same effect. She is not taking any medication, denies any palpitations, but complains of fatigue and has dyspnea after playing ball with her son for 10 or 15 minutes.

Despite the patient's denial of injury or trauma, the neck and shoulder should be screened for any possible musculoskeletal or neurologic origin of symptoms. Your observation of the woman indicates that she is 30 to 40 lb overweight. She confides that she is under physical and emotional stress by the daily demands made by seven people in her house. She is not involved in any kind of exercise program outside of her play activities with the children. These two factors (obesity and stress) could account for her chronic fatigue and dyspnea, but that determination must be made by a physician. Even if you can identify a musculoskeletal basis for this patient's symptoms, the past medical history of rheumatic heart disease and absence of medical follow-up would support your recommendation that the patient should go to a physician for a medical check-up.

How do you rule out the possibility that this pain is not associated with a mitral valve prolapse and is caused instead by true cervical spine or shoulder pain?

It should be pointed out here that the physical therapist is not equipped with the skills, knowledge, or expertise to determine that the mitral valve prolapse is the cause of the patient's symptoms. However, a thorough subjective and objective evaluation can assist the therapist both in making a determination regarding the patient's musculoskeletal condition and in providing clear and thorough feedback for the physician upon referral.

Screening for Mitral Valve Prolapse

- Pain of a mitral valve must be diagnosed by a physician
- Mitral valve may be asymptomatic
- Patient has a positive history for rheumatic fever
- Carefully ask the patient about a history of possible neck or shoulder pain, which the patient may not mention otherwise

- Musculoskeletal pain associated with the neck or shoulder is more superficial than cardiac pain
- Total body exertion causing shoulder pain may be secondary to angina or myocardial ischemia and subsequent infarction, whereas movements of just the upper extremity causing shoulder pain are more indicative of a primary musculoskeletal lesion

  Does your shoulder pain occur during exercise, such as walking, climbing stairs, mowing the lawn, or during any other physical or sexual activity that doesn't require the use of your arm or shoulder?
- Presence of associated signs and symptoms, such as dyspnea, fatigue, or heart palpitations
- X-ray findings, if available, may confirm osteophyte formation with decreased intraforaminal spaces, which may contribute to cervical spine pain
- History of neck injury or overuse
- History of shoulder injury or overuse
- Results of objective tests to clear or rule out the cervical spine and shoulder as the cause of symptoms
- Presence of other neurologic signs to implicate the cervical spine or thoracic outlet type of symptoms (e.g., abnormal deep tendon reflexes, subjective report of numbness and tingling, objective sensory changes, muscle wasting or atrophy)
- Pattern of symptoms: A change in position may relieve symptoms associated with a cervical disorder

CASE STUDY

References

Andreoli, K.G., Fowkes, V.H., Zipes, D.P., and Wallace, A.G.: Comprehensive Cardiac Care, 4th ed. St. Louis, C.V. Mosby, 1979.

Andreoli, K.G., Zipes, D.P., Wallace, A.G., et al: Comprehensive Cardiac Care, 6th ed. St. Louis, C.V. Mosby, 1987.

Andreoli, T.E., Carpenter, C.J., Plum, F., and Smith, L.H.: Cecil's Essentials of Medicine. Philadelphia, W.B. Saunders Company, 1986.

Arthritis Foundation: Arthritis: Medical information series. Raynaud's phenomenon. Atlanta, GA, Arthritis Foundation, 1985.

Barnard, C., and Evans, P.: Your Healthy Heart. United Kingdom, Multimedia Publications, 1985.

Barnes, A.R., and Burchell, H.B.: Acute pericarditis simulating acute coronary occlusion. Am. Heart J., *23*:247, 1942.

Bauwens, D.B., and Paine, R.: *In* Thoracic pain. Blacklow, R.S. (ed): MacBryde's Signs and Symptoms, 6th ed. Philadelphia, J.B. Lippincott, 1983, pp. 139–164.

Berkow, R. (ed): The Merck Manual, 15th ed. New Jersey, Merck Sharp & Dohme Research Lab, 1987.

Capps, J.A., and Coleman, G.H.: An Experimental and Clinical Study of Pain in the Pleura, Pericardium and Peritoneum. New York, Macmillan, 1932.

Cella, J., and Watson, J.: Nurses' Manual of Laboratory Tests, 1st ed. Philadelphia, F.A. Davis, 1989.

Dawber, T.R., Meadors, G.F., and Moore, F.E., Jr.: Epidemiological approaches to heart disease: The Framingham study. Am. J. Public Health, *41*:279, 1951.

Fell, G., and Strandness, D.E.: Management of vascular disease. *In* Kotke, F.J., Stillwell, G.K., and Lehmann, J.F. (eds): Krusen's Handbook of Physical Medicine and Rehabilitation, 3rd ed. Philadelphia, W.B. Saunders Company, 1982, pp. 809–814.

Forshee, T.: Systemic origins of chest pain. Nurs 87, *17*:30, 1987.

Friedman, M., and Rosenman, R.H.: Type A Behavior and Your Heart. New York, Fawcett Crest, 1974.

Gasner, D., and McCleary, E.H.: The AMA Straight-Talk, No-Nonsense Guide to HEARTCARE. New York, Random House, 1984.

Hindle, P., and Wallace, A.G.: Complications of coronary artery disease. *In* Andreoli, K.G., Zipes, D.R., Wallace, A.G., et al (eds): Comprehension Cardiac Care, 6th ed. St. Louis, C.V. Mosby, 1987, pp. 114–129.

Hurst, J.W. (ed): The Heart, Vols. 1 and 2. New York, McGraw-Hill, 1986.

Juergens, J.L., Spittell, J.A., Jr., and Fairbairn, J.F., II:

Allen-Barker-Hines Peripheral Vascular Diseases, 5th ed. Philadelphia, W.B. Saunders Company, 1980.

Kavanagh, J.M.: Assessment of the cardiovascular system. *In* Phipps, W., Long, B., and Woods, N.: Medical-Surgical Nursing: Concepts and Clinical Practice. St. Louis, C.V. Mosby, 1987, pp. 1065–1192.

Kisner, C., and Colby, L.A.: Therapeutic Exercise: Foundation and Techniques. Philadelphia, F.A. Davis, 1985.

Layzer, R.B.: Neuromuscular Manifestations of Systemic Disease. Philadelphia, F.A. Davis, 1985.

Massie, E., and Kleiger, R.E.: Palpitation and tachycardia. *In* Blacklow, R.S. (ed): MacBryde's Signs and Symptoms, 6th ed. Philadelphia, J.B. Lippincott, 1983, pp. 295–315.

Miller, B.F., and Keane, C.B.: Encyclopedia and Dictionary of Medicine, Nursing and Allied Health, 4th ed. Philadelphia, W.B. Saunders, 1987.

Nursing 82: Giving Cardiac Care. Springhouse, PA, Intermed Communications, 1982.

Nursing 84: Cardiovascular Disorders. Springhouse, PA, Intermed Communications, 1984.

Pinckney, C., and Pinckney, E.R.: The Patient's Guide to Medical Tests. New York, Facts on File Publications, 1986.

Smith, R.B.: Thoracic outlet syndrome. *In* Hurst, J.W. (ed): The Heart, Vols. 1 and 2. New York, McGraw-Hill, 1986, pp. 916–918.

Stollerman, G.H.: Acute rheumatic fever and its management. *In* Hurst, J.W.: The Heart, Vols. 1 and 2. New York, McGraw-Hill, 1986, pp. 1306–1313.

Travell, J.G., and Simons, D.G.: Myofascial Pain and Dysfunction: The Trigger Point Manual. Baltimore, Williams & Wilkins, 1983.

Walsh, E., and Woloszyn, C.: Interventions for persons with problems of the peripheral vascular system. *In* Phipps, W., Long, B., and Woods, N.: Medical-Surgical Nursing: Concepts and Clinical Practice. St. Louis, C.V. Mosby, 1987, pp. 1193–1222.

Wenger, N.K., and Schlant, R.C.: *In* Hurst, J.W. (ed): The Heart, Vols. 1 and 2. New York, McGraw-Hill, 1986, pp. 817–838.

Young, J.R.: Diseases of the peripheral arteries. *In* Hurst, J.W. (ed): The Heart, Vols. 1 and 2. New York, McGraw-Hill, 1986, pp. 1339–1354.

Zipes, D.P., and Maloy, L.B.: Arrhythmias. *In* Andreoli, K.G., Zipes, D.P., Wallace, A.G., et al (eds): Comprehensive Cardiac Care, 6th ed. St. Louis, C.V. Mosby, 1987, pp. 131–202.

Bibliography

Amundsen, L.R.: Cardiac Rehabilitation. New York, Churchill Livingstone, 1981.

Fardy, P.S., Bennett, J.L., Reitz, N.L., and Williams, M.A.: Cardiac Rehabilitation. St. Louis, C.V. Mosby, 1980.

Irwin, S., and Tecklin, J.S.: Cardiopulmonary Physical Therapy, Vol. 1. St. Louis, C.V. Mosby, 1985.

Kostis, J.B., and DeFelice, E.A.: Beta Blockers in the Treatment of Cardiovascular Disease. New York, Raven Press, 1985.

Pollock, M.L., and Schmidt, D.H.: Heart Disease and Rehabilitation. New York, John Wiley & Sons, 1979.

Ross, J.J., and O'Rourke, R.A.: Understanding the Heart and Its Diseases. New York, McGraw-Hill, 1976.

Wyngaarden, J.B., and Smith, L.H., Jr., (eds): Cecil's Textbook of Medicine, 18th ed. Philadelphia, W.B. Saunders Company, 1988.

Chapter 4

Overview of Pulmonary Signs and Symptoms

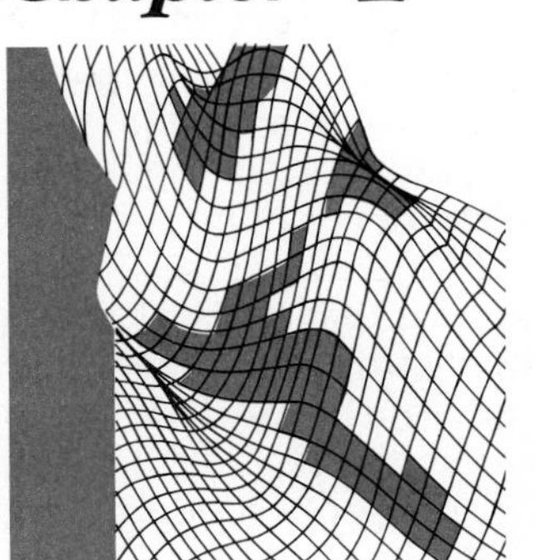

☐ ***Clinical Signs and Symptoms of:***

- Acute Bronchitis
- Chronic Bronchitis
- Emphysema
- Asthma
- Pneumonia
- Bronchiectasis
- Tuberculosis
- Lung Cancer
- Brain Metastasis
- Metastasis to the Spinal Cord
- Cystic Fibrosis
- Deep Venous Thrombosis
- Pulmonary Embolism
- Cor Pulmonale
- Pleurisy
- Spontaneous Pneumothorax
- Respiratory Acidosis
- Respiratory Alkalosis

Pulmonary pain patterns are usually localized in the substernal or chest region over involved lung fields that may include the anterior chest, side, or back. However, pulmonary pain can radiate to the neck, upper trapezius, costal margins, thoracic back, scapulae, or shoulder. Shoulder pain may radiate along the medial aspect of the arm mimicking other neuromuscular causes of neck or shoulder pain. Pulmonary pain usually increases with inspiratory movements, such as laughing, coughing, sneezing, or deep breathing, and the patient notes the presence of associated symptoms, such as dyspnea (exertional or at rest), persistent cough, fever, and chills.

In the case of pleuropulmonary disorders, the patient's recent personal medical history may include a previous or recurrent upper respiratory infection, or pneumonia. Central nervous system (CNS) symptoms, such as muscle weakness, muscle atrophy, headache, loss of lower extremity sensation, and localized or radicular back pain may be associated with lung cancer and must be investigated by a physician for diagnosis.

For the patient presenting with neck, shoulder, or back pain, it may be necessary to consider the possibility of a pulmonary cause requiring medical referral. The material in this chapter will assist the physical therapist treating both the patient with a known pulmonary problem and the patient presenting with musculoskeletal signs and symptoms that may have an underlying systemic basis.

For example, a 67-year-old woman with a known diagnosis of rheumatoid arthritis has been treated, when required, in a physical therapy clinic for the last 8 years. She has occasionally had chest pain that she describes as "coming on suddenly, like a knife pushing from the inside out — it takes my breath away." She missed 2 days of treatment due to illness, and when she returned to the clinic, the physical therapist noticed that she had newly developed a cough and that her rheumatoid arthritis was much worse. She says that she missed her appointments because she had the "flu." Further questioning to elicit the potential development of chest pain on inspiration, the presence of ongoing fever and chills, and the changes in breathing pattern would be warranted if the patient continues to complain of persistent symptoms. Positive findings beyond the reasonable period for influenza (7 to 10 days) or increase in pulmonary symptoms would lead the physical therapist to suggest that the patient should seek medical attention.

This actual clinical case points out the fact that patients currently undergoing physical therapy for a known musculoskeletal problem may be describing to the physical therapist signs and symptoms of systemic disease. The alert professional should recognize the need for medical follow-up.

PULMONARY PHYSIOLOGY

The primary function of the respiratory system is to provide oxygen and to remove carbon dioxide from cells in the body. The act of breathing, in which the oxygen and carbon dioxide exchange occurs, involves the two interrelated processes of ventilation and respiration. Ventilation is the movement of air from outside the body to the alveoli of the lungs. Respiration is the process of oxygen uptake and carbon dioxide elimination between the body and the outside environment (Brucia, 1987).

The structures involved in the act of breathing are divided into two main categories — upper airway and lower airway. The upper airway consists of the nose, sinuses, pharynx, tonsils, and larynx, and the lower airway consists of the conducting airways (trachea, right and left mainstem bronchi) and respiratory units (respiratory bronchioles, alveolar ducts, and alveoli). The structures of the upper airway function to warm, moisten, and filter the air that enters the lungs.

The larynx forms the upper portion of the trachea and consists of several cartilaginous structures held together by muscles and ligaments. The chief functions of the larynx are to serve as an airway between the trachea and pharynx and to protect the vocal cords. The epiglottis, a leaf-shaped lid of fibrocartilage, closes the entrance to the larynx during swallowing, thus food and fluid are not aspirated (inhaled) into the trachea. The closing of the entrance into the trachea (glottis) also allows for an increase in intrathoracic pressure needed for lifting and coughing (Brucia, 1987).

The conducting airway structures have three primary functions: filtering, warming, and humidifying air. Air inspired through a normal respiratory tree is filtered of all particles before reaching the alveoli. This filtration occurs because goblet cells in the epithelial layer of the airways secrete copious amounts of mucus that coat the airways and trap foreign particles. In addition, cilia, which are found as far into the respiratory tree as the bronchi, then propel the mucus up the airway so that the foreign material can be removed by coughing, sneezing, or swallowing.

Respiration occurs within the alveoli (minute sacs that arise from the walls of the respiratory bronchioles) and within the alveolar ducts. The alveoli consist of a single layer of squamous epithelium and an elastic basement membrane. These two layers in conjunction with the layers of capillary endothelium form the alveolar-capillary membrane across which diffusion of oxygen and carbon dioxide occur.

The alveoli, in addition to respiratory function, produce surfactant, which is a substance that prevents lung collapse.

The right lung is divided into three lobes: upper, middle, and lower; the left lung has only two lobes: upper and lower. The right bronchus (airway leading to the lung) is wide and short and extends from the trachea at a straighter angle than does the left bronchus. The left bronchus is narrower and lies at more of an angle from the trachea (Brucia, 1987).

The lungs lie in and are protected by the thoracic cavity, which consists of the sternum and ribs anteriorly, and the ribs, scapulae, and vertebral column, posteriorly. The thoracic cavity is lined with pleura or serous membrane. One surface of the pleura lines the inside of the rib cage (parietal pleura), and the other surface, the visceral pleura, covers the lungs (Brucia, 1987).

Pulmonary Ventilation

Air moves in and out of the lungs as a result of changes in pressure. At the beginning of inspiration, the atmospheric air pressure is greater than alveolar pressure, thus air moves into the alveoli. When the alveolar pressure is greater than atmospheric pressure, expiration occurs and air moves out of the lungs. The pressure gradient between the atmosphere and the alveoli is created by changes in the size of the thoracic cavity. As the thorax increases in size, pressure in the thorax decreases and air flows in from the atmosphere. The size of the thorax increases by contraction of the diaphragm and the external intercostal muscles. As the thorax expands, it pulls the lungs with it because the moist surfaces of the lungs and chest wall are bound together. Expiration is a passive process that is caused by the elastic recoil of the lungs and thoracic muscles (Brucia, 1987).

Gas Movement

Oxygen diffuses across the alveolar-capillary membrane from the alveoli into the blood because the pressure of oxygen of the alveolar air is greater than that of venous blood. Carbon dioxide diffuses in the opposite direction because the pressure of carbon dioxide in the venous blood is greater than the pressure of carbon dioxide in the alveolar air. Diffusion of oxygen can be decreased by the following factors (Brucia, 1987)

- Decreased atmospheric oxygen
- Decreased alveolar ventilation
- Decreased alveolar-capillary surface area
- Increased alveolar-capillary membrane thickness

Breathing is an automatic process by which sensors detecting changes in the levels of carbon dioxide continuously direct data to the medulla. The medulla then directs respiratory muscles that adjust ventilation. Breathing patterns can be altered voluntarily when this automatic response is overridden by conscious thought. The major sensors mentioned here are the central chemoreceptors (located near the medulla) and the peripheral sensors (located in the carotid body and aortic arch). The central chemoreceptors respond to increases in carbon dioxide and decreases in pH in cerebrospinal fluid. As carbon dioxide increases, the medulla signals a response to increase respiration. The peripheral chemoreceptor system responds to low arterial blood oxygen and is believed to function only in pathologic situations, such as when there are chronically elevated carbon dioxide levels (e.g., chronic obstructive pulmonary disease [COPD]).

PULMONARY PATHOPHYSIOLOGY

Chronic Obstructive Pulmonary Disease

COPD occurs in patients with chronically obstructed airways. This disease is most commonly caused by chronic bronchitis and emphysema and is less often attributed to bronchiectasis, asthma, and cystic fibrosis. COPD is an inclusive term for long-term pulmonary diseases, characterized by increased resistance to airflow, and usually refers to a combination of chronic bronchitis and emphysema. Predisposing factors to COPD include cigarette smoking, air pollution, occupational exposure to irritating dusts or gases, familial hereditary factors, infection, allergies, aging, and potentially harmful drugs and chemicals. COPD rarely occurs in nonsmokers. Air pollution, combined with the effects of cigarette smoking, exacerbates COPD by inducing bronchospasm and muscosal edema, which in turn, increases airway resistance (Nursing 84, 1984).

In all forms of COPD, narrowing of the airways obstructs airflow to and from the lungs (Table 4–1). This narrowing impairs ventilation by trapping air in the bronchioles and alveoli. The obstruction increases the resistance to airflow. Trapped air hinders normal gas exchange and causes distention of the alveoli. Other pathology of COPD varies with each form of the disease (Nursing 84, 1984).

Bronchitis

Acute. Acute bronchitis is an inflammation of the trachea and bronchi (tracheobronchial tree) that is selflimiting and of short duration with few pulmonary signs. Acute bronchitis may result from chemical irritation (e.g., smoke, fumes, gas) or may occur with infections such as influenza, measles, chickenpox, or whooping cough. These predisposing conditions may become apparent during the subjective examination (i.e., *Personal/Family History* form or the *Physical Therapy Interview*). Although bronchitis is usually mild, it can become complicated in elderly patients and in patients with chronic lung or heart disease. Pneumonia is a critical complication (Berkow, 1987).

CLINICAL SIGNS AND SYMPTOMS OF ACUTE BRONCHITIS

- Mild fever from 1 to 3 days
- Malaise
- Back and muscle pain
- Sore throat
- Cough with sputum production followed by wheezing
- Possibly laryngitis

Chronic. Chronic bronchitis is a condition associated with prolonged exposure to nonspecific bronchial irritants and is accompanied by mucous hypersecretion and by structural changes in the bronchi (large air passages leading into the lungs) (Berkow,

Table 4–1. RESPIRATORY DISEASES: SUMMARY OF DIFFERENCES

Disease	Primary Area Affected	Result
Bronchitis	Membrane lining bronchial tubes	Inflammation of lining
Bronchiectasis	Bronchial tubes (bronchi or air passages)	Bronchial dilation with inflammation
Pneumonia	Alveoli (air sacs)	Causative agent invades alveoli with resultant outpouring from lung capillaries into air spaces and continued healing process
Emphysema	Air spaces beyond terminal bronchioles (alveoli)	Breakdown of alveolar walls Air spaces enlarged
Asthma	Bronchioles (small airways)	Bronchiole obstructed by muscle spasm, swelling of mucosa, thick secretions
Cystic fibrosis	Bronchioles	Bronchioles become obstructed and obliterated. Later, larger airways become involved. Plugs of mucus cling to airway walls leading to bronchitis, bronchiectasis, atelectasis, pneumonia, or pulmonary abscess

1987). This irritation of the tissue usually results from exposure to cigarette smoke, long-term dust inhalation, or air pollution and causes hypertrophy of mucous-producing cells in the bronchi. The swollen mucous membrane and thick sputum obstruct the airways causing wheezing, and the patient develops a cough to clear the airways. The clinical definition of a patient with chronic bronchitis is anyone who coughs for at least 3 months per year for 2 consecutive years without having had a precipitating disease.

In bronchitis, partial or complete blockage of the airways from mucous secretions causes insufficient oxygenation in the alveoli. This combination of cyanosis from insufficient arterial oxygenation and edema from ventricular failure may result in the patient known as a "blue bloater" (Fig. 4–1).

CLINICAL SIGNS AND SYMPTOMS OF CHRONIC BRONCHITIS

- Persistent cough with production of sputum (worse in the morning and evening than at mid-day)
- Reduced chest expansion
- Wheezing
- Fever
- Dyspnea (shortness of breath)
- Cyanosis (blue discoloration of skin and mucous membranes)
- Pulmonary edema

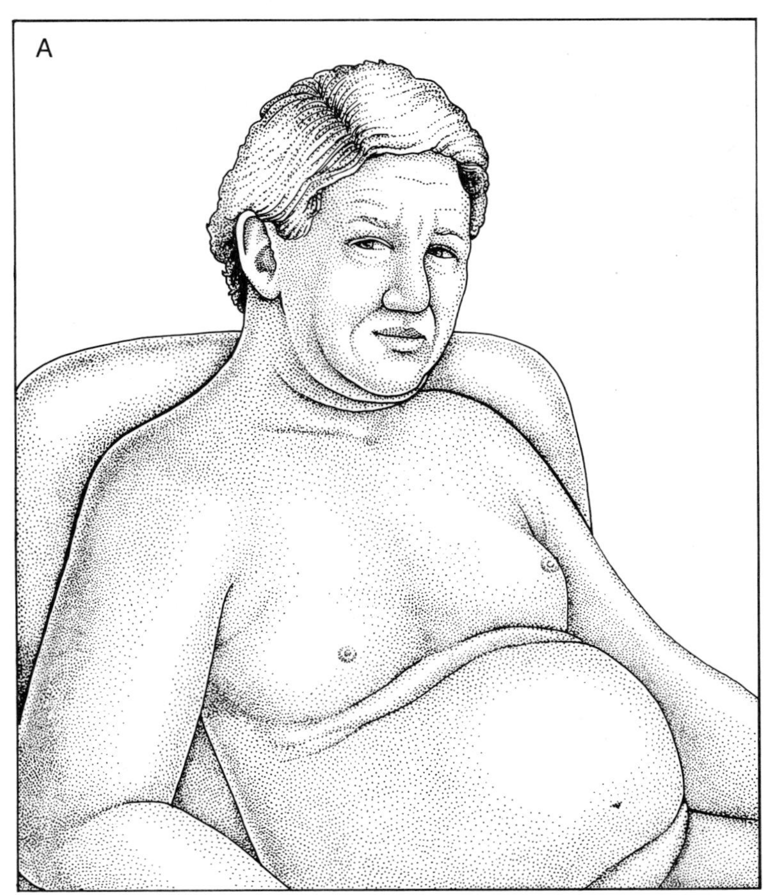

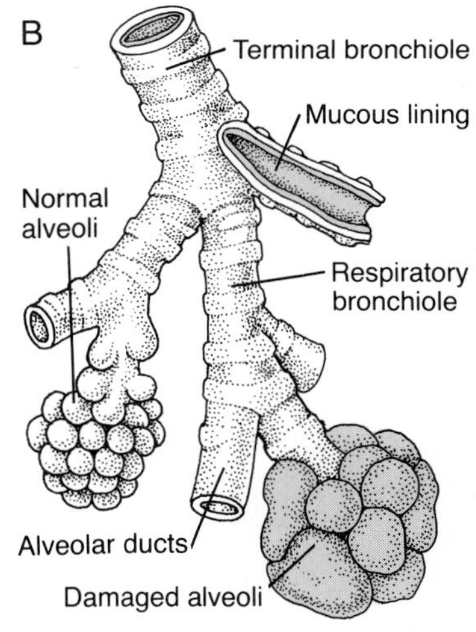

Figure 4–1. *A*, The patient with chronic bronchitis may develop cyanosis and pulmonary edema causing a characteristic look called "the blue bloater." *B*, Chronic bronchitis may lead to the formation of the misshapen or large alveolar sacs with reduced space for oxygen and carbon dioxide exchange.

Emphysema

Emphysema may develop after a long history of chronic bronchitis, during which air becomes trapped in the alveoli because mucus blocks the small terminal bronchioles and airway walls have collapsed (Nursing 84, 1984). Emphysema is thus an accumulation of air in the lungs resulting from abnormal enlargement or overinflation of air sacs (alveoli) in the lungs with destruction of lung tissue. When the air spaces become overinflated, the alveolar walls rupture and the alveolar capillary bed is destroyed (Ford, 1987). This irreversible destruction reduces the elasticity of the lungs, and the effort to exhale trapped air causes dyspnea on exertion or eventually, dyspnea at rest. The combined effects of trapped air and alveolar distention change the size and shape of the patient's chest causing a barrel chest, increased expiratory effort, and the characteristic name: "pink puffer" (Fig. 4–2).

Centrilobular emphysema (see Fig. 4–2) is one of two primary types of emphysema. It occurs when several bronchioles break down

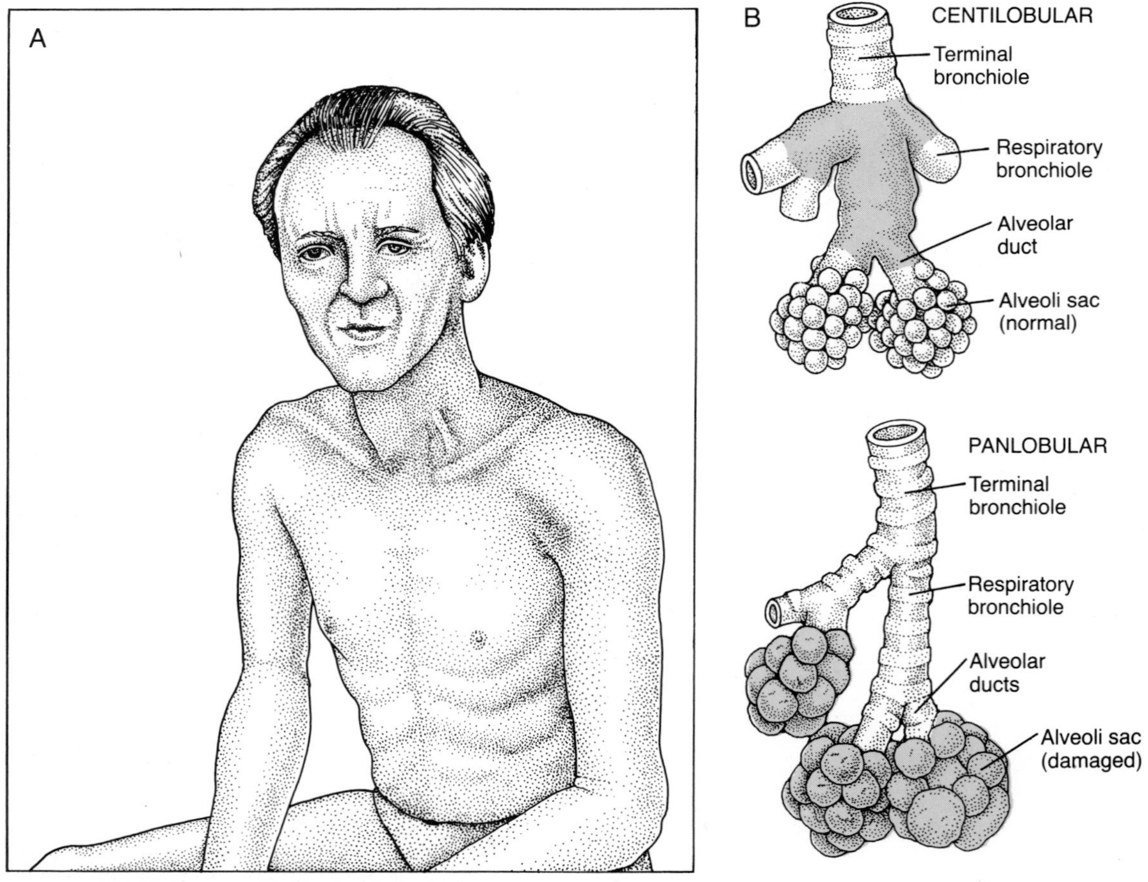

Figure 4–2. *A*, The patient with emphysema develops trapped air in the lungs so that cyanosis is not a problem, but rather, expelling air becomes increasingly difficult. The resultant physical features may be referred to as "the pink puffer." *B*, Centrilobular emphysema affects the upper airways and produces destructive changes in the bronchioles. Panlobular emphysema affects the lower airways and is more diffusely scattered throughout the alveoli.

to form an airspace, whereas, panlobular (or panacinar) emphysema occurs when the more distal alveolar walls are destroyed. This destruction of alveolar walls may occur secondary to infection or to irritants (most commonly, cigarette smoke). As the disease progresses, there is a loss of surface area available for gas exchange. In the final stages of emphysema, the overloaded heart reaches its limit of muscular compensation and begins to fail (cor pulmonale). The most important factor in the treatment of chronic bronchitis and emphysema is cessation of smoking.

Pursed-lip breathing causes resistance to outflow at the lips, which in turn maintains intrabronchial pressure and improves the mixing of gases in the lungs. This type of breathing should be encouraged to help the patient to get rid of the stale air trapped in the lungs. Cardiac complications, especially enlargement and dilatation of the right ventricle with resultant right-sided heart failure (cor pulmonale) may develop from pulmonary emphysema (Miller and Keane, 1987).

CLINICAL SIGNS AND SYMPTOMS OF EMPHYSEMA

- Shortness of breath
- Dyspnea on exertion
- Orthopnea (only able to breathe in the upright position) immediately after assuming the supine position
- Chronic cough
- Barrel chest
- Weight loss
- Malaise
- Use of accessory muscles of respiration
- Prolonged expiratory period (with grunting)
- Wheezing
- Pursed-lip breathing
- Increased respiratory rate
- Peripheral cyanosis

INFLAMMATORY/INFECTIOUS DISEASES

Allergies

Allergy refers to the abnormal hypersensitivity that takes place when a foreign substance (allergen) is introduced into the body of a person prone to allergies. The body fights these invaders by producing a special antibody called immunoglobulin E(IgE). This antibody, a chemical released into the blood, helps the body to attack and destroy foreign materials. *Atopy* refers to people who have a genetic predisposition to produce large quantities of IgE causing this state of clinical hypersensitivity or allergy. Allergy is a reflection of the individual's production of this IgE antibody. The reaction between the allergen and the susceptible person (i.e., allergy-prone host) results in the development of a number of typical signs and symptoms usually involving the gastrointestinal tract, respiratory tract, or skin.

Clinical signs and symptoms of allergies vary from one patient to another according to the allergies present. Each patient should be asked what known allergies are present and what the specific reaction to the allergen would be for that particular patient. The physical therapist can then be alert to any of these warning signs during treatment and can take necessary measures, whether that means grading exercise to patient tolerance or appropriately using prescribed medications.

Asthma

Asthma, a medical term, which comes from the Greek word for "panting" and means "shortness of breath," (Gershwin and Klingelhofer, 1986) is actually a collection of respiratory symptoms caused by infections, hypersensitivity to irritants (e.g., pollutants, allergens), psychologic stress, cold air, exercise, or drug use (Nursing 84, 1984). Bronchospasms of the smooth muscle lining the bronchial tubes cause narrowing of the airways, and

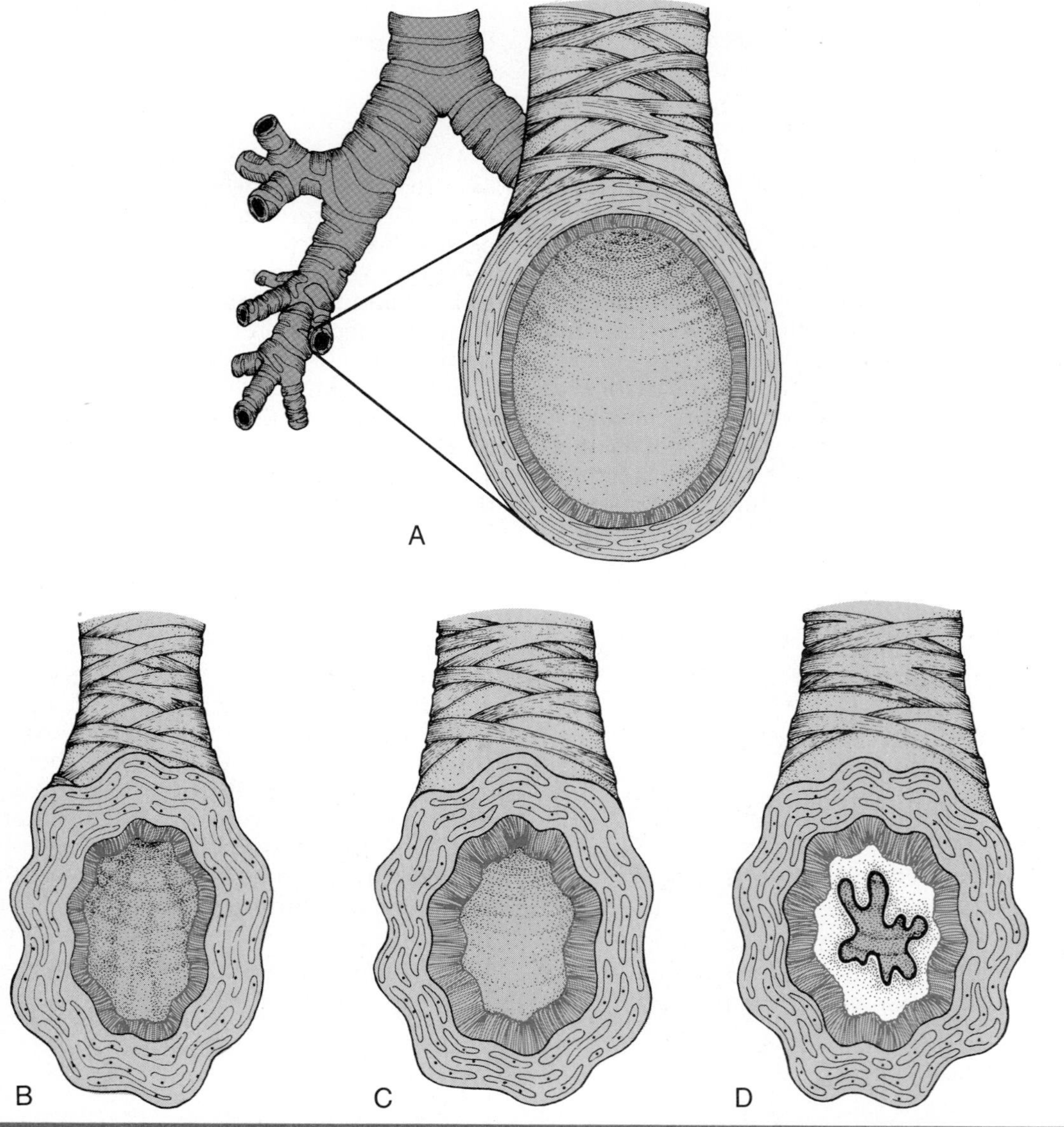

Figure 4–3. *A*, Cross-section of a normal bronchus, with mucous membrane in color. *B*, Bronchospasm: The smooth muscle surrounding the bronchus contracts and causes narrowing of the airway. *C*, Edema of the mucous membrane further narrows the airway. *D*, Increased mucous secretion by the submucosal glands. (From Foster, R.L., Hunsberger, M.M., and Anderson, J.J.: Family-Centered Nursing Care of Children. Philadelphia, W.B. Saunders Company, 1989.)

these spasms are accompanied by edema (Fig. 4–3).

Hypersecretion of mucus causes airway obstruction with resultant wheezing on expiration, and a cough develops to eliminate mucus. This narrowing of airways is diffuse, but uneven, thus some alveoli are overventilated and others are underventilated, which leads to hypoxia (decreased oxygen in the arterial blood).

Asthma may occur at any age, although it is likely to occur for the first time before 5 years of age. In childhood, it is three times more common and more severe in males; however, after puberty, the incidence in the sexes is equal. Ten to fifteen million Americans endure various degrees of asthma, from occasional bouts of shallow breathing to episodes severe enough to cause hypoxia (reduction of oxygen in body tissues) and cyanosis. According to the National Center for Health Statistics (NCHS), asthma is the leading cause of morbidity (illness resulting in loss of time at work or school) in the United States. It is found more often in urban, industrialized settings, in colder climates, and among the urban disadvantaged, especially blacks. The effects of asthma are reversible with treatment.

Asthma may be categorized according to the precipitating cause(s): *extrinsic* bronchial asthma (or allergic asthma) refers to attacks that follow exposure to allergens, such as airborne pollens, molds, dust, and animal dander (skin and hair shedding). It is associated with high serum levels of the special antibody called IgE, which is a hereditary allergic mechanism, and represents a true allergic reaction. These patients are still likely to wheeze after exertion or exercise.

Intrinsic bronchial asthma (or infective asthma) follows or can be made worse by infection, psychologic or emotional stress, and changes in environment or climate. Physical exertion is a well-known trigger for asthma and causes exercise-induced asthma. The attack typically comes a few minutes after the workout, when the body's output of adrenaline (which dilates the airways) subsides. In most persons, both allergenic and nonallergenic factors are significant and cause a *mixed* asthma of both extrinsic and intrinsic elements (Gershwin and Klingelhofer, 1986).

CLINICAL SIGNS AND SYMPTOMS OF ASTHMA

Clinical signs and symptoms of asthma differ in degree (Table 4–2) and frequency among patients, but the primary symptoms are:

- Episodes of dyspnea
- Prolonged expiration
- Cough with or without sputum production, especially 5 or 10 minutes after exercise begins
- Skin retraction (clavicles, ribs, sternum)
- Abnormal fatigue
- Tickle in the back of the throat accompanied by a cough
- Tickle occasionally at the back of the neck
- Wheezing (advanced asthma)
- Nostril flaring (advanced)

The patient prefers to sit upright or leans forward, using accessory muscles of respiration. Sternocleidomastoid retraction and intercostal retractions are evident during inspiration along with nasal flaring. As the airway obstruction becomes more severe, the patient may become anxious, which, in turn, increases the body's metabolic demands inducing fatigue and further respiratory distress (Nursing 84, 1984).

Physical therapists working with known asthmatics should encourage patients to main-

Table 4–2. STAGES OF ASTHMA

Mild	Moderate	Severe
Symptoms reverse with cessation of activity	Audible wheezing Use of accessory muscles of respiration Leaning forward to catch breath	Blue lips/fingernails Tachypnea (30–40/min) despite cessation of activity Cyanotic-induced seizures Skin and rib retraction

tain hydration by drinking fluids to prevent mucous plugs from hardening and to take prescribed medications (e.g., antihistamines, bronchodilators) before exercising in order to minimize exercise-induced attacks. Exercise or hyperventilation-induced asthma can be potentially prevented by exercising in a moist, humid environment and by grading exercise per patient tolerance using diaphragmatic breathing.

Pneumonia

Pneumonia is an inflammation of the lungs and can be caused by a bacterial, viral, or mycoplasmal infection. It may be primary or secondary (a complication of another disease) and may involve one or both lungs at the level of the lobe (lobular pneumonia) or more distally at the bronchioles and alveoli (bronchopneumonia). Bronchopneumonia is seen more frequently than lobular pneumonia and is common in patients postoperatively and in patients with chronic bronchitis, particularly when these two situations coexist (Gaskell and Webber, 1980). Infectious agents responsible for pneumonia are typically present in the upper respiratory tract and cause no harm unless resistance is lowered severely by some other factor, such as a severe cold, disease, alcoholism, or generally by poor health (e.g., poorly controlled diabetics, patients with chronic renal problems). The elderly or bedridden patients are particularly at risk due to physical inactivity and immobility. This limited mobility causes normal secretions to pool in the airways and thus facilitates bacterial growth (Miller and Keane, 1987).

CLINICAL SIGNS AND SYMPTOMS OF PNEUMONIA

Clinical signs and symptoms of pneumonia depend on the type of pneumonia but may include:

- Sudden and sharp pleuritic chest pain that is aggravated by chest movement
- Hacking productive cough (rusty or green, purulent sputum)
- Dyspnea
- Tachypnea (rapid respirations associated with fever or pneumonia) accompanied by decreased chest excursion on the affected side
- Cyanosis
- Headache
- Fever and chills
- Generalized aches and myalgia that may extend to the thighs and calves
- Fatigue

Bronchiectasis

Bronchiectasis is a chronic pulmonary condition that occurs after infections, such as childhood pneumonia or cystic fibrosis. The prevalence of this disease has fallen greatly since the introduction of antibiotics (West, 1977). It is characterized by abnormal dilatation of the large air passages leading into the lungs (bronchi) and by destruction of bronchial walls. Bronchiectasis is caused by repeated damage to bronchial walls. The resultant destruction and bronchial dilatation reduce bronchial wall movement so that secretions cannot be removed effectively from the lungs, and the patient is predisposed to frequent respiratory infections (Ford, 1987). Ventilation is eventually obstructed, and advanced bronchiectasis may cause pneumonia, cor pulmonale, or right-sided ventricular failure (Nursing 84, 1984).

CLINICAL SIGNS AND SYMPTOMS OF BRONCHIECTASIS

Clinical signs and symptoms of bronchiectasis vary widely depending on the extent of the disease and on the presence of complicating infection, but may include:

- Chronic, "wet" cough with copious foul-smelling secretions; generally worse in the morning after being recumbent for a length of time

- Hemoptysis (bloody sputum)
- Occasional wheezing sounds
- Dyspnea
- Sinusitis (inflammation of one or more paranasal sinuses)
- Weight loss
- Anemia
- Malaise
- Recurrent fever and chills

Tuberculosis

Tuberculosis (TB) is a bacterial infectious disease transmitted by the gram-positive, acid-fast bacillus, *Mycobacterium tuberculosis.* TB most often involves the lungs, but can also occur in the kidneys, bones, lymph nodes, and meninges and can be disseminated throughout the body (Lewis, 1983). The mycobacterium is usually spread by airborne droplet nuclei, which are produced when infected persons sneeze, speak, or cough. Once released into the atmosphere, the organisms are dispersed and can be inhaled by a susceptible host. Brief exposure to a few bacilli rarely causes an infection. More commonly, it is spread with repeated close contact with an infected person.

After the bacilli are inhaled, they pass into the respiratory system and implant themselves on the bronchioles or alveoli. After implantation, the organisms multiply with no initial resistance from the host. While a cellular immune response is being activated, the bacilli can spread via lymph channels to circulating blood and thus throughout the body so that significant spread can occur before the body can mount a defense. Eventually, acquired cell-mediated immunity limits further multiplication and a characteristic tissue reaction called an epithelioid cell tubercle results. The central portion of this lesion undergoes necrosis and can produce a cavity in the bronchi. Tubercular material may then enter the bronchial system and can be transmitted via airborne droplets.

This lesion heals and calcification and scarring take place. These changes can be seen by x-ray. When the lesion heals, the infection enters a latent period in which it may persist without producing a clinical illness. The infection may remain dormant or may develop into a clinical disease if persistent organisms begin to rapidly multiply (Lewis, 1983). Certain individuals are at higher risk for clinical disease, including those who are immunosuppressed, diabetics, children less than 2 years of age, and adolescents. Clinical TB can also occur as an opportunistic infection in human immunodeficiency virus (HIV) infected (i.e., acquired immunodeficiency syndrome [AIDS]) patients who are also infected with the tubercle bacillus. The incidence of TB has risen for the first time in recent history, most prominently in areas of the country where there are many patients infected with HIV (MMWR, 1987).

Clinical signs and symptoms are absent in the early stages of TB. Many cases are found incidentally when routine chest x-rays are done for other reasons. When systemic manifestations of active disease initially present, the clinical signs and symptoms listed below may appear.

CLINICAL SIGNS AND SYMPTOMS OF TUBERCULOSIS

- Fatigue
- Malaise
- Anorexia
- Weight loss
- Low-grade fevers (especially in late afternoon)
- Night sweats
- Frequent, productive cough
- Dull chest pain or discomfort

Tuberculin skin testing is done to determine if the body's immune response has been activated by the presence of the bacillus. A positive reaction develops 3 to 10 weeks after the initial infection. A positive skin test reaction indicates the presence of a tuberculous infection, but does not show whether the infection is dormant or is causing a clinical illness. Chest x-rays and sputum cultures are done as a follow-up to positive skin tests. All cases of active disease are treated, and certain cases of inactive disease are treated prophylactically.

NEOPLASTIC DISEASE

Lung Cancer (Bronchogenic Carcinoma) (Nursing 84, 1984)

Lung cancer is the leading cause of cancer death in American men and women (now surpassing breast cancer as being the most common cancer in women). There is a close correlation between the number of cigarettes smoked and the development of cancer of the lung and larynx with an estimated 120,000 new cases of bronchogenic cancer per year in the United States. The majority of these people die within 5 years after diagnosis. Eighty per cent of all patients who are diagnosed as having lung cancer are smokers (Loehnen, 1989). Informed opinion now accepts the viewpoint that 85 to 90% of lung cancers result from cigarette smoking (Morgan and Hales, 1983). The 5-year survival rate (number of patients who are alive 5 years after the initial diagnosis of lung cancer) is only 8% for men and 12% for women. Cigarette smoking multiplies the risk of lung cancer when combined with exposure to occupational respiratory carcinogens, such as asbestos.

Clinical signs and symptoms of lung cancer remain silent until the disease process is at an advanced stage. The patient may have a vague aching in the chest associated with lung cancer. Depending on the type of cancer, the patient may have pleuritic pain on inspiration that limits lung expansion.

EARLY SYMPTOMS OF LUNG CANCER

- Hemoptysis (coughing or spitting up blood due to ulceration of blood vessels)
- Dyspnea (shortness of breath)
- Wheezing (due to obstruction of the bronchus)
- Seizures
- Recurrent pneumonia
- Sudden, unexplained weight loss

More specific symptoms are related to the locations of the primary tumor and of tumor metastases (transfer of disease from one organ to another not directly connected with it). Metastatic tumors may involve the chest wall, pleura, pulmonary parenchyma, or bronchi. Tumor spread to these structures may occur via the blood stream or lymphatic channels or by direct extension. The lungs are the most frequent site of metastases because any tumor cells dislodged from a primary neoplasm into the circulation or lymphatics are usually filtered by the lungs. Carcinoma of the kidney, breast, pancreas, colon, and uterus are especially likely to metastasize to the lungs (Morgan, 1983).

Central tumors cause increased cough, dypsnea, and diffuse chest pain that can refer pain to the scapulae and upper back. This pain is the result of peribronchial or perivascular nerve involvement. Other symptoms may include postobstructive pneumonia with fever, chills, malaise and anorexia, hemoptysis, and fecal breath odor (secondary to infection within a necrotic tumor mass). If these tumors extend to the pericardium, the patient may develop a sudden onset of dysrhythmia (tachycardia or atrial fibrillation), weakness, anxiety, and dyspnea.

Apical (Pancoast's) tumors of the lung apex do not usually cause symptoms while confined to the pulmonary parenchyma. They can extend into surrounding structures and frequently involve the eighth cervical and first thoracic nerves within the brachial plexus. This nerve involvement produces (sharp) neuritic pain in the axilla, shoulder, and subscapular area on the affected side with atrophy of the upper extremity muscles.

Trigger points of the serratus anterior muscle (see Fig. 3–10) also mimic the distribution of pain caused by eighth cervical nerve root compression. Trigger points may be ruled out by palpation or lack of neurologic deficits and may be confirmed by elimination with appropriate physical therapy treatment (e.g., stretching, neuroprobe, spray, and stretch) (Reynolds, 1981). Further local tumor growth may erode the first and second ribs and associated vertebrae, causing bone pain and paravertebral pain associated with involvement of sympathetic nerve ganglia.

Peripheral tumors are most often asymptomatic until the tumor extends through visceral and parietal pleura to the chest wall. Irritation of the nerves causes localized sharp pleuritic pain that is aggravated by inspiration. Metastases to the mediastinum (tissues and organs between the sternum and the vertebrae including the heart and its large vessels, trachea, esophagus, thymus, lymph nodes) may cause hoarseness or dysphagia secondary to vocal cord paralysis as a result of entrapment or compression of the laryngeal nerve.

SYMPTOMS OF BRAIN METASTASIS

About 10% of all patients with lung cancer have CNS involvement at the time of diagnosis. Major clinical symptoms of brain metastasis result from increased intracranial pressure and include:

- Headache
- Nausea and vomiting
- Malaise
- Anorexia
- Weakness
- Alterations in mental processes

SIGNS AND SYMPTOMS OF METASTASIS TO THE SPINAL CORD

Metastases to the spinal cord produces signs and clinical symptoms of cord compression including:

- Back pain (localized or radicular)
- Muscle weakness
- Loss of lower extremity sensation
- Bowel and bladder incontinence
- Diminished or absent lower extremity reflexes (unilateral or bilateral)

GENETIC DISEASE OF THE LUNG

Cystic Fibrosis

Cystic fibrosis (CF) is an inherited disease of the exocrine (or "outward-secreting") glands primarily affecting the digestive and respiratory systems. Abnormally thick, sticky mucous secretions obstruct ducts in the pancreas, liver, and lungs. Obstruction of the bronchioles by mucous plugs and trapped air predisposes the patient to infection, which starts a destructive cycle of increased mucous production with increased bronchial obstruction and damage and eventually destroys lung tissue.

The course of CF varies from one patient to another depending on the degree of pulmonary involvement. Deterioration is inevitable, leading to debilitation and eventually to death. Complications of CF include hemoptysis and spontaneous pneumothorax (accumulation of gas or air in the pleural cavity resulting in collapse of the lung on the affected side) (Gaskell and Webber, 1980). The prognosis has improved steadily during the last four decades due to more aggressive treatment before the onset of irreversible pulmonary changes. The median survival age is 20 years; today, half of the people with CF live beyond 21 years of age (Cystic Fibrosis Foundation, 1987).

CLINICAL SIGNS AND SYMPTOMS OF CYSTIC FIBROSIS

Clinical signs and symptoms of cystic fibrosis in the early or undiagnosed stages

- Persistent coughing and wheezing
- Recurrent pneumonia
- Excessive appetite but poor weight gain
- Salty, skin/sweat
- Bulky, foul-smelling stools (undigested fats due to a lack of amylase and tryptase enzymes)

SIGNS AND SYMPTOMS OF PULMONARY INVOLVEMENT

- Tachypnea (very rapid breathing)
- Sustained chronic cough with mucous production and vomiting
- Barrel chest (caused by trapped air)
- Use of accessory muscles of respiration and intercostal retraction
- Cyanosis and digital clubbing
- Exertional dyspnea with decreased exercise tolerance

Further complications include:

- Pneumothorax
- Hemoptysis
- Right-sided heart failure secondary to pulmonary hypertension

The patient may develop further pulmonary complications, such as pneumothorax, hemoptysis, and right-sided heart failure secondary to pulmonary hypertension (Berkow, 1987).

PLEUROPULMONARY DISORDERS

Pulmonary Embolus

Pulmonary embolus (PE) caused by a dislodged blood clot that travels to the lungs may cause shortness of breath, tachypnea (very rapid breathing), tachycardia, and chest pain. In almost all cases, pulmonary embolism originates as deep venous thrombosis (DVT) in the proximal deep venous system of the lower legs. The embolism causes an area of blockage, which then results in a localized area of ischemia known as a *pulmonary infarct.* The infarct may be caused by small emboli that extend to the lung surface (pleura) and result in acute pleuritic pain. Hemoptysis occurs in 50% of the cases.

CLINICAL SIGNS OF DEEP VENOUS THROMBOSIS

- Most episodes are clinically silent (Dalen and Alpert, 1986)
- Unilateral leg swelling in most cases

A careful review of the *Personal/Family History* form (outpatient) or hospital medical chart (inpatient) may alert the therapist to the presence of factors that predispose a patient to have a PE. These factors include (Miller and Keane, 1987):

Stasis of blood flow (e.g., immobilization due to bed rest, such as with burn patients, obstetric and gynecologic patients, the elderly, or obese populations)

Venous injury (e.g., secondary to surgical procedures, trauma, or fractures of the legs or pelvis)

Malignancy

Use of oral contraceptives

Cardiovascular disease

Chronic lung disease

Diabetes mellitus

CLINICAL SIGNS AND SYMPTOMS OF PULMONARY EMBOLISM (Ford, 1987)

- Pleuritic chest pain
- Diffuse chest discomfort
- Tachypnea (increased respiratory rate)
- Tachycardia
- Hemoptysis (bloody sputum)
- Anxiety, restlessness, apprehension
- Dyspnea, persistent cough

Cor Pulmonale

When a PE has been sufficiently massive to obstruct 60 to 75% of the pulmonary circulation, the patient may have central chest pain and acute cor pulmonale occurs. This condition is an enlargement of the right ventricle in response to increased cardiac output to compensate for pulmonary congestion. As cor pulmonale progresses, edema and other signs of right-sided heart failure develop (Nursing 84, 1984).

CLINICAL SIGNS AND SYMPTOMS OF COR PULMONALE

Early clinical signs and symptoms of cor pulmonale may include:

- Chronic cough
- Either exertional dyspnea or dyspnea at rest
- Fatigue
- Wheezing
- Weakness

Pleurisy

Pleurisy is an inflammation of the pleura or serous membrane enveloping the lungs. The membranous pleura that encases each lung consists of two close-fitting layers: the visceral layer encasing the lungs and the parietal layer lining the inner chest wall. A lubricating fluid lies between these two layers. If the fluid content remains unchanged by the disease, the pleurisy is said to be dry. If the fluid increases abnormally, it is a wet pleurisy or pleurisy with effusion (pleural effusion). If the wet pleurisy becomes infected with formation of pus, the condition is known as purulent pleurisy or empyema (Miller and Keane, 1987).

CLINICAL SIGNS AND SYMPTOMS OF PLEURISY

- Chest pain
- Cough
- Dyspnea
- Fever, chills
- Tachypnea (rapid, shallow breathing)

The chest pain is sudden and may vary from vague discomfort to an intense stabbing or knifelike sensation in the chest. The pain is aggravated by breathing, coughing, laughing, or other similar movements associated with deep inspiration. The visceral pleura is insensitive; pain results from inflammation of the parietal pleura. Because the latter is innervated by the intercostal nerves, chest pain is usually felt over the site of the pleuritis, but pain may be referred to the lower chest wall, abdomen, neck, upper trapezius muscle, and shoulder due to irritation of the central diaphragmatic pleura (Fig. 4–4) (Berkow, 1987).

Pleurisy may occur as a result of many factors including pneumonia, tuberculosis, lung abscess, influenza, systemic lupus erythematosus (SLE), rheumatoid arthritis, and pulmonary infarction. Pleurisy, with or without effusion associated with SLE, may be accompanied by acute pleuritic pain and dysfunction of the diaphragm (Gaskell and Webber, 1980).

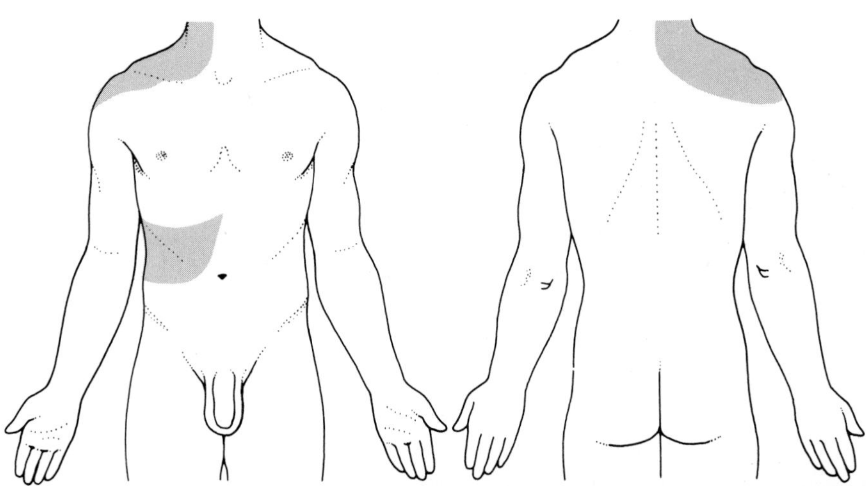

Figure 4–4. Chest pain over the site of pleuritis is usually perceived by the patient (not shown). Referred pain (*light red*) associated with pleuritis may occur on the same side as the pleuritic lesion affecting the shoulder, upper trapezius muscle, neck, lower chest wall, or abdomen.

Spontaneous Pneumothorax

Spontaneous pneumothorax or free air in the pleural cavity between the visceral and parietal pleurae may occur secondary to pulmonary disease or as a result of trauma and subsequent perforation of the chest wall. When the pneumothorax is small, the lung often expands again in several days. If the lung fails to expand again or collapses further, air must be withdrawn from the pleural cavity through the use of a chest tube (Gaskell and Webber, 1980).

CLINICAL SIGNS AND SYMPTOMS OF SPONTANEOUS PNEUMOTHORAX

- Dyspnea
- Sudden, sharp chest pain
- Shoulder pain
- Weak and rapid pulse
- Fall in blood pressure
- Dry, hacking cough

Symptoms of spontaneous pneumothorax vary depending on the size of the pneumothorax and on the extent of lung disease. When air enters the pleural cavity, the lung collapses, producing dyspnea and a shift of tissues and organs to the unaffected side. The patient may have severe pain in the upper and lateral thoracic wall, which is aggravated by any movement and by the cough and dyspnea that accompany it (Bauwens and Paine, 1983). The pain may be referred to the ipsilateral shoulder (corresponding shoulder on the same side as the pneumothorax), across the chest, or over the abdomen (Fig. 4–5). The patient may be most comfortable when sitting in an upright position.

PULMONARY PAIN PATTERNS

(Bauwens and Paine, 1983)

As discussed earlier in the section on chest pain in Chapter 3, the parietal pleura is sensitive to painful stimulation, but the visceral pleura is insensitive. Within the pulmonary system, the trachea and large bronchi are innervated by the vagus trunks, whereas, the finer bronchi and lung parenchyma appear to be free of pain innervation. Tracheobronchial pain is referred to sites in the neck or anterior chest at the same levels as the points of irritation in the air passages (Fig. 4–6). This irrita-

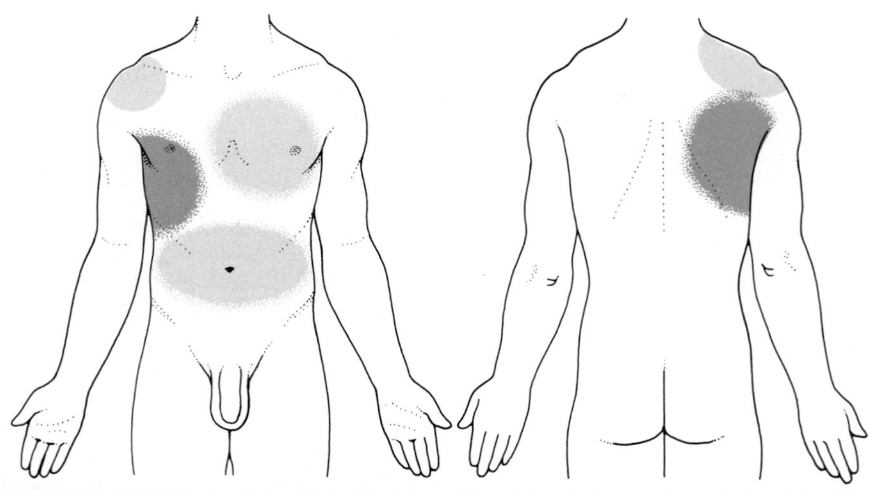

Figure 4–5. Possible pain patterns associated with spontaneous pneumothorax: upper and lateral thoracic wall with referral to ipsilateral shoulder, across the chest, or over the abdomen.

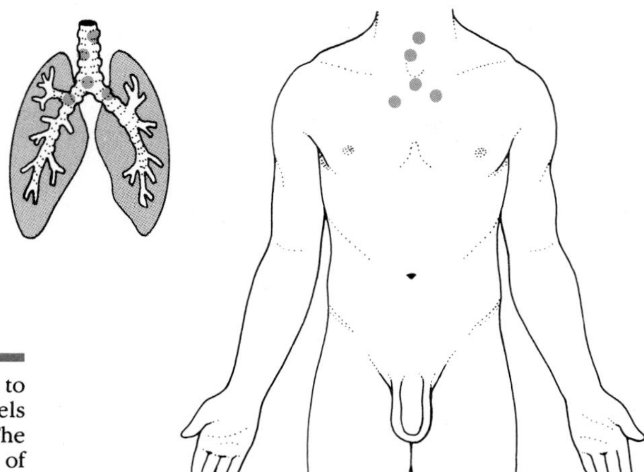

Figure 4–6. Tracheobronchial pain is referred to sites in the neck or anterior chest at the same levels as the points of irritation in the air passages. The points of pain are on the same side as the areas of irritation.

tion may be caused by inflammatory lesions, irritating foreign materials, or cancerous tumors.

Extensive disease may occur in the periphery of the lung without occurrence of pain until the process extends to the parietal pleura. Pleural irritation then results in sharp, localized pain that is aggravated by any respiratory movement. Patients usually note that the pain is alleviated by lying on the affected side, which diminishes the movement of that side of the chest ("autosplinting") (Heimer and Scharf, 1983). Debate continues concerning the mechanism by which pain occurs in the parietal membrane. It has been long held that friction between the two pleural surfaces (when the membranes are irritated and covered with fibrinous exudate) causes sharp pain. Other theories suggest that intercostal muscle spasm due to pleurisy or stretching of the parietal pleura causes this pain.

Pleural pain is present in pulmonary disease processes including pleurisy, pneumonia, pulmonary infarct (when it extends to the pleural surface thus causing pleurisy), tumor (when it invades the parietal pleura), and spontaneous pneumothorax. Tumor, especially bronchogenic carcinoma, may be accompanied by severe, continuous pain when the tumor tissue, extending to the pleurae through the lung, constantly irritates the pain nerve endings in the pleura.

The diaphragmatic pleura receives dual pain innervation through the phrenic and intercostal nerves. Damage to the phrenic nerve produces paralysis of the corresponding half of the diaphragm. The phrenic nerves are sensory and motor from both surfaces of the diaphragm. Stimulation of the peripheral portions of the diaphragmatic pleura results in sharp pain felt along the costal margins, which can be referred to the lumbar region by the lower thoracic somatic nerves. Stimulation of the central portion of the diaphragmatic pleura results in sharp pain referred to the upper trapezius muscle and shoulder on the ipsilateral side to the stimulation (see Fig. 3–9). Pain of cardiac and diaphragmatic origin is often experienced in the shoulder because the heart and diaphragm are supplied by the C_5-C_6 spinal segment, and the visceral pain is referred to the corresponding somatic area (Heimer and Scharf, 1983).

Diaphragmatic pleurisy secondary to pneumonia is common and refers sharp pain along the costal margins or upper trapezius, which is aggravated by any diaphragmatic motion, such as coughing, laughing, or deep breathing. There may be tenderness to palpation along the costal margins, and sharp pain occurs when the patient is asked to take a deep breath. A change in position (side bending or rotation of the trunk) does not reproduce the symptoms, which would be the case with a true intercostal lesion or tear. Forceful, repeated coughing can result in an intercostal lesion in the presence of referred intercostal pain from diaphragmatic pleurisy, which can make differentiation between these two entities impossible without a medical referral and further diagnostic testing.

OVERVIEW OF PULMONARY PAIN PATTERNS

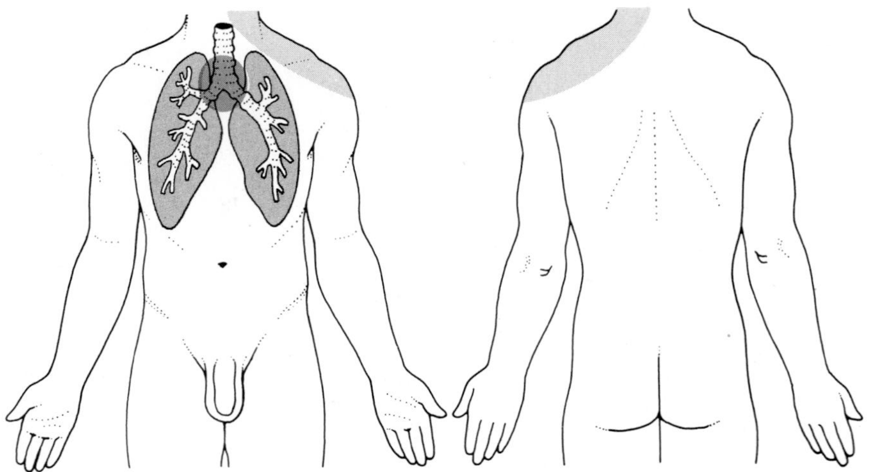

Figure 4-7. Primary pain patterns (***dark red***) associated with pleuropulmonary disorders, such as pulmonary embolus, cor pulmonale, pleurisy, or spontaneous pneumothorax, may vary, but usually include substernal or chest pain. Pain over the involved lung fields (anterior, lateral, or posterior) may occur (not shown). Pain may radiate (***light red***) to the neck, upper trapezius muscle, ipsilateral shoulder, costal margins, or upper abdomen (the latter two areas are now shown).

Pleuropulmonary Disorders

Location (Fig. 4-7):	Substernal or chest over involved lung fields—anterior, side, and back
Referral:	Often well localized (patient can point right to the exact site of pain) without referral
	May radiate to neck, upper trapezius muscle, shoulder, costal margins, or upper abdomen
	Thoracic back pain occurs with irritation of the posterior parietal pleura (Hall, 1983)

Description:	Sharp ache, stabbing, anginalike pressure, or crushing pain with pulmonary embolism
	Anginalike chest pain with severe pulmonary hypertension
Intensity:	Moderate
Duration:	Hours to days
Associated Signs and Symptoms:	Preceded by pneumonia or upper respiratory infection
	Wheezing
	Dyspnea (exertional or at rest)
	Hyperventilation
	Tachypnea (increased respirations)
	Fatigue, weakness
	Tachycardia (increased heart rate)
	Fever, chills
	Edema
	Apprehension or anxiety, restlessness
	Persistent cough or cough with blood (hemoptysis)
	Dry hacking cough (occurs with the onset of spontaneous pneumothorax)
	Medically determined signs and symptoms (e.g., by chest auscultation and chest x-ray)
Relieving Factors:	Sitting
	Some relief when at rest, but most comfortable position varies (pneumonia)
	Pleuritic pain may be relieved by lying on the affected side
Aggravating Factors:	Breathing at rest
	Increased inspiratory movement (e.g., laughter, coughing, sneezing)
	Symptoms accentuated with each breath

Lung Cancer

Location:	Anterior chest
Referral:	Scapulae, upper back, ipsilateral shoulder radiating along the medial aspect of the arm
	First and second ribs and associated vertebrae and paravertebral muscles (apical or Pancoast's tumors)
Description:	Localized, sharp pleuritic pain (peripheral tumors)
	Dull, vague aching in the chest
	Neuritic pain of shoulders/arm (apical or Pancoast's tumors)

	Bone pain due to metastases to adjacent bone or to the vertebrae
Intensity:	Moderate to severe
Duration:	Constant
Associated Signs and Symptoms:	Hemoptysis (coughing or spitting up blood)
	Dyspnea or wheezing
	Fever, chills, malaise, anorexia, and weight loss
	Fecal breath odor
	Tachycardia or atrial fibrillation (palpitations)
	Muscle weakness or atrophy (e.g., Pancoast's tumor may involve the shoulder and the arm of the affected side)
	Associated CNS symptoms: Headache Nausea Vomiting Malaise
	Signs of cord compression: Localized or radicular back pain Weakness Loss of lower extremity sensation Bowel/bladder incontinence
	Hoarseness, dysphagia (peripheral tumors)
Relieving Factors:	None without medical intervention
Aggravating Factors:	Inspiration: deep breathing, laughing, coughing

ACID-BASE REGULATION

The proper balance of acids and bases in the body is essential to life. This balance is very complex and must be kept within the narrow parameters of a pH of 7.35 to 7.45 in the extracellular fluid (Table 4–3). This number (or pH value) represents the *hydrogen ion* concentration in body fluid. A reading of less than 7.35 is considered "acidosis," and a reading greater than 7.45 is called "alkalosis." Life cannot be sustained if the pH values are less than 7.0 or greater than 7.8 (Soltis and Cassmeyer, 1987).

There are two ways in which hydrogen ions (or acids) circulate throughout the body:

- Volatile hydrogen of carbonic acid
- Nonvolatile hydrogen in organic acids, such as lactic, sulfuric, pyruvic, and phosphoric acids

Normal body metabolism results in the production of many of these acids. The lungs excrete a large amount of the *volatile* hydrogen in the carbonic acid as carbon dioxide (CO_2) and water (H_2O); and the lungs excrete a smaller amount of the nonvolatile acids (Soltis and Cassmeyer, 1987).

Living human cells are extremely sensitive to alterations in body fluid pH (hydrogen ion concentration), thus there are various mechanisms in operation to keep the pH at a relatively constant level. Acid-base regulatory mechanisms include chemical buffer systems, the respiratory system, and the renal system.

Table 4–3. LABORATORY VALUES: UNCOMPENSATED AND COMPENSATED RESPIRATORY ACIDOSIS AND ALKALOSIS

	Normal pH Level	Normal P_{CO_2} Level	Normal HCO_3 Level
Arterial Blood	pH(7.35–7.45)	P_{CO_2}(35–45 mm Hg)	HCO_3(22–26 meq/l)
Respiratory Acidosis (uncompensated)	<7.35	>45	Normal
Compensated	Normal	>45	>26
Respiratory Alkalosis (uncompensated)	>7.45	<35	Normal
Compensated	Normal	<35	<22

These systems interact very closely to maintain a normal acid-base ratio of 20 parts of bicarbonate to 1 part of carbonic acid and thus to maintain normal body fluid pH.

The carbonic-acid/bicarbonate system is the primary extracellular fluid (ECF) chemical buffer system. This system responds immediately to changes in ECF pH. Carbonic acid is formed by the combination of CO_2 and H_2O. When a strong base is added to body fluids, it is buffered by carbonic acid. When a strong acid is added to the system, a bicarbonate buffer changes it to a salt and carbonic acid. The carbonic acid then further dissociates into CO_2 and H_2O and is excreted by the lungs.

The respiratory control center in the brain responds to increases in CO_2 and hydrogen ions in the body fluids by increasing or decreasing the rate and depth of respiration. When the body pH decreases or becomes more acid, respiratory rate and depth increase so that the lungs can increase the breakdown of carbonic acid to CO_2 and H_2O and can then exhale both the CO_2 and hydrogen. With increased respiratory rate, less CO_2 is available for the formation of carbonic acid. Conversely, when the pH rises or becomes more alkaline, the rate and depth of respiration decrease so that CO_2 is retained and more carbonic acid is formed.

However, long-term correction of acid-base disturbances is controlled by the renal excretion of hydrogen and by the renal production of bicarbonate. Even though this mechanism occurs more slowly (hours to days) than buffer (immediate) or respiratory changes (minutes to hours), renal action is more thorough and selective than is that of the other acid-base regulators. The primary mechanism of renal control in acid-base balance is the increase or decrease in the production of bicarbonate.

Respiratory Acidosis

Any condition that decreases pulmonary ventilation increases the retention and concentration of CO_2, hydrogen, and carbonic acid, which then results in an increase in the amount of circulating hydrogen, and is called respiratory acidosis. If ventilation is severely compromised, CO_2 levels become extremely high and respiration is depressed even further causing hypoxia as well. During respiratory acidosis, potassium moves out of cells into the ECF to exchange with circulating hydrogen. This results in hyperkalemia (abnormally high potassium concentration in the blood) and cardiac changes that can result in cardiac arrest.

Respiratory acidosis can result from pathologies that decrease the efficiency of the respiratory system. These pathologies can include damage to the medulla, which controls respiration, obstruction of airways (e.g., neoplasm, foreign bodies, pulmonary disease, such as COPD, pneumonia), loss of lung surface ventilation (e.g., pneumothorax, pulmonary fibrosis), weakness of respiratory muscles (e.g., poliomyelitis, spinal cord injury, Guillain-Barré syndrome), or overdose of respiratory depressant drugs (Soltis and Cassmeyer, 1987).

CLINICAL SYMPTOMS OF RESPIRATORY ACIDOSIS

- Decreased ventilation
- Confusion
- Sleepiness and unconsciousness
- Diaphoresis
- Shallow rapid breathing
- Restlessness
- Cyanosis

As hypoxia becomes more severe, the latter four signs and symptoms may appear. Cardiac arrhythmias may also be present as the potassium level in the blood serum rises.

Treatment is directed at restoration of efficient ventilation. If the respiratory depression and acidosis is severe, injection of intravenous sodium bicarbonate and use of a mechanical ventilator may be necessary. Any patient with symptoms of inadequate ventilation or CO_2 retention needs immediate medical referral.

Respiratory Alkalosis

Increased respiratory rate and depth decrease the amount of available CO_2 and hydrogen and create a condition of increased pH or alkalosis. By increasing pulmonary ventilation, CO_2 and hydrogen are eliminated from the body too quickly and are not available to buffer the increasing alkaline environment.

Respiratory alkalosis is usually due to *hyperventilation.* Rapid, deep respirations are often caused by neurogenic or psychogenic problems, including anxiety, pain, and cerebral trauma or lesions. Other causes can be related to conditions that greatly increase metabolism (e.g., hyperthyroidism) or overventilation of patients with a mechanical ventilator.

CLINICAL SYMPTOMS OF RESPIRATORY ALKALOSIS

- Lightheadedness
- Dizziness
- Numbness and tingling of the face, fingers, and toes
- Syncope (fainting)

If the alkalosis becomes more severe, muscular tetany and convulsions can occur. Cardiac arrhythmias due to serum potassium loss through the kidneys may also occur. The kidneys keep hydrogen in exchange for potassium.

Treatment of respiratory alkalosis includes reassurance, assistance in slowing breathing and facilitating relaxation, sedation, pain control, CO_2 administration, and use of a rebreathing device such as a rebreathing mask or paper bag. A rebreathing device allows the patient to inhale and "rebreathe" the exhaled CO_2.

Respiratory alkalosis related to hyperventilation is a relatively common condition and might be present more often in the physical therapy setting than respiratory acidosis. Pain and anxiety are common causes of hyperventilation, and treatment needs to be focused toward reduction of both of these interrelated elements. If hyperventilation continues in the absence of pain or anxiety, serious systemic problems may cause this problem and immediate physician referral is necessary.

If either respiratory acidosis or alkalosis persist for hours to days in a chronic, non–life-threatening manner, the kidneys then begin to assist in the restoration of normal body fluid pH by selective excretion or retention of hydrogen ions or bicarbonate. This process is called "renal compensation." When the kidneys compensate effectively, blood pH values are within normal limits (7.35 to 7.45) even though the underlying problem may still cause the respiratory imbalance.

SUMMARY

When patients have chest pain, they usually fall into two categories: those who demonstrate chest pain associated with pulmonary symptoms and those who have true musculoskeletal problems, such as intercostal strains and tears, myofascial trigger points, fractured ribs, or myalgias secondary to overuse.

Patients with chronic, persistent cough, whether that cough is productive or dry and hacking, may develop sharp, localized intercostal pain similar to pleuritic pain. Both intercostal and pleuritic pain are aggravated by respiratory movements, such as laughing, coughing, deep breathing, or sneezing.

The physical therapist will want to rule out systemic origin of symptoms through a series of questions to elicit the presence of associated systemic (pulmonary) signs and symptoms. Aggravating and relieving factors may provide further clues that can assist in making treatment or referral decisions. To assist the physical therapist in appropriate questioning and possible patient referral, this chapter has emphasized:

- Pulmonary disorders including COPD, inflammatory/infectious diseases, neoplastic disease, and genetic disease of the lung
- Pleuropulmonary disorders including PE, cor pulmonale, pleurisy, and spontaneous pneumothorax
- Overview and discussion of pulmonary pain patterns
- Discussion of basic acid-base regulation

Systemic Signs and Symptoms Requiring Physician Referral

Anorexia
Apprehension
Arthralgias, myalgias
Anxiety
Barrel chest
Bowel/bladder incontinence
Bulky, foul-smelling stools
Chest pain
Chronic laryngitis
Cough with sputum
Cyanosis
Digital clubbing
Dysphagia
Dyspnea
Fecal breath odor
Fever, chills
Hacking cough
Headache
Hemoptysis
Hoarseness
Malaise, fatigue
Muscle weakness
Nausea, vomiting
Orthopnea
Pursed-lip breathing
Restlessness
Salty skin and sweat
Skin rash, pigmentation
Sore throat
Syncope
Tachypnea
Unexplained weight loss
Wheezing

SUBJECTIVE EXAMINATION

Special Questions to Ask

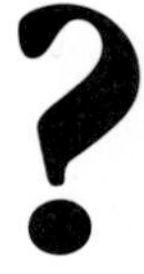

□ Have you ever had trouble with breathing?

□ Are you having difficulty in breathing now?

□ Do you ever have shortness of breath or breathlessness or can't quite catch your breath?

If yes, when does this happen? When you rest? When you lie flat, walk on level ground, or walk up stairs?

Subjective Exam

Special Questions to Ask

When are you under stress or tension and how long does it last?

What do you do to get your breathing back to normal?

- □ How far can you walk before you feel breathless?
- □ What symptom stops your walking (e.g., shortness of breath, heart pounding, or weak legs)?
- □ Do you have any breathing aids (e.g., oxygen, nebulizer, humidifier, or intermittent positive pressure breathing)?
- □ Do you have a cough? (Note whether the patient smokes, for how long and how much: Do you have a smoker's hack?)

  If yes, to cough separate from smoker's cough, when did it start?

  Do you cough anything up? If yes, please describe the color, amount, and frequency.

  Are you taking anything to prevent this cough? If yes, does it seem to help?
- □ Are there occasions when you can't seem to stop coughing?
- □ Do you ever cough up blood?

  If yes, what color is it? (Bright red = fresh blood; brown or black = older blood)

  If yes, has this condition been treated?
- □ Have you strained a muscle from coughing?
- □ Have you ever injured your chest?
- □ Does it hurt to touch your chest or to take a deep breath (e.g., coughing, sneezing, sighing, or laughing)?
- □ Have you ever been treated for a lung problem?

  If yes, please describe what this problem was, when it occurred, and how it was treated?
- □ Have you ever had a blood clot in your lungs?

  If yes, when did it occur and how was it treated?
- □ Have you had a chest x-ray taken in the last 5 years?

  If yes, when and where was it done? Give the results.
- □ Do you work around asbestos, coal, dust, chemicals, or fumes?

  If yes, please describe.

  Do you wear a mask at work? If yes, approximately how much of the time do you wear a mask?
- □ If the patient is a farmer, ask what kind of farming: Some agricultural products may cause respiratory irritation.
- □ Have you ever had tuberculosis?

  If yes, when did it occur and how was it treated? What is your current status?

Subjective Exam

Special Questions to Ask

- □ When was your last test for tuberculosis? Was the result normal?
- □ (If the person indicated *asthma* on the Personal/Family History form): How can you tell when you are having an asthma attack?

  What triggers an asthma attack for you? (Correlate this question with the core interview questions in the physical therapy interview concerning stressors and stress levels.)

  Do you use medications during an attack?

  If yes, which ones?

  Do you exercise?

  If yes, determine the amount and the intensity of exercise.

  Do you have trouble with asthma during exercise?

  Do you time your medications with your exercise to prevent an asthma attack during exercise?

- □ Have you gained or lost a lot of weight recently?

  Gained **(Pulmonary edema, congestive heart failure, fat deposits under the diaphragm in the obese patient reduces ventilation)**

  Lost **(Emphysema, cancer)**

- □ Do your ankles swell? **(Congestive heart failure)**
- □ Have you been unusually tired lately? **(Congestive heart failure, emphysema)**
- □ Have you noticed a change in your voice? **(Pathology of left hilum or trachea)**
- □ Have you ever broken your nose or been told that you have a deviated septum (nasal passageway)?

  If yes, does this seem to affect your breathing? **(Hypoxia)**

- □ Do you have nasal polyps?

  If yes, does this seem to affect your breathing?

- □ Have you ever had lung or heart surgery?

  If yes, what and when? (Decreased vital capacity)

PHYSICIAN REFERRAL

It is more common for a physical therapist to be treating a patient with a previously diagnosed musculoskeletal problem who now has chronic, recurrent pulmonary symptoms than to be the primary evaluator and caretaker of a patient with pulmonary symptoms. In either case, the physical therapist needs to know what further questions to ask and which of the patient's responses represent serious symptoms that require medical follow-up. Additionally, some patients occasionally require medical referral. These patients either have shoulder or back pain referred from diseases of the diaphragmatic or parietal pleura, secondary to metastatic lung cancer. Patients who have intercostal pain secondary to insidious trauma or repetitive movements, such as coughing, can benefit from physical therapy treatment. In all of these situations, the referral of a patient to a physician is based on the family history of pulmonary disease, the presence of pulmonary symptoms of a systemic nature, or the absence of substantiating objective findings indicating a musculoskeletal lesion.

CASE STUDY

Referral

A 65-year-old man has come to you for an evaluation of low back pain, which he attributes to lifting a heavy box 2 weeks ago. During the course of the medical history, you notice that the patient has a persistent cough and that he sounds hoarse. After reviewing the *Personal/Family History* form, you note that the patient smokes two packs of cigarettes each day and that he has smoked at least this amount for the last 50 years. (One pack per day for one year is considered "one pack year.") This patient has smoked an estimated 100 pack years; any patient who has smoked for 20 "pack years" or more is considered to be at risk for the development of serious lung disease. What questions will you ask to decide for yourself whether this back pain is systemic?

Introduction to patient. It is important for me to make certain that your back pain is not caused by other health problems, such as prostate problems or respiratory infection, thus I will ask a series of questions that may not seem to be related to your back pain, but I want to be very thorough and to cover every possibility in order to obtain the best and most effective treatment for you.

Pain

From your intake form I see that you associate your back pain with lifting a heavy box 2 weeks ago. When did you first notice your back pain (sudden or gradual onset)?

Have you ever hurt your back before or have you ever had pain similar to this episode in the past? (Systemic disease: recurrent and gradually increases over time)

Please describe your pain (supply descriptive terms if necessary)

How often do you have this pain?

FUPs: How long does it last when you have it?

Have you noticed any changes in your pain/symptoms since they first started up to the present time?

Do you have any numbness in the groin or pelvis? (Saddle anesthesia: cauda equina)

What aggravates your pain/symptoms?

What relieves your pain/symptoms?

How does rest affect your pain?

Pulmonary

I notice you have quite a cough and you sound hoarse to me. How long have you had this cough and hoarseness and when did it first begin?

CASE STUDY

Do you have any back pain associated with this cough? Any other pain associated with your cough?
If yes, have the patient describe where, when, intensity, aggravating and relieving factors.

How does it feel when you take a deep breath? Does your low back hurt when you laugh or take a deep breath?

When you cough, do you produce phlegm or mucus?
If yes, have you ever noticed any red streaks or blood in it?

Does your coughing or back pain keep you awake at night?

Have you been examined by a physician for either your cough or your back pain?

Have you had any recent chest or spine x-rays taken?

If yes, when and where. What were the results?

General Systemic

Have you had any nightsweats, daytime fevers, or chills?

Do you have difficulty in swallowing or experience recurrent laryngitis? **(Oral cancer)**

Urology

Have you ever been told that you have a prostate problem or prostatitis? If yes, determine when this occurred, how it was treated, and whether the patient had the same symptoms at that time that he is now describing to you.

Have you noticed any change in your bladder habits?
For example, have you had any difficulty in starting to urinate?
Or if you start urinating, does the flow start and stop without you being able to control it?
Is there any burning or discomfort on urination?
Have you noticed any blood in your urine?
Have you recently had any difficulty with kidney stones or bladder or kidney infections?

Gastrointestinal

Have you noticed any change in your bowel pattern?
Have you had difficulty having a bowel movement or find that you have soiled yourself without even realizing it? (**Cauda equina lesion**—this would require immediate referral to a physician)
Does your back pain begin or increase when you are having a bowel movement?
Is your back pain relieved after having a bowel movement?

Have you noticed any association between when you eat and when your pain/symptoms increase or decrease?

Final Question

Is there anything about your current back pain or your general health that we have not discussed that you think is important for me to know?

CASE STUDY

Refer to **Special Questions to Ask** at the end of this chapter for other questions that may be pertinent to this patient, depending on his answers to these questions.

Physician Referral

As always, correlation of findings is important in making a decision regarding medical referral. If the patient has a positive family history for respiratory problems (especially lung cancer) and if clinical findings indicate pulmonary involvement, the patient should be strongly encouraged to see a physician for a medical check-up. If there are positive systemic findings, such as difficulty in swallowing, persistent hoarseness, shortness of breath at rest, night sweats, fevers, bloody sputum, recurrent laryngitis, or upper respiratory infections *either in addition to or in association with* the low back pain, the patient should be advised to see a physician, and the physician should receive a copy of your findings. This guideline covers the patient who has a true musculoskeletal problem but also has other health problems, as well as the patient who may have back pain of a systemic origin that is unrelated to the lifting injury 2 weeks ago.

References

Bauwens, D.B., and Paine, R.: Thoracic pain. *In* Blacklow, R.S. (ed): MacBryde's Signs and Symptoms, 6th ed. Philadelphia, J.B. Lippincott, 1983, pp. 139–164.

Berkow, R. (ed): The Merck Manual, 15th ed. Rahway, NJ, Merck Sharp & Dohme Research Laboratories, 1987.

Brucia, J.: Assessment of the Respiratory System. *In* Phipps, W., Long, B., and Woods, N. (eds): Medical-Surgical Nursing: Concepts and Clinical Practice. St. Louis, C.V. Mosby, 1987, pp. 1259–1287.

Centers for Disease Control: Human Immunodeficiency virus infection in the United States: A review of current knowledge. MMWR, 36 (Suppl. S–6): 8, 1987.

Cystic Fibrosis Foundation: The Genetics of Cystic Fibrosis. Bethesda, MD, Cystic Fibrosis Foundation, 1987.

Dalen, J.E., and Alpert, J.: Pulmonary embolism. *In* Hurst, J.W. (ed): The Heart, Vols. 1 and 2. New York, McGraw-Hill, 1986, pp. 1105–1118.

Ford, R.D.: Patient Teaching Manual. 1. Springhouse, PA, Springhouse Corporation, 1987.

Gaskell, D.V., and Webber, B.A.: The Brompton Hospital Guide to Chest Physiotherapy, 4th ed. Oxford, Blackwell Scientific Publications, 1980.

Gershwin, M.E., and Klingelhofer, E.L.: Asthma. Reading, MA, Addison-Wesley Publishing Co, Inc., 1986.

Hall, A.: Back pain. *In* Blacklow, R.S. (ed): MacBryde's Signs and Symptoms, 6th ed. Philadelphia, J.B. Lippincott, 1983, pp. 195–209.

Heimer, D., and Scharf, S.M.: History and physical examination. *In* Baum, G.L., and Wolinsky, E. (eds): Textbook of Pulmonary Diseases, 3rd ed. Boston, Little Brown, 1983, pp. 223–233.

Lewis, S.: Nursing role in management of lower respiratory problems. *In* Lewis, S. and Collier, I. (eds): Medical-Surgical Nursing: Assessment and Management of Clinical Problems, 1st ed. New York, McGraw-Hill Book Co., 1983, pp. 457–506.

Loehnen, C.P.: Lecture material presented to senior physical therapy students in "Clinical Medicine" course. Missoula, MT, University of Montana, 1989.

Miller, B.F., and Keane, C.B.: Encyclopedia and Dictionary of Medicine, Nursing and Allied Health, 4th ed. Philadelphia, W.B. Saunders Company, 1987.

Morgan, V.K.C.: Tumors of the lung other than bronchogenic carcinoma. *In* Baum, G.L., and Wolinsky, E. (eds): Textbook of Pulmonary Diseases, 3rd ed. Boston, Little Brown, 1983, pp. 1087–1104.

Morgan, V.K.C., and Hales, M.R.: Bronchogenic carcinoma. *In* Baum, G.L., and Wolinsky, E. (eds): Textbook of Pulmonary Diseases, 3rd ed. Boston, Little Brown, 1983, pp. 1045–1086.

Nursing 84: Respiratory Disorders. Springhouse, PA, Springhouse Corporation, 1984.

Reynolds, M.D.: Myofascial trigger point syndromes in the practice of rheumatology. Arch. Phys. Med. Rehabil. *62*:111, 1981.

Soltis, B., and Cassmeyer, V.: Fluid and electrolyte balance. *In* Phipps, W., Long, B., and Woods, N.: Medical-Surgical nursing: Concepts and Clinical Practice. St. Louis, C.V. Mosby, 1987, pp. 215–253.

West, J.B.: Pulmonary Pathophysiology: The Essentials. Baltimore, Williams & Wilkins, 1977.

Bibliography

Farber, S.M., and Wilson, R.H.L.: Chronic obstructive emphysema. CIBA, Clinical Symposia, *20*:35, 1968.

Haas, F., and Haas, S.: The Essential Asthma Book. New York, Scribner Book Companies, 1987.

Kuida, H.: Pulmonary hypertension and pulmonary heart disease. *In* Hurst, J.W. (ed): The Heart, Vols. 1 and 2. New York, McGraw-Hill, 1986, pp. 1091–1099.

Light, K.E.: Review of aged respiratory system. Phys. Occupational Ther. Geriatrics, *3*:5, 1983.

Lister M.J. (ed): Respiratory Care. Phys. Ther., 61:1703, 1981.

Pulmonary Problems in Infants and Children. Am. J. Nurs., 81:509, 1981.

Ray, C.S., Sue, D.Y., and Bray, C.: Effects of obesity on respiratory function. Am. Rev. Respir. Dis., *128*:501, 1983.

Weiss, E.B.: Bronchial Asthma. CIBA, Clinical Symposia, *27*:3, 1975.

Wieczorek, R.R., and Horner-Rosner, B.: The asthmatic child: Preventing and controlling attacks. Am. J. Nurs., 79:258, 1979.

Young, P.: Asthma and Allergies: An Optimistic Future. U.S. Department of Health and Human Services, NIH, March 1980.

Chapter 5

Overview of Hematology: Signs and Symptoms

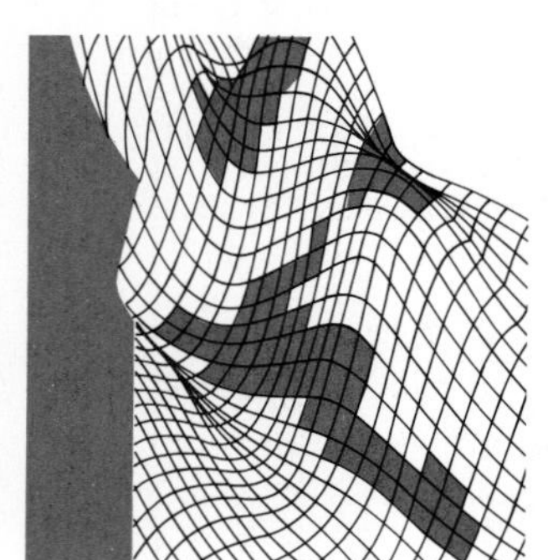

☐ ***Clinical Signs and Symptoms of:***

Anemia
Polycythemia
Sickle Cell Anemia
Leukocytosis
Leukopenia
Thrombocytopenia
Acute Hemarthrosis
Muscle Hemorrhage
Gastrointestinal Involvement

Hematology is defined as the study of blood. The blood consists of two major components: plasma, a pale yellow or gray-yellow fluid; and formed elements, erythrocytes (red blood cells or RBCs), leukocytes (white blood cells or WBCs), and platelets (thrombocytes). Blood is the circulating tissue of the body; the fluid and its formed elements circulate through heart, arteries, capillaries, and veins.

The erythrocytes carry oxygen to tissues and remove carbon dioxide from them. Leukocytes act in inflammatory and immune responses. The plasma carries antibodies and nutrients to tissues and removes wastes from tissues. Coagulation factors in plasma, together with platelets, control the clotting of blood.

Primary hematologic diseases are uncommon, but hematologic manifestations secondary to other diseases are common (Purtilo and Purtilo, 1989).

Blood Composition

The total blood volume in an adult is about 6 liters (5.5 q) or about 7.5% of the body weight. Approximately 45% of blood consists of formed elements: erythrocytes, leukocytes, and platelets (thrombocytes). The remaining 55% of the blood is the fluid portion, which is called plasma. Approximately 90% of plasma consists of water. The remaining 10% consists of proteins (albumin, immunoglobulin and other globulins, and fibrinogen), carbohydrates, vitamins, hormones, enzymes, lipids, and salts.

The proteins exert a powerful osmotic pull so that water can move from tissues into the blood. The globulins (alpha, beta, and gamma) transport other proteins; gamma globulin (consisting primarily of immunoglobulins) functions as antibodies and specifically gives the body immunity from disease. Fibrinogen is a protein in the plasma that is converted into fibrin (also known as clotting factor I) and used in the formation of a blood clot.

The term, hematopoiesis means the production of blood cells. The hematopoietic system consists of the circulating blood, the bone marrow, the spleen, the thymus, and the lymph nodes, supplemented by the reticuloendothelial (capable of engulfing or phagocytosing particles) cells lining blood sinuses and found in most organs of the body.

Blood Formation

Stem cells are precursor or mother cells for blood cells with the capacity for both blood cell replication and differentiation. Stem cells are the precursor cells for various morphologically different blood cells through a process called differentiation. The stem cell is stimulated to change into clearly recognizable forms of the various cell types (Table 5–1).

Blood cells must go through stages of development in the same way that a human matures during development. In a healthy person, only mature adult cells are seen in the blood, whereas in many diseases, the immature and abnormal forms of the cells may be present. In the human embryo, hematopoiesis begins within 2 weeks after conception. Initially, the primitive stem cells arise in blood islands within the yolk sac of the embryo. Later (still during the gestational period), hematopoiesis takes place at different times in the liver, spleen, thymus, lymph nodes, and bone marrow. At birth, and continuing during life, hematopoiesis is confined to the bone marrow.

Table 5–1. FORMATION OF BLOOD CELLS

Stem Cells (Precursors)	Mature Cells
Monoblasts or promonocytes	Monocytes
Monocytes	Macrophages
Erythroblasts	Erythrocytes
Myeloblasts	Granulocytes
Lymphoblasts	Lymphocytes
Megakaryocytes	Platelets

In the child, hematopoietic (red) bone marrow is located in the flat bones of the skull, clavicle, sternum, ribs, pelvis, and also in the long bones of the extremities and vertebrae. By 18 years of age (and for the remainder of adult life), the red bone marrow is normally confined to the flat bones only.

Control of Hematopoiesis

Erythrocyte, leukocyte, and platelet production are all thought to be controlled by hormones and feedback mechanisms that maintain an ideal number of cells. The number of individual blood cells is controlled by specific hormones. Erythropoietin governs erythrocyte production; thrombopoietin governs platelet production; and leukopoietin theoretically controls granulocyte production (Brown, 1980; Purtilo and Purtilo, 1989).

Erythropoiesis, for example, is controlled by the oxygen concentration in the kidneys. The main function of the erythrocyte is to carry hemoglobin, which transports oxygen to the tissues. When an individual's hemoglobin level is below normal, the tissues do not receive an adequate supply of oxygen and a state of hypoxia exists. This condition stimulates the kidneys to produce a hormone, erythropoietin, in response to this lowered oxygen concentration in the blood. Erythropoietin is released from the kidneys and stimulates bone marrow stem cells to produce new erythrocytes.

Normally, the rate of production of erythrocytes determines the hemoglobin level or erythrocyte count in the peripheral blood and shows little variation among normal individuals.

Production of erythrocytes can be limited by the availability of essential nutrients (e.g., iron, protein, folate, vitamins B_{12} and B_6). Deficiency of these essential nutrients prevents normal maturation of the primitive red blood cells (erythroblasts) into erythrocytes resulting in a nutritional deficiency anemia.

Erythrocytes

Erythrocytes outnumber leukocytes by 600 to 1. The average number of erythrocytes per cubic millimeter of circulating blood is about five million. Women are a few per cent below this value, and men are a few per cent above it (Guyton, 1986). This difference in erythrocyte values between men and women may be due to the erythropoietic stimulation that androgenic hormones have on the bone marrow. In addition, the altitude at which the person lives and the person's level of exercise also affect the number of erythrocytes produced.

At high altitudes, where the quantity of oxygen in the air is decreased, insufficient amounts of oxygen are carried to the tissues, and erythrocytes are produced rapidly so that the number of erythrocytes available for oxygen transport increases. The degree of a person's physical activity also helps to determine the rate at which erythrocytes are produced. The athlete may have an erythrocyte count as high as 6.5 million per cubic millimeter, whereas a sedentary person may have a count as low as 3 million per cubic millimeter (Guyton, 1986).

Five days are required to produce new erythrocytes from stem cell to mature erythrocyte. These erythrocytes live approximately 120 days in the bloodstream before being filtered through the spleen into the liver, where damaged erythrocytes are engulfed by reticuloendothelial cells. The mature erythrocyte consists primarily of hemoglobin and functions to supply oxygen to the tissues, removing carbon dioxide. Because of its biconcave disklike shape and flexibility, the erythrocyte is capable of squeezing through the narrow capillaries without rupturing. Abnormalities in either the shape or flexibility of erythrocytes are important components of some blood disorders, such as sickle cell anemia. Disorders of erythrocytes are classified as follows:

- Anemia (too few erythrocytes)
- Polycythemia (too many erythrocytes)
- Poikilocytosis (abnormally shaped erythrocytes)
- Anisocytosis (abnormal variations in size of erythrocytes)
- Hypochromia (deficient in hemoglobin)

Hemoglobin

Hemoglobin consists of an iron-containing molecule, heme, and the protein, globin. Synthesis of hemoglobin begins in the mitochondria and continues in the cytoplasm of the cell. No hemoglobin synthesis takes place in the mature erythrocyte. The hemoglobin molecule within the erythrocyte is responsible for supplying the tissues with oxygen. The normal hemoglobin molecule has an attraction for oxygen as the oxygen binds to the iron in the hemoglobin. However, the iron of heme bonds more readily with carbon monoxide than with oxygen; a bond that is so tight that none of the body's chemistry can break it up (Page, 1981). Carbon monoxide poisoning and iron deficiency (e.g., in diet) are the two primary factors that can adversely affect hemoglobin's ability to bind with oxygen.

Leukocytes

Blood contains three major groups of leukocytes:

- Lymphoid cells (lymphocytes, plasma cells)
- Monocytes
- Granulocytes (neutrophils, eosinophils, and basophils)

Lymphocytes produce antibodies and react with antigens, thus initiating the immune response to fight infection. *Monocytes* are the largest circulating blood cells and represent an immature cell until they leave the blood and travel to the tissues. Once migrated, monocytes form macrophages when activated by foreign substances such as bacteria. The monocytes are active phagocytes. *Granulocytes* (granular leukocytes) contain within their granules, lysing agents capable of digesting various foreign materials. Granulocytes assist in initiating the inflammatory response and defend the body against infectious agents by phagocytosing bacteria and other infectious substances.

Generally, the *neutrophils* (granulocytes) are the first phagocytic cells to reach an infected area, followed by monocytes that then work together with the neutrophils to phagocytize all foreign material present. The capacity of corticosteroids or ethanol to diminish the accumulation of neutrophils in inflamed areas may be due to their ability to reduce cell adherence. *Eosinophils* carry approximately one third of the blood histamine present. Eosinophils become active in the later stages of inflammation and are also active in allergic reactions and parasitic infections (Brown, 1980). Causes of eosinophilia (abnormally large number of eosinophils in the blood) follow (Reich, 1984):

- Allergic disorders
- Hodgkin's disease
- Idiopathic
- Inherited
- Leukemia, eosinophilic
- Malignancy
- Myelocytic leukemia (chronic)
- Necrosis of tissue
- Parasitic infections
- Pernicious anemia
- Skin diseases
- Tropical eosinophilia
- Vasculitis
- Radiation therapy

Basophils have a high content of heparin and histamine and have an important role in acute, systemic, allergic reactions. In the presence of bacteria or other infectious agents, the basophils erupt and distribute chemicals that trigger inflammation. At this point, neutrophils, eosinophils, or monocytes arrive to engulf or phagocytize the alien particle. Little else is known of the function of basophil cells.

The leukocyte count denotes the number of leukocytes in 1 cu mm of whole blood. The leukocyte in a normal, healthy individual is usually between 5 to 10,000 leukocytes per cu mm. The leukocyte count may be elevated *(leukocytosis)* in bacterial infections, appendicitis, leukemia, pregnancy, hemolytic disease of the new born, uremia, ulcers, and normally at birth. The leukocyte count may drop below normal values *(leukopenia)* in viral diseases (e.g., measles), brucellosis, typhoid fever, infectious hepatitis, rheumatoid arthritis, cirrhosis of the liver, and lupus erythematosus. Radiation or chemotherapy may also lower the leukocyte count.

Laboratory Procedures for Detecting Leukocyte Abnormalities. There are only a small number of laboratory procedures useful for diagnosing abnormalities of leukocytes—total leukocyte count, leukocyte differential, peripheral blood morphology, and bone marrow morphology.

A differential leukocyte count is often done to determine whether a person has an infection or disease of the blood, such as leukemia. A differential count of 100 leukocytes in an adult normally shows neutrophils numbering 60 to 70%, lymphocytes up to 20 to 40%, monocytes up to 4 to 8%, eosinophils up to 2 to 6%, and basophils from zero to 1%.

Platelets (Thrombocytes)

Platelets are the smallest formed element in blood, formed from megakaryocytes in the bone marrow. Platelets function primarily in hemostasis (stopping bleeding) and in maintaining capillary integrity (Brown, 1980). They are important in the coagulation (blood clotting) mechanism by forming hemostatic plugs in small ruptured blood vessels or by adhering to any injured lining of larger blood vessels. A number of substances derived from the platelet that function in blood coagulation have been labeled "platelet factors." Platelets survive approximately 8 to 10 days in circulation and are then removed by the reticuloendothelial cells. *Thrombocytosis* refers to a condition in which the number of platelets is abnormally high, whereas, *thrombocytopenia* refers to a condition in which the number of platelets is abnormally low.

Platelets are affected by anticoagulant drugs including aspirin and heparin, by diet (presence of lecithin preventing coagulation or vitamin K from promoting coagulation), by exercise that boosts the production of chemical activators that destroy unwanted clots, and by liver disease that affects the supply of vitamin K. Platelets are also easily suppressed by radiation and chemotherapy.

Normal Hemostasis and Coagulation (Bithell, 1987; Reich, 1984)

Hemostasis may be defined as the process that arrests the flow of blood from vessels containing blood under pressure (i.e., the process that keeps the blood within the circulatory system). Hemostasis is initiated by vascular injury and results in the formation of a firm platelet-fibrin barrier that prevents the escape of blood from the damaged vessel. In humans, hemostasis is the result of three interrelated phenomena:

- Various reactions intrinsic to blood vessels
- The formation of platelet plugs
- The formation of fibrin, the result of the processes of blood coagulation

The process of platelet aggregation and blood coagulation are intrinsically "self-propagating." They constitute a threat to the organism if they extend beyond the wound site into the general circulation. This process normally does not happen because of homeostatic regulatory phenomena.

Vascular Phase

The vascular phenomenon associated with normal hemostasis and coagulation in humans is not clearly understood. The endothelium may release or secrete several substances that are active in the vascular phase of the hemostatic process. These substances include:

- Tissue factor (activates the extrinsic pathway of coagulation)
- Adenosine diphosphate (ADP; mediates platelet aggregation)
- Bradykinin (vasodilator; important in inflammation)

The first step in the vascular phase is the constriction of arterioles at the edges of the wound while platelets clump together (platelet phase) to form a clot or thrombi, which in turn applies mechanical pressure by plugging the site of bleeding and by preventing further bleeding.

Platelet Phase

After vascular injury, ADP is released from injured tissues or erythrocytes as the major factor in the initiation of the platelet phase. Platelets are first seen to adhere to exposed subendothelial structures, particularly collagen fibers. This phenomenon called *platelet adhesion* produces biochemical activation of the platelets. Various prostaglandins (fatty acids) and thromboxanes, which induce platelet aggregation and constrict arterial smooth muscle, are then synthesized. Other substances from storage sites within the platelet are released into the external environment to aid in vasoconstriction. Activated platelets become "sticky" and attach to each other to form clumps or plugs that increase progressively in size *(platelet aggregation).*

Plugs consisting entirely of platelets may stop bleeding in small injuries but permanent hemostasis requires the presence of fibrin, which is the protein end-product of blood coagulation.

Coagulation Phase

The coagulation of blood involves the interaction of several plasma coagulation factors that leads to the conversion of a plasma protein, fibrinogen, into fibrin. The fibrin forms a mesh that then traps platelets and erythrocytes to plug blood vessels (Purtilo and Purtilo, 1989). By international agreement and common usage, the coagulation proteins are designated by Roman numerals (Reich, 1984):

- Factor I (fibrinogen)
- Factor II (prothrombin)
- Factor V
- Factors VII through XII

Numerals III, IV, and VI are not used. The numeric order does not reflect reaction sequence.

Plasma clotting factors are inactive until substances released by injured tissues trigger activation of these factors. For example, fibrin is a strong polymer (protein) that is the physical basis of permanent hemostatic plugs formed in all blood clots. Thrombin (an enzyme) converts circulating fibrinogen into fibrin polymers. Thrombin generation occurs through two different reaction sequences, the intrinsic and extrinsic coagulation pathways that are not discussed in further detail in this text. The reader is referred to a more comprehensive hematologic textbook for a more definite understanding of these pathways (see Bibliography).

CLASSIFICATION OF BLOOD DISORDERS

Erythrocytes

Anemia

Anemia is a reduction in the oxygen-carrying capacity of the blood due to an abnormality in the quantity or quality of erythrocytes. Anemia is not a disease, but is instead a symptom of any of a number of different blood disorders. It can be caused by factors such as poor diet (nutritional anemia), blood loss, exposure to industrial poisons such as chlorine gas, or diseases of the bone marrow (Miller and Keane, 1987). Anemias are classified usually on the basis of erythrocyte appearance (morphology) or etiology of the disease. Most anemias are caused by

1. Loss of erythrocytes
2. Hemolysis (increased destruction of erythrocytes)
3. Decreased production of erythrocytes

Anemias are usually classified on the basis of erythrocyte appearance (morphology) or etiology of the disease as follows (Purtilo and Purtilo, 1989):

- Acute or chronic loss of blood
  - Hemorrhage
  - Excessive menstruation
  - Bleeding hemorrhoids
  - Bleeding peptic ulcers
  - Renal failure (hemodialysis)
- Destruction of erythrocytes
  - Mechanical or autoimmune hemolysis
- Decreased production of erythrocytes due to nutritional deficiency
  - Iron, B_{12}, folic acid deficiency
- Molecular defects in proteins
  - Hereditary spherocytosis*
  - Thalassemia†
  - Sickle cell disease
  - Enzyme deficiencies
- Miscellaneous
  - Endocrine diseases, such as hypothyroidism
  - Marrow failure, such as leukemia
  - Aplastic anemia
  - Chronic inflammatory diseases
  - Malignant diseases
  - Decreased production of erythropoietin in end-stage renal disease

Deficiency in the oxygen-carrying capacity of blood may result in disturbances in the function of many organs and tissues. These disturbances may lead to various symptoms that can also differ from one patient to another. Slowly developing anemia in young, otherwise healthy individuals is well tolerated, and there may be no symptoms until hemoglobin concentration and hematocrit fall below 50%

* Erythrocytes have small spheres instead of the normal flexible biconcave disk shapes. These spheres rupture easily.

† Hemolytic anemia marked by a decreased rate of synthesis of one or more hemoglobin polypeptide chains.

of normal. This person will probably make an appointment with a physician because a friend or many people have commented on the person's pale appearance. However, anemia of rapid onset may result in additional symptoms of dyspnea and palpitations before hemoglobin/hematocrit fall below 50% (Shattil and Cooper, 1983).

CLINICAL SIGNS AND SYMPTOMS OF ANEMIA

- Skin pallor (palms of hands, nail beds)
- Fatigue and listlessness
- Dyspnea on exertion accompanied by heart palpitations and rapid pulse (more severe anemia)

Although anemia is not the most common cause of weakness and fatigue, rapid onset of listlessness characterized by weakness and fatigue is an early sign of anemia and reflects the lack of oxygen transport to the lungs and muscles. Many patients can have moderate-to-severe anemia without these symptoms. Because of the wide normal variations in skin color, changes in skin color, oral mucosa, and conjunctiva are more important than just pale skin. Changes in the hands and fingernail beds (Table 5–2) are more reliable signs in observing anemia than facial skin. Although there is no difference in normal blood volume associated with severe anemia, there is a redistribution of blood so that organs most sensitive to oxygen deprivation (e.g., the brain, heart, and muscles) receive more blood than, for example, the hands and kidneys (Shattil and Cooper, 1983).

During the inspection/observation portion of the objective examination, the physical therapist should look for pale palms with normal-colored creases (severe anemia: pale creases as well). Observation of the hands should be done at the patient's heart level and with warm hands because cold hands look pale due to vasoconstriction. The physician should also look at the conjunctivae, mouth, pharynx, and lips for paleness or yellow color as additional confirming signs of anemia. Specific skin and nail changes are shown in Table 5–2.

Systolic blood pressure may not be affected, but diastolic pressure may be lower than normal with an associated increase in the resting pulse rate. Resting cardiac output is usually normal in patients with anemia, but cardiac output increases with exercise more than in nonanemic persons. As the anemia becomes more severe, resting cardiac output increases and exercise tolerance progressively decreases until dyspnea, tachycardia, and palpitations occur at rest (Shattil and Cooper, 1983).

A blood test is required to medically diagnose anemia. It is difficult to define the bor-

Table 5–2. CHANGES ASSOCIATED WITH HEMATOLOGIC DISORDERS*

Skin Changes	Causes
Light, lemon-yellow tint	Untreated pernicious anemia
White, waxy appearance	Severe anemia secondary to acute hemorrhage
Gray-green yellow	Chronic blood loss
Gray tint	Leukemia
Pale hands or palmar creases	Anemia
Nail Bed	
Brittle	Long-standing iron deficiency anemia
Concave (rather than convex)	Long-standing iron deficiency anemia
Oral Mucosa/Conjunctiva	
Pale, yellow color	Anemia

* From Reich, P.R.: Hematology: Physiopathologic Basis for Clinical Practice, 2nd ed. Boston, Little, Brown, 1984.

derline between normal blood and anemia. The World Health Organization (WHO) has defined anemia in terms of the level of hemoglobin, using 13 grams per deciliter (g/dl) for men and 12 g/dl for women as the lower limit of normal. These measures must take into consideration the variation in values among normal healthy subjects, and the overlap between ranges of optimal and suboptimal hemoglobin values (Callender, 1986). Treatment is determined according to the cause of the anemia.

Polycythemia (Callender, 1986; Miller and Keane, 1987)

Polycythemia (also referred to as erythrocytosis) is defined as an increase in the total erythrocyte mass of the blood, characterized by an excessive number of erythrocytes so that the hematocrit (volume of packed erythrocytes) is above normal (Table 5–3). Patients with polycythemia have increased whole blood viscosity and increased blood volume. The increased erythrocyte production results in this thickening of the blood and an increased tendency toward clotting. The viscosity of the blood limits its ability to flow easily, diminishing the supply of blood to the brain and to other vital tissues. Increased platelets in combination with the increased blood viscosity may contribute to the formation of intravascular thrombi. In the normal, healthy person, the number of erythrocytes is maintained at a stable level corresponding to the oxygen demand of the tissues. Any factors that reduce the supply of oxygen stimulate the production of the hormone, erythropoietin, which is responsible for the control of erythrocyte production. The resultant increase in erythrocytes enables the blood to carry more oxygen to the tissues.

There are two distinct forms of polycythemia:

Table 5–3. LABORATORY VALUES ASSOCIATED WITH POLYCYTHEMIA

	Men	Women
Hemoglobin	>17.5 g/dl	>15.5 g/dl
Erythrocytes	$>6.0 \times 10^{12}/l$	$>5.5 \times 10^{12}/l$
Hematocrit	42–52%	37–47%

- Primary (also known as polycythemia vera)
- Secondary polycythemia

Polycythemia Vera. This disorder is one of a group of disorders collectively called myeloproliferative diseases. In this condition, production of erythrocytes is no longer under the control of erythropoietin. Although the effects of this form of polycythemia are well known: hyperplasia of the cell-forming tissues of the bone marrow with resultant elevation of the erythrocyte count and hemoglobin level and increase in the number of leukocytes and platelets, the etiology is unknown.

Polycythemia vera is a blood disorder that occurs in older people who are between 50 and 60 years of age, and it is rarely diagnosed before 40 years of age. Men and women are affected equally. The increase in blood volume may be two to three times that of normal. Because of the increased concentration of erythrocytes and the resultant increased blood viscosity, the patient shows increased skin coloration and elevated blood pressure. Gout is sometimes a complication of this form of polycythemia, and a typical attack of acute gout may be the first symptom.

Secondary Polycythemia. This disorder is a physiologic condition resulting from a decreased oxygen supply to the tissues caused by situations such as normal acclimatization to high altitudes, heavy tobacco smoking, or in association with severe, chronic lung and heart disorders, especially congenital heart defects. The body attempts to compensate for the reduced oxygen by manufacturing more hemoglobin and more erythrocytes. In some conditions the production of erythropoietin is inappropriately increased, resulting in polycythemia. This occurs particularly in association with any kidney abnormalities, because the kidney is the main site of erythropoietin production.

CLINICAL SIGNS AND SYMPTOMS OF POLYCYTHEMIA

Clinical signs and symptoms of polycythemia (whether primary or secondary) are directly related to the increase in blood viscosity described earlier and may include:

- Headache
- Dizziness
- Irritability
- Blurred vision
- Fainting
- Decreased mental acuity
- Feeling of fullness in the head
- Disturbances of sensation in the hands and feet
- General malaise and fatigue
- Weight loss
- Easy bruising
- Intolerable pruritus (skin itching) **(polycythemia vera)***
- Cyanosis (blue hue to the skin)
- Clubbing of the fingers
- Splenomegaly (enlargement of spleen)
- Gout
- Hypertension

The symptoms of this disease are often insidious in onset with vague complaints, and the patient may only be diagnosed secondary to a sudden complication (e.g., a stroke or thrombosis). Blockage of the capillaries supplying the digits of either hands or feet may cause a peripheral vascular neuropathy with decreased sensation, burning, numbness, or tingling. This small blood vessel occlusion can also contribute to the development of cyanosis and clubbing. If the underlying disorder is not recognized and treated, the patient may develop gangrene and have subsequent loss of tissue.

Treatment. Because of the threat of complications from a thrombosis or hemorrhage, treatment is essential and directed toward reducing erythrocytes and platelets to normal values and suppressing the overactive bone marrow. In secondary polycythemia, successful treatment of the causative condition relieves the polycythemia. Mild cases can be treated with periodic phlebotomy (removal of excess blood), although this does not stop the rapid regeneration of erythrocytes and may cause iron deficiency. More serious cases require myelosuppressive therapy with radioactive agents. Injected into a vein, these agents localize in the bone marrow and irradiate the overactive marrow cells. The prognosis is good for 15 to 20 years after diagnosis, but enlargement of the spleen and replacement of the bone marrow by fibrous tissue results eventually in a condition called myelofibrosis, which may develop into an atypical leukemia-like disorder.

Sickle Cell Anemia (Maugh, 1981)

Sickle cell disease is a serious, hereditary, chronic disease in which the erythrocytes are rigid and crescent-shaped or sickle-cell-shaped when they are deoxygenated. Most of these cells, however, simply assume distorted shapes and become extremely rigid. Because these erythrocytes must be flexible enough to pass through capillary blood vessels smaller than they are, rigid erythrocytes wedge in the capillaries and block normal blood flow.

The sickle cell defect occurs in hemoglobin, the oxygen-carrying constituent of erythrocytes. Normal adult hemoglobin (HbA) consists of two paired polypeptide chains (alpha and beta chains). Sickle cell anemia occurs when one amino acid is substituted for another in one of the polypeptide chains.* Thalassemias (another group of hemolytic anemias) occur where there is a genetically determined imbalance in the production of alpha and beta chains (Callender, 1986).

The mutant gene coding for hemoglobin S (HbS) occurs on one chromosome in about 8 to 10% of American blacks and in as many as 20% of black Africans, although it can also

* This condition of skin itching is particularly related to warm conditions, such as in bed at night or in a bath and is called the "hot bath sign" (Callender, 1986).

* Specifically, the substitution of valine for glutamic acid at the sixth position of the beta-globin chain.

occur in persons of Mediterranean ancestry. Individuals with the mutant gene from only one parent are said to have sickle cell trait. About 40% of the hemoglobin in these individuals is HbS. Under normal circumstances, there appear to be no clinical signs and symptoms associated with this amount of HbS. Sickle cell disease occurs when the individual inherits the mutant gene from each parent, thus almost all the hemoglobin is HbS. Approximately 50,000 individuals have sickle cell disease in the United States, and there is a correspondingly higher number in Africa.

Researchers postulate that in the arterial system, the erythrocytes contain an oxygenated solution of HbS (Mozzarelli et al, 1987). When the cell squeezes through a narrow capillary to reach the venous system, it releases its oxygen to the tissues. The sickle hemoglobin transports oxygen normally, but when it loses its oxygen, the hemoglobin molecules align themselves in such a way that the erythrocytes become stiff and sickle-cell-shaped. For a time, this "sickling" is reversible because the cells are reoxygenated in arterial blood; however, eventually, the change becomes irreversible. In the process of sickling and unsickling, the erythrocyte membrane becomes damaged. In addition, the abnormally stiff cells do not pass easily through capillaries and veins and tend to cause obstruction to the blood flow (Callender, 1986). Under stress, oxygen is released too soon and the cell sickles while it is in the capillary, thus blocking this small vessel. Oxygen deprivation takes place, and damage to tissue occurs. The sooner that the oxygen is released, the more severe (clinically) is the sickle cell disease. This release time can be shortened even more by the presence of acidosis, dehydration, trauma, strenuous physical exertion, emotional stress, pregnancy, extremes of heat and cold, and increased body temperatures (fever).

Sickle cell anemia is characterized by a series of "crises" that result from early destruction of the abnormal cells and obstruction of blood flow to the tissues. Stress from viral or bacterial infection, hypoxia, dehydration, emotional disturbance, extreme temperatures, or fatigue may precipitate a crisis. Clinical crises in sickle cell disease can be either acute or chronic and usually fit into one of three categories based on mechanism (Thomas and Holbrook, 1987):

- Vaso-occlusion
- Infection
- Erythrocyte destruction or sequestration

Clinical symptoms may be observed in the first year of life (Ahulu-Konotey, 1974).

CLINICAL SIGNS AND SYMPTOMS OF SICKLE CELL ANEMIA

- Pain
    - Abdominal
    - Chest
    - Headaches
- Bone and joint crises from the ischemic tissue lasting for hours to days and subsiding gradually
    - Low-grade fever
    - Extremity pain
    - Back pain
    - Periosteal pain
    - Joint pain, especially in the shoulder and hip
- Vascular complications
    - Cerebrovascular accidents (affects children and young adults most often)
    - Chronic leg ulcers
    - Avascular necrosis of the femoral head
    - Bone infarcts
- Pulmonary crises
    - Bacterial pneumonia
    - Pulmonary infarction (less common)
- Neurologic manifestations:
    - Convulsions
    - Drowsiness
    - Coma
    - Stiff neck
    - Paresthesias
    - Cranial nerve palsies
    - Blindness
    - Nystagmus

- Hand-foot syndrome
    - Fever
    - Pain
    - Dactylitis (painful swelling of the dorsum of hands and feet)
- Splenic sequestration crisis (occurs before adolescence)
    - Liver and spleen enlargement due to trapped erythrocytes
    - Subsequent spleen atrophy due to repeated blood vessel obstruction
- Renal complications
    - Enuresis (bed-wetting)
    - Nocturia (excessive urination at night)
    - Hematuria (blood in the urine)
    - Pyelonephritis
    - Renal papillary necrosis
    - End-stage renal failure (elderly population)

The vaso-occlusive crises (painful episodes of ischemic tissue damage) typically last for 5 or 6 days. Older patients more often report extremity and back pain during vascular crises. Compared with hand-foot syndrome, the pain is usually asymmetric and is not associated with swelling. Sickle cell disease in a young child often presents as the hand-foot syndrome in a symmetric pattern. Occlusion of small vessels supplying the metacarpal and metatarsal bones causes painful swelling, which is often accompanied by a low-grade fever. Vaso-occlusive crises other than hand-foot syndrome are less common in children under 5 years of age (Vichinsky et al, 1988).

Cerebrovascular accidents (CVAs) are a frequent and severe manifestation of sickle cell anemia, and they affect 6 to 12% of patients, most commonly children. Recovery may be complete in some cases, or serious neurologic damage may result. A second CVA occurs in up to 70% of patients who have the initial neurologic insult.

Prognosis and Treatment. The prognosis for persons with sickle cell disease is poor. Some people with the disease have only a few symptoms, whereas others are affected severely and have a short life span. Very few people who are affected severely live beyond the age of 20, and some people die in infancy or in early childhood (Miller and Keane, 1987). Early diagnosis, especially newborn screening for the abnormal hemoglobins, is important in the long-term preventative care of these patients.

Although there is no cure for sickle cell anemia, significant decreases in morbidity and mortality have been achieved by early diagnosis, intensive medical supervision, and advances in the treatment of complications (Vichinsky et al, 1983, 1988). Treatment is symptomatic, and preventive measures are used to reduce the incidence of crises and to avoid dehydration and infections. When the crisis is due to inflammatory changes, medications such as corticosteroids are sometimes administered to relieve musculoskeletal pain (Miller and Keane, 1987). Specific physical therapy treatment of the patient with sickle cell disease (whether a child or an adult) was documented by McLaurin (1985).

Leukocytes

Leukocytosis

Leukocytosis characterizes many infectious diseases and has a leukocyte count of more than 10,000 leukocytes per cubic millimeter. It can be associated with an increase in circulating neutrophils (neutrophilia). Leukocytosis is a common finding and may be caused by the following (Griffin, 1986):

- Bacterial infections
- Inflammation or tissue necrosis (e.g., infarction, myositis, vasculitis)
- Metabolic intoxications (e.g., uremia, eclampsia, acidosis, gout)
- Neoplasms (especially bronchogenic carcinoma, lymphoma, melanoma)
- Acute hemorrhage
- Postsplenectomy
- Acute appendicitis
- Pneumonia

- Intoxication by chemicals
- Acute rheumatic fever

CLINICAL SIGNS AND SYMPTOMS OF LEUKOCYTOSIS

These clinical signs and symptoms are usually associated with symptoms of the conditions listed earlier and may include:

- Fever
- Symptoms of localized or systemic infection
- Symptoms of inflammation or trauma to tissue

Leukopenia

Leukopenia, or reduction of the number of leukocytes in the blood below 5,000 per microliter, is often caused by viral infections. Leukopenia may also occur secondary to failure of bone marrow (aplastic anemia) in the patient with leukemia or malignancies after treatment with radiotherapy or chemotherapy. Infection in the immunosuppressed patient is a major problem after treatment for cancer, prompting the reminder of the importance of good handwashing practices when treating any of these patients.

CLINICAL SIGNS AND SYMPTOMS OF LEUKOPENIA (Reich, 1984)

- Sore throat
- High fever, chills
- Ulcerations of mucous membranes (mouth, rectum, vagina)

Treatment. Treatment is directed toward elimination of the chemical causing the reduced leukocytes or control of the precipitating infection.

Leukemia

Although leukemia is a disease arising from the bone marrow and involves the uncontrolled growth of blood cells, a complete discussion of this cancer can be found in Chapter 10.

Platelets

Thrombocytosis

Thrombocytosis is a platelet count of more than one million per microliter. It is usually temporary and may occur as a compensatory mechanism after severe hemorrhage, surgery, and splenectomy, in iron deficiency, in polycythemia vera, and as a manifestation of an occult (hidden) neoplasm (e.g., lung cancer). It is associated with a tendency to clot as well as a tendency to bleed. These manifestations can occur simultaneously because the excessive concentration of platelets is thought to interfere with the production of thromboplastin, which is necessary for normal coagulation (Aaron, 1988). Blood viscosity is increased by the very high platelet count resulting in intravascular clumping (or thrombosis) of the sludged platelets (Reich, 1984).

Thrombocytopenia

Thrombocytopenia, a decrease in the number of platelets (less than 150,000 cu mm) in circulating blood can result from decreased or defective platelet production or from an accelerated platelet destruction. A major concern with this disorder is the prevention of excessive bleeding from trauma to the mucous membranes, skin, and underlying tissues (Miller and Keane, 1987). Severe bleeding may occur from any mucous membrane including the nose, uterus, gastrointestinal tract, urinary tract, and respiratory tract. Causes of thrombocytopenia include (Griffin, 1986):

- Bone marrow infiltration by malignant cells (e.g., leukemia, metastatic carcinoma)
- Viral infections
- Prosthetic heart valves
- Nutritional deficiency
- Drugs (e.g., cytotoxic agents, gold, sulfonamides, ethanol/alcohol)

- Hemorrhage
- Disseminated intravascular coagulation (DIC): widespread formation of thromboses primarily in the capillaries
- Hypersplenism (condition of exaggerated hemolytic processes within the spleen)
- Aplastic anemia (deficiency of erythrocytes because of arrested development of erythrocytes in the bone marrow)
- Autoantibody-mediated platelet injury (e.g., systemic lupus erythematosus, secondary to drugs such as quinidine, quinine, and sulfonamides)

CLINICAL SIGNS AND SYMPTOMS OF THROMBOCYTOPENIA

- Bleeding after minor trauma
- Spontaneous bleeding
    - Petechiae (small red dots)
    - Ecchymoses (bruises)
    - Purpura spots (bleeding under the skin
- Menorrhagia (excessive menstruation)
- Bleeding of the gums and nose

Severe thrombocytopenia results in the appearance of multiple petechiae, most often observed on the lower legs. Gastrointestinal bleeding and bleeding into the central nervous system associated with severe thrombocytopenia may be life-threatening manifestations of thrombocytopenic bleeding. These severe consequences of thrombocytopenia are not usually encountered by the physical therapist, and this disorder does not cause massive bleeding into the tissues or the joints. Medical treatment of thrombocytopenia varies, depending on the precipitating cause.

Coagulation Disorder

Hemophilia (Cotta et al, 1986)

Hemophilia is a hereditary blood clotting disorder caused by an abnormality of functional plasma-clotting proteins known as factor VIII or IX. In most cases, the hemophiliac has normal amounts of the deficient factor circulating, but it is in a functionally inadequate state. Persons with hemophilia bleed longer than those with normal levels of functioning factors VIII or IX, but the bleeding is not any faster than would occur in a normal person with the same injury.

This disease is sex-linked recessive with bleeding manifested only in men; women carry and transmit the abnormal genes. The disease affects approximately one in 10,000 men from all races and socioeconomic groups. A man with hemophilia cannot transmit the disease to his sons, but all of his daughters will be genetic carriers of the disease. Although in most cases of hemophilia, there is a known family history, this disorder can occur in families without a previous history of blood clotting disorders.

The most common form of hemophilia is hemophilia A (classic hemophilia), which affects the factor VIII gene, and hemophilia B (Christmas disease), which affects the factor IX gene. Both forms produce similar clinical bleeding patterns, but hemophilia A is the most common type affecting approximately 80% of all hemophiliacs. Another clotting disorder is von Willebrand's disease, which is a rare deficiency or defect of a glycoprotein (von Willebrand factor)* and is frequently confused with hemophilia A. Von Willebrand's disease can also affect women.

Hemophilia can be described as being mild, moderate, or severe based on the amount of active clotting factor present in the blood. The level of severity remains constant throughout a person's life. The level of clotting factor and clinical symptoms present are usually similar among family members. Normal concentrations of coagulation factors are between 50 and 150%.

Persons with *mild hemophilia* have a clot-

* For further information, refer to Hilgartner, M., and Montgomery, R.: Understanding von Willebrand's Disease. New York, The National Hemophilia Foundation, 1985.

ting activity level of 5 to 50%. Spontaneous hemorrhages are rare, and joint and deep muscle bleeding is uncommon. These people bleed with surgical or other major trauma and must then be treated like people with severe hemophilia. Hemophiliacs who are classified as *moderate* in severity have clotting factor levels greater than 1%, but less than 5%. Spontaneous bleeding is usually not a problem with these patients; however, they can still have major bleeding episodes after minor trauma. *Severe hemophilia* is defined as having factor level activity in the blood less than 1% of normal. These persons are likely to bleed spontaneously or with only slight trauma.

Over time, the hemophiliac may develop an inhibitor for administered factor VIII or IX, which is an acquired circulating antibody that destroys these factors when the replacement clotting factors are infused as a method of treatment. An inhibitor is found in approximately 10 to 20% of people with factor VIII deficiency and in 2 to 3% of those people with factor IX deficiency. Inhibitors usually develop in severe hemophiliacs before the age of 20 and often result in complications in treatment.

Clinical Manifestations

Bleeding into the joint spaces (hemarthrosis) is the most common clinical manifestation of hemophilia most often affecting the knee, elbow, ankle, hip, and shoulder (in order of most common appearance). Recurrent hemarthrosis results in hemophiliac arthopathy (joint disease). Bleeding may result from an identifiable trauma or stress or may be spontaneous (most common with the severe hemophiliac). Hemarthroses are not common in the first year of life, but increase in frequency as the child begins to walk. The severity of the hemarthrosis may vary (depending on the degree of injury) from mild pain and swelling, which resolves without treatment within 1 to 3 days, to severe pain with an excruciatingly painful, swollen joint that persists for several weeks and resolves slowly with treatment.

CLINICAL SIGNS AND SYMPTOMS OF AN ACUTE HEMARTHROSIS

- Aura or prickling sensation
- Stiffening into the position of comfort
- Decreased range of motion
- Pain
- Swelling
- Tenderness
- Heat

Bleeding into the joints eventually results in chronic joint changes with a progressive loss of motion, muscle atrophy, and flexion contractures. This type of affected joint is susceptible particularly to being injured again, setting up a cycle of vulnerability to trauma and repeated hemorrhages.

Bleeding into the muscles is the second most common site of bleeding in persons with hemophilia. Muscle hemorrhages can be more insidious and massive compared with joint hemorrhages. They may occur anywhere, but are common in the flexor muscle groups, predominantly the iliopsoas, gastrocnemius, and flexor surface of the forearm, and result in deformities such as hip flexion contractures, equinus position of the foot, or Volkmann's deformity of the forearm.

CLINICAL SIGNS AND SYMPTOMS OF MUSCLE HEMORRHAGE

- Gradually intensifying pain
- Protective spasm of the muscle
- Limitation of movement at the surrounding joints
- Muscle assumes the position of comfort

Gastrointestinal bleeding involvement may occur gradually or suddenly and may last for several weeks.

CLINICAL SIGNS AND SYMPTOMS OF GASTROINTESTINAL INVOLVEMENT

- Abdominal pain and distention
- Melena (blood in stool)
- Hematemesis (vomiting blood)
- Fever
- Low abdominal/groin pain due to bleeding into wall of large intestine or iliopsoas muscle
- Flexion contracture of the hip due to spasm of the iliopsoas muscle secondary to retroperitoneal hemorrhage

Over time, the following complications may occur:

- Vascular compression causing localized ischemia and necrosis
- Replacement of muscle fibers by nonelastic fibrotic tissue causing shortened muscles and thus producing joint contractures
- Peripheral nerve lesions from compression of a nerve that travels in the same compartment as the hematoma, most commonly affects the femoral, ulnar, and median nerves
- Pseudotumor formation with bone erosion

Treatment. Effective treatment is based on an accurate diagnosis of the deficient clotting factor and its level in the blood. This requires a battery of common blood tests for bleeding time, partial thromboplastin time, factor assays, and a battery of common blood tests to monitor the liver, kidney, immune function, and hepatitis status. Current treatment relies on human plasma-derived clotting factor that is produced using one of several processing methods. Although transmission of the human immunodeficiency (HIV) virus (precursor for the acquired immunodeficiency syndrome [AIDS]) has almost been eliminated, the transmission of the hepatitis virus is still a problem. With the advent of genetic engineering, scientists have been developing methods of gene splitting that may eventually allow laboratory synthesis of clotting factors to eliminate even this potential complication (Garrett, 1988).

Comprehensive medical management of hemophilia may involve the use of drugs to control pain in acute bleeding and chronic arthropathies. The common pain reliever, aspirin, and any of its derivatives cannot be used by persons with hemophilia because it inhibits platelet function. Anti-inflammatory nonsteroidal drugs can contain derivatives of aspirin and must be used cautiously. Corticosteroids are used occasionally for the treatment of chronic synovitis.

Physical therapy treatment has been effective in preventing spontaneous bleeding through the protective strengthening of the musculature surrounding affected joints and through patient education. Physical therapy is used during episodes of acute hemorrhage to control pain and additional bleeding and to maintain positioning and prevent further deformity (Cotta et al, 1986).

SUMMARY

This chapter has included a brief discussion of blood composition and formation, normal hemostasis and coagulation, and then a description of blood disorders involving erythrocytes, leukocytes, platelets, and coagulation disorders. The conditions included are limited to the hematologic disorders that are most commonly encountered in a physical therapy practice, whether on an inpatient or an outpatient basis. In the course of this discussion, we have attempted to provide an overview of:

- Anemia
- Polycythemia
- Sickle cell anemia
- Leukocytosis
- Leukopenia
- Thrombocytosis
- Thrombocytopenia
- Hemophilia

Systemic Signs and Symptoms Requiring Physician Referral

Any patient who has any of the following generalized symptoms without obvious or already known cause should be further evaluated by a physician. At the very least, these signs and symptoms should be documented and a copy should be sent to the physician.

- Abdominal/chest/back pain
- Blurred vision
- Changes in hands and fingernails
- Changes in skin color
- Cyanosis
- Dactylitis
- Decreased mental acuity
- Digital clubbing
- Disturbances of sensation in hands/feet
- Dizziness
- Dyspnea on exertion
- Easy bruising
- Evidence of hemarthrosis/muscle hemorrhage
- Fainting
- Fever
- Fatigue and listlessness
- Feeling of fullness in head
- Headache
- Irritability
- Palpitations
- Petechiae
- Pruritus
- Palpitations
- Rapid pulse
- Weakness
- Weight loss

SUBJECTIVE EXAMINATION

Special Questions to Ask

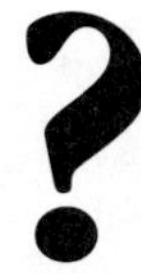

- □ Is there a known history of anemia in your family?
- □ Have you recently had a serious blood loss (possibly requiring transfusion)? **(Anemia)**
- □ Do you experience shortness of breath or heart palpitations with slight exertion (e.g., climbing stairs) or even just at rest? **(Anemia)**
- □ **For patients at elevations above 3,500 feet:** Have you recently moved from one geographical location to another? **(Polycythemia)**
- □ Have you ever been told that you have a congenital heart defect (also chronic lung/heart disorders)? **(Polycythemia: also possible with history of heavy tobacco use)**
- □ Do you ever have episodes of dizziness, blurred vision, headaches, fainting, or feeling of fullness in your head? **(Polycythemia)**
- □ Do you have a history of bruising easily or excessive blood loss? **(Polycythemia, hemophilia, thrombocytopenia)**

  For example, do you ever notice tiny, round (nonraised) red spots on your skin that later change color to blue or yellow? **(Petechiae associated with thrombocytopenia)**

  For example, do you usually notice excessive bruising, bleeding, or bleeding into the joints spontaneously or after minor trauma, surgery, or dental procedures?
- □ Do you have recurrent infections and low-grade fever, such as colds, influenzalike symptoms, other upper respiratory infections? **(Abnormal leukocytes)**

Subjective Exam

Special Questions to Ask

□ Do you tend to have frequent nose bleeds? (Epistaxis)

If yes to either of the last two questions, ask more about the initial onset of these bleeding episodes.*

□ Do you have black, tarry stools **(bleeding into the gastrointestinal tract)** or blood in urine **(genitourinary tract)?**

□ Has any previous bleeding been severe enough to require blood transfusions?

□ Have you been exposed to occupational or industrial gases, such as chlorine gas, mustard gas, agent orange, napalm (chemical and biologic warfare)?

□ **For women (Anemia, thrombocytopenia):** Do you frequently have prolonged or excessive bleeding in association with your menstrual flow? (Excessive may be considered to be measured by the use of more than 4 tampons each day; prolonged menstruation usually refers to more than 5 days—both of these measures are subjective and must be considered along with other factors, such as the presence of other symptoms, personal menstrual history, placement in the life cycle [i.e., in relation to menopause].)

* Symptoms beginning in infancy or childhood suggest a congenital hemostatic defect, whereas symptoms beginning later in life indicate an acquired disorder, such as secondary to drug-induced defect of platelet function, a common cause of easy bruising and excessive bleeding. This bruising or bleeding occurs usually in association with trauma, menstruation, dental work, or surgical procedures. Drug-induced bruising or bleeding may also occur with use of aspirin, and aspirin-containing compounds, nonsteroidal anti-inflammatory agents like ibuprofen (Motrin), fenoprofen (Nalfon), naproxen (Naprosyn), and penicillins because these drugs inhibit platelet function to some extent (Reich, 1984).

PHYSICIAN REFERRAL

Understanding the components of a patient's past medical history that can affect hematopoiesis can provide the physical therapist with valuable insight into the patient's present symptoms, which are usually already well known to the attending physician. For example, the effects of certain drugs, exposure to radiation, or recent cytotoxic cancer chemotherapy can all affect bone marrow. Whenever uncertain, the physical therapist is encouraged to contact the physician by telephone for discussion and clarification of the patient's medical symptoms.

A history of excessive menses, a folate poor diet, alcohol abuse, drug ingestion, family history of anemia, and family roots in geographical areas where red blood cell enzyme or hemoglobin abnormalities are prevalent represent some important findings that may correlate with objective findings to alert the physical therapist to the need for medical referral when the patient is not already under the care of a physician.

CASE STUDY

Referral

You are working in a hospital setting and you have received a physician's referral to "evaluate and treat" a patient who was involved in a serious automobile accident 10 days ago. The patient had internal injuries that required immediate abdominal surgery and 600 ml of blood transfused within 24 hours postoperatively. His condition is considered to be medically "stable."

What specific medical information should you look for in the patient's chart before beginning your evaluation?

Patient's name, age, and occupation

Past medical history:	Previous myocardial infarcts, history of heart disease, diabetes (type)
Surgical report:	Type of surgery, location of scar, any current contraindications
Were there any other injuries?	If yes, what were these and what is the current status of each injury?
Body weight	
Pulmonary status:	Is the patient a cigarette or pipe smoker? Is the patient currently receiving oxygen or respiratory therapy? What is the patient's current pulmonary status after the accident and postoperatively?
Laboratory report:	Hematocrit/hemoglobin levels Anemia?
Current status:	Nursing reports of the patient's complaints of any kind (e.g., symptoms of dyspnea or heart palpitations from rapid loss of blood)
Vital signs:	Blood pressure Presence of fever Resting pulse rate
Current medications:	Be aware of the purpose for each medication and its potential side effects. Has the patient been up at all yet? If yes, when? How far did he walk? How much assistance was required? Did he have symptoms of orthostatic hypotension? Does the patient have any gastrointestinal symptoms? Patient's orientation to time, place, and person. Are there any dietary or fluid restrictions while the patient is in the physical ther-

CASE STUDY

Are there any known discharge plans at this time?

apy department? Is he on an intravenous line?

References

Aaron, M.J.: Hemorrhagic disorders and abnormalities of platelet and vascular functions. *In* Beeson, P., and McDermott, W. (eds): Cecil's Textbook of Medicine, 18th ed. Philadelphia, W.B. Saunders Company, 1988, pp. 1042–1060.

Ahulu-Konotey, F.I.D.: The sickle cell diseases. Arch. Intern. Med., *133*:611, 1974.

Bithell, T.C.: Normal hemostasis and coagulation. *In* Thorup, O.A. (ed): Leavell and Thorup's Fundamentals of Clinical Hematology, 5th ed. Philadelphia, W.B. Saunders Company, 1987, pp. 126–162.

Brown, B.A.: Hematology: Principles and Procedures, 3rd ed. Philadelphia, Lea & Febiger, 1980.

Callender, S.T.: Blood Disorders. Oxford, Oxford University Press, 1986.

Cotta, S., Jutra, M., and McQuarrie, A: Physical Therapy in Hemophilia. New York, The National Hemophilia Foundation, 1986.

Garrett, A.: Personal Communication. New York, The National Hemophilia Foundation, Dec. 28, 1988.

Griffin, J.P.: Hematology and Immunology. Norwalk, CT, Appleton-Century-Crofts, 1986.

Guyton, A: Textbook of Medical Physiology, 7th ed. Philadelphia, W.B. Saunders Company, 1986.

Hofrichter, J., and Ross, P.D.: Personal Communication. Bethesda, MD, National Institute of Arthritis and Musculoskeletal and Skin Diseases (NIAMSD), Jan 1989.

Maugh, T.H.: New understanding of sickle cell emerges. Science, *211*:265, 1981.

McLaurin, S.E.: Sickle cell disease: A need for physical therapy intervention. Clin. Management, *6*:12, 1985.

Miller, B.F., and Keane, C.B.: Encyclopedia and Dictionary of Medicine, Nursing, and Allied Health, 4th ed. Philadelphia, W.B. Saunders Company, 1987.

Mozzarelli, A., Hofrichter, J., and Eaton, W. A.: Delay time of hemoglobin S polymerization prevents most cells from sickling in vivo. Science, 237:500, 1987.

Page, J.: Blood: The river of life. Washington, DC, U.S. News Books, 1981.

Purtilo, D.T., and Purtilo, R. B.: A Survey of Human Diseases, 2nd ed. Boston, Little, Brown, 1989.

Reich, P.R.: Hematology: Physiopathologic Basis for Clinical Practice, 2nd ed. Boston, Little, Brown, 1984.

Shattil, S.J., and Cooper, R.A.: Anemia, weakness, and pallor. *In* Blacklow, R.S. (ed): MacBryde's Signs and Symptoms, 6th ed. Philadelphia, J.B. Lippincott, 1983, pp. 563–589.

Thomas, R., and Holbrook, T.: Sickle cell disease. Postgrad. Med., *81*:265, 1987.

Vichinsky, E. P., Hurst, D., and Lubin, B.: Sickle cell disease: Basic Concepts. Hosp. Med., Sept. 1983, pp. 128–158.

Vichinsky, E. P., Hurst, D., and Lubin, B.: Update on sickle cell disease. Hosp. Med., Feb. 1988, pp. 131–149.

Bibliography

Aronstram, A: Haemophilic Bleeding. Philadelphia, W.B. Saunders Company, 1985.

Bryant, N.J.: An Introduction to Immunohematology, 2nd ed. Philadelphia, W.B. Saunders Company, 1982.

Hilgartner, M., and Montgomery, R.: Understanding von Willebrand's Disease. New York, The National Hemophilia Foundation, 1985.

Hoffbrand, A.V., and Pettit, J.E.: Clinical Hematology. Philadelphia, W.B. Saunders Company, 1988.

McCollough, N.C. (ed): Musculoskeletal Disorders in Hemophilia. Washington, DC, National Academy of Sciences, 1973.

Nathan, D.G., and Oski, F.A.: Hematology of Infancy and Childhood, 3rd ed. Philadelphia, W.B. Saunders Company, 1987.

Oski, F.A., and Naiman, J.L.: Hematologic Problems in the Newborn, 3rd ed. Philadelphia, W.B. Saunders Company, 1982.

Stamatoyannopoulos, G., Nienhuis, A.W., Leder, P., and Majerus, P.W.: The Molecular Basis of Blood Diseases. Philadelphia, W.B. Saunders Company, 1987.

Sun, N.C.J.: Hematology: An Atlas and Diagnostic Guide. Philadelphia, W.B. Saunders Company, 1987.

Thorup, O.A. (ed): Leavell and Thorup's Fundamentals of Clinical Hematology, 5th ed. Philadelphia, W.B. Saunders Company, 1987.

Williams, W.J., Beutler, E., Erslev, A.J., and Lichtman, M.A.: Hematology, 3rd ed. New York, McGraw-Hill, 1983.

Wintrobe, M.M. (ed): Clinical Hematology, 8th ed. Philadelphia, Lea & Febiger, 1981.

Chapter 6

Overview of Gastrointestinal Signs and Symptoms

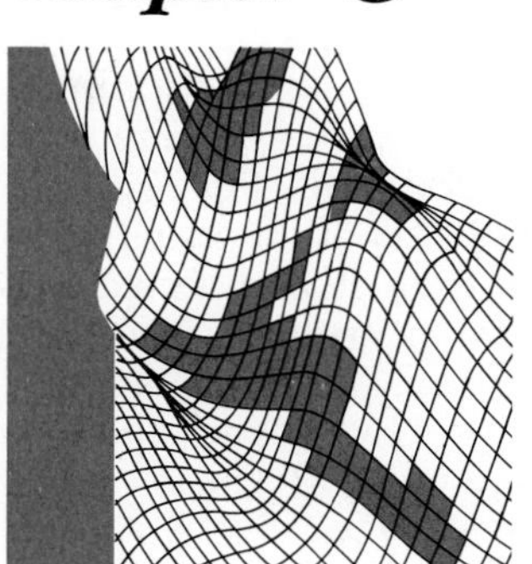

☐ ***Clinical Signs and Symptoms of:***

Ulcerative Colitis and Regional Enteritis

Irritable Bowel Syndrome

Gastrointestinal (GI) disorders can refer pain to the sternal region, shoulder, scapular region, midback, lower back, and hip. This pain can mimic primary musculoskeletal lesions causing confusion for the physical therapist or for the physician assessing the patient's chief complaints. Although these musculoskeletal symptoms can occur alone, the patient usually has other systemic signs and symptoms associated with GI disorders. A careful interview to screen for systemic illness is essential when assessing the patient who has musculoskeletal pain of unknown etiology. The physical therapy interview should include a few important questions concerning the patient's history and the presence of any associated signs or symptoms to immediately alert the physical therapist with regard to the need for medical follow-up.

The most common intra-abdominal diseases to refer pain to the musculoskeletal system occur as a result of ulceration or infection of the mucosal lining. Although pain can be experienced in an area that is far from the actual site of the disorder, the GI system offers patterns of pain and accompanying symptoms that should give the physical therapist who does a thorough investigation some grounds for suspicion.

The most clinically meaningful GI symptoms and the most common underlying causes of those symptoms are presented in this chapter.

GASTROINTESTINAL PHYSIOLOGY (Long, 1987)

The upper GI tract consists of structures that aid in the ingestion and digestion of food, namely, the mouth, esophagus, stomach, and duodenum (Fig. 6–1). The lower GI tract consists of the small and large intestines. Digestion is completed in the small intestine, and most of the nutrients are absorbed in this organ. The large intestine serves primarily to absorb water and electrolytes and to eliminate the waste products of digestion.

Esophagus

The esophagus is a hollow tube, the upper one third of which consists of skeletal muscle and the remainder of smooth muscle. It is lined with mucous membrane that secretes a mucoid substance for protection. Swallowing consists of three phases: a voluntary phase in which the tongue forces the bolus of food into the pharynx, an involuntary pharyngeal phase in which the food moves into the upper esophagus, and an esophageal phase during which food moves from the pharynx and down into the stomach. The cardiac sphincter prevents reflux (backward flow) of the contents of the stomach back into the lower esophagus. Food is prevented from passing into the trachea by the closing of the trachea and the opening of the esophagus.

Stomach

The stomach and the remainder of the GI tract are made up of five layers of smooth muscle that have two types of contractions: tonus contractions and rhythmic contractions. These

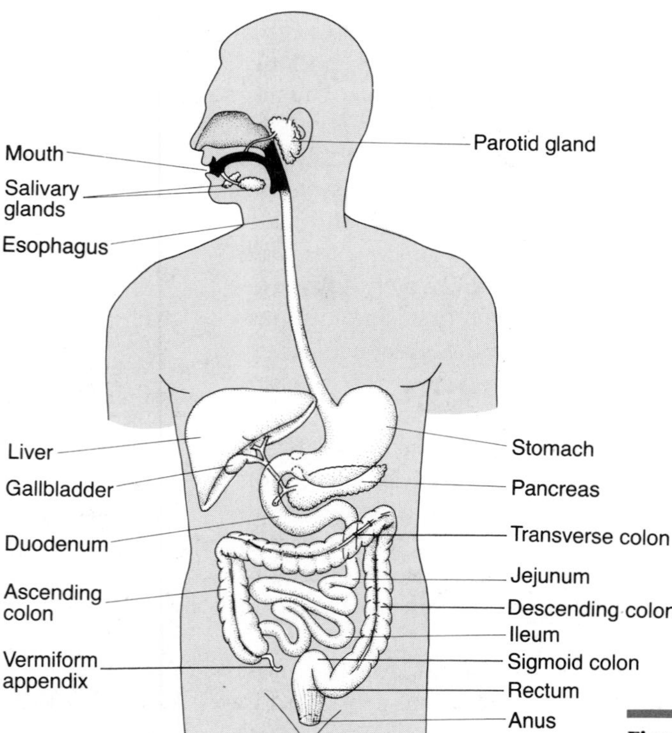

Figure 6–1. Organs of the digestive system. (From Guyton, A.C.: Textbook of Medical Physiology, 7th ed. Philadelphia, W.B. Saunders Company, 1989.)

contractions assist the peristaltic movement of food and are responsible for the mixing of the food. The food bolus enters the stomach and continues to move through the stomach and intestines by peristalsis (muscular contraction that causes a wave to push food along). As the food moves toward the pyloric sphincter, peristaltic waves increase in force and intensity. The fluid mass now becomes known as chyme (semifluid mass of partly digested food). Chyme is pumped through the pyloric sphincter into the duodenum.

Intestines

The small intestine is about 2.5 cm (1 in.) wide and 6 m (20 ft) long and fills most of the abdomen. It consists of three parts—the duodenum, which connects to the stomach; the jejunum or middle portion; and the ileum, which connects to the large intestine.

The large intestine is about 6 cm (2.5 in.) wide and 1.5 m (5 ft) long. It consists of three parts—the cecum, which connects to the small intestine; the colon; and the rectum. The ileocecal valve prevents backward flow of fecal contents from the large intestine to the small intestine. The vermiform appendix, which has no function, is an appendage close to the ileocecal valve. The colon consists of four parts—the ascending, transverse, descending, and sigmoid colons. The rectum is 17 to 20 cm (7 to 8 in.) long, ending in the 2- to 3-cm anal canal. The opening (anus) is controlled by a smooth muscle internal sphincter and by a striated muscle external sphincter.

Contents of the small intestine (chyme) are propelled toward the anus by peristaltic movement, which also mixes the intestinal contents. Chyme moves slowly and normally takes 3 to 10 hours to move from the stomach to the ileocecal valve. The major portion of digestion occurs in the small intestine by the action of pancreatic and intestinal secretions and by bile (liver secretion that breaks down fats). Ninety per cent of absorption of nutrients occurs within the small intestine. Reabsorption of water, electrolytes, and the bile salts occurs predominantly in the ascending colon. The colon has the capacity to absorb six to eight times more fluid than is delivered to it daily.

Pancreas (Miller and Keane, 1987)

The pancreas is a large, elongated gland that is located transversely behind the stomach between the spleen and the duodenum (Fig. 6–2). The pancreas is both an exocrine gland and an endocrine gland. Its function in diges-

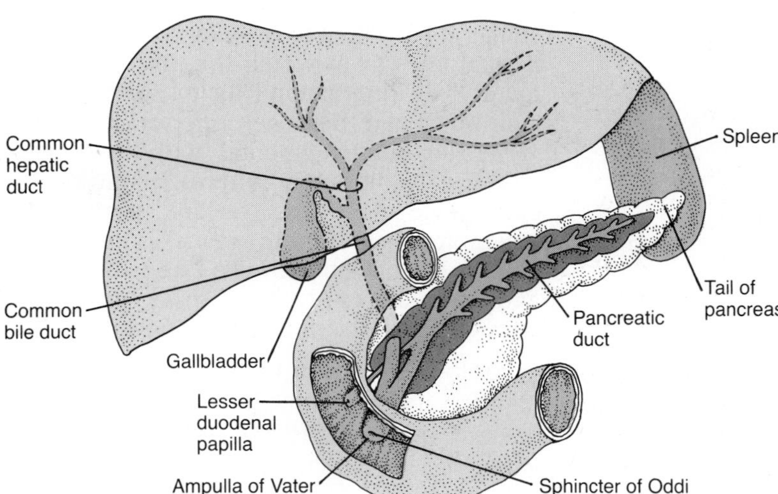

Figure 6–2. Anatomic relationship between the liver, gallbladder, and pancreas.

tion is primarily an exocrine activity. The pancreas secretes digestive enzymes and pancreatic juice that are transported through the hepatic duct to the duodenum where proteins, carbohydrates, and fats are broken down. Bicarbonate ions in the pancreatic secretion help to neutralize the acidic chyme that is passed along from the stomach to the duodenum.

Because of the pancreas's dual function as both an exocrine and endocrine gland, the pancreas and the disorders of the pancreas including diabetes mellitus, digestive disorders, pancreatic carcinoma, pancreatitis, and cystic fibrosis are discussed in various chapters throughout the text. This chapter focuses primarily on the digestive disorders associated with the pancreas.

ABDOMINAL PAIN (Bauwens and Paine, 1983; Travell and Simons, 1983; Way, 1983)

Pain is a subjective sensation resulting from the central transmission of peripherally received noxious stimuli (Way, 1983). It usually indicates damage to tissue unless the stimulus is removed. Afferent nerve impulses transmit pain from the esophagus to the spinal cord by small, unnamed sympathetic nerves. Visceral afferent nerves from the liver, diaphragm, and pericardium are derived from dermatomes C_3 to C_5 and reach the central nervous system (CNS) via the phrenic nerve. Afferent nerves from the gallbladder, stomach, pancreas, and small intestine travel through the celiac plexus (network of ganglia and nerves supplying the abdominal viscera) and the greater splanchnic nerves and enter the spinal cord from T_6 to T_9. Afferent stimuli from the colon, appendix, and pelvic viscera enter the 10th and 11th thoracic segments through the mesenteric plexus and lesser splanchnic nerves. Finally, the sigmoid colon, rectum, ureters, and testes are innervated by fibers that reach T_{11} to L_1 segments through the lower splanchnic nerve.

Stimuli for Abdominal Pain

The abdominal viscera are ordinarily insensitive to many stimuli, such as cutting, tearing, or crushing, which, when applied to the skin, evoke severe pain. These stimuli do not cause perceptible pain when applied to the abdominal viscera. Visceral pain fibers are sensitive only to stretching or tension in the wall of the gut from neoplasm, distention, or forceful muscular contractions secondary to bowel obstruction or spasm. The rate that tension develops must be rapid enough to produce pain; gradual distention, such as with malignant obstruction, may be painless unless ulceration occurs. Inflammation may produce visceral pain and ischemia (deficiency of blood) that subsequently produces pain by increasing the concentration of tissue metabolites in the region of the sensory nerve. Pain associated with ischemia is steady pain, whether this ischemia is secondary to vascular disease or due to obstruction causing strangulation of tissue. Other causes of abdominal pain are shown in Table 6-1.

Types of Abdominal Pain

Visceral

Visceral pain (internal organs) occurs in the midline because the abdominal organs receive sensory afferents from both sides of the spinal cord. The site of pain corresponds to dermatomes from which the diseased organ receives its innervation (Fig. 6-3). Pain is not well localized because innervation of the viscera is multisegmental with few nerve endings. Additionally, although the viscera experience pain, the visceral peritoneum (membrane enveloping organs) is insensitive to pain. It is possible to have extensive disease without pain until the disease progresses enough to involve the parietal peritoneum.

Location (Fig. 6-4): Midline
Dermatomal levels

Referral: Poorly localized (the patient cannot point to the specific site)

Table 6-1. CAUSES OF ABDOMINAL PAIN*

Intra-Abdominal	Extra-Abdominal
Generalized Peritonitis	***Thoracic***
Perforated viscus: peptic ulcer	Pneumonitis
Primary bacterial peritonitis	Pulmonary embolism
Pneumococcal	Pneumothorax
Streptococcal	Empyema
Enteric bacillus	Myocardial ischemia
Tuberculosis	Myocarditis
Nonbacterial peritonitis	Endocarditis
Ruptured ovarian cyst	Esophagitis
Ruptured follicle cyst	Esophageal spasm
	Esophageal rupture
***Localized Peritonitis*†**	
Appendicitis	***Neurogenic***
Cholecystitis	Radiculitis
Peptic ulcer	Spinal cord tumors
Regional enteritis (Crohn's disease)	Peripheral nerve tumors
Colitis: ulcerative, amebic, bacterial	Spinal arthritis
Abdominal abscess	Herpes zoster
Postoperative	Tabes dorsalis
Hepatic	
Pancreatic	***Metabolic***
Splenic	Uremia
Tubo-ovarian	Diabetes mellitus
Pancreatitis	Acute adrenal insufficiency
Hepatitis: viral, toxic	
Pelvic inflammatory disease	***Miscellaneous***
Endometriosis	Muscular contusion
Lymphadenitis	Hematoma
	Tumor
Pain from Increased Visceral Tension	
Intestinal obstruction	
Adhesions	
Hernia	
Tumor	
Fecal impaction	
Intestinal hypermotility	
Irritable colon	
Gastroenteritis	
Biliary obstruction	
Gallstone	
Stricture	
Tumor	
Parasites	
Ureteral obstruction: calculi (kidney stone)	
Hepatic capsule distention	
Acute hepatitis (toxic or viral)	
Common duct obstruction	
Renal capsule distention	
Pyelonephritis	
Ureteral obstruction	
Uterine obstruction	
Neoplasm	
Pregnancy/childbirth	
Ruptured ectopic pregnancy	
Aortic aneurysm	

Table 6–1. CAUSES OF ABDOMINAL PAIN* Continued

Intra-Abdominal	Extra-Abdominal
Ischemia	
Intestinal angina or infarction	
Arterial stenosis	
Embolism	
Polyarteritis	
Splenic infarction	
Torsion	
Gallbladder	
Spleen	
Ovarian cyst	
Testicle	
Appendix	
Hepatic infarction: toxemia	
Tumor necrosis: uterine fibroid	
Retroperitoneal Neoplasms	

* From Sleisenger, M.H. and Fortran, J.S. (eds): Gastrointestinal Disease, 2nd ed. Philadelphia, W.B. Saunders Company, 1983.

† Many types of local peritonitis may become generalized by rupture into the free peritoneal cavity.

No specific referral patterns

Description: Cramping, burning, and gnawing

Intensity: Dull

Duration: Constant

Associated Signs and Symptoms: Sweating
Pallor
Restlessness
Nausea
Emesis (vomiting)

Parietal

Parietal (somatic) relates to the wall of any cavity, such as the chest or pelvic cavities. Whereas the visceral peritoneum is insensitive to pain, the parietal peritoneum is well supplied with pain nerve endings. Parietal pain may be unilateral (rather than midline only), because at any given point the parietal peritoneum obtains innervation from only one side of the nervous system.

Location: Midline or unilateral pelvic region

Localized more precisely to the site of the lesion than visceral pain

Referral: Pelvic cavity: Wide variety of pain patterns depending on the organs involved—referred to abdomen, lower back, or legs

Description: Knifelike, cutting, stabbing

Intensity: More intense than visceral pain

Duration: Constant

Associated Signs and Symptoms: Aggravated by coughing or by respiratory movement

Referred

Location: Pain occurs in *remote areas* supplied by the same neurosegment as the diseased organ by way of shared central pathways for afferent neurons.

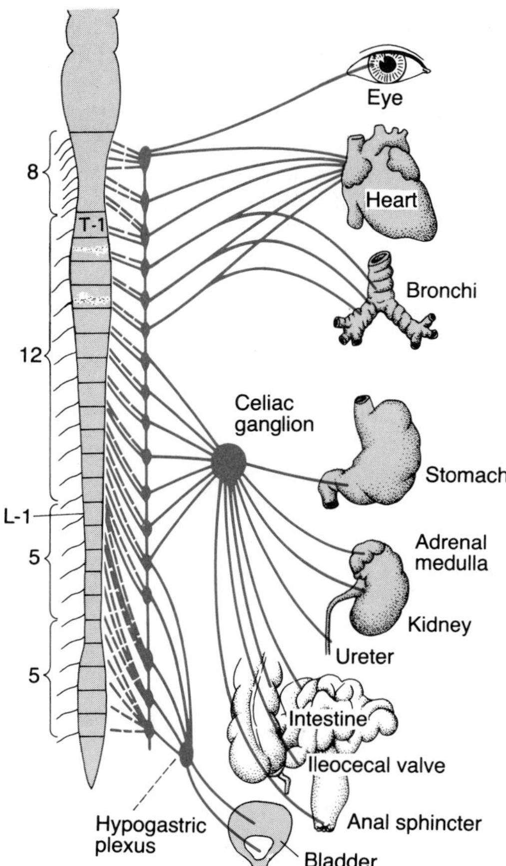

Figure 6–3. Diagram of the autonomic nervous system. The visceral afferent fibers mediating pain travel with the sympathetic nerves, except for those from the pelvic organs that follow the parasympathetics of the pelvic nerve. Sympathetics are represented here by ***solid lines;*** parasympathetics are represented by ***dashed lines.*** (From Guyton, A.C.: Textbook of Medical Physiology, 7th ed. Philadelphia, W.B. Saunders Company, 1989.)

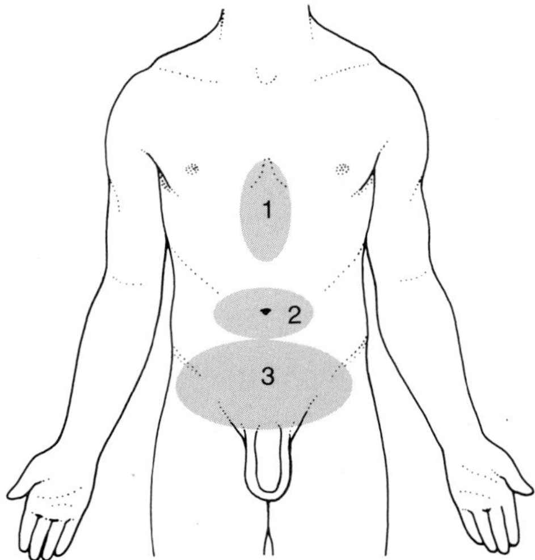

Figure 6–4. Visceral pain: (1) epigastric region; (2) the periumbilical region; and (3) the lower midabdominal region.

	Pain may be felt in skin or deeper tissues.
	Patient can point precisely to the area that hurts (well-localized).
Referral:	Referred pain occurs *when noxious visceral stimulus becomes more intense.*
	Referred pain *can occur alone* (without accompanying visceral pain), but usually visceral pain precedes the development of referred pain.
	Hyperesthesia (excessive sensibility to sensory stimuli) of skin and *hyperalgesia* (excessive sensibility to painful stimuli) of muscle may develop in the referred pain distribution
Description:	Tenderness, burning, aching
Intensity:	Dull to exquisite
Duration:	Constant
Associated Signs and Symptoms:	Muscle spasm
	Vasoconstriction
	Radial pulse difficult to palpate
	Increased pulse rate
	Increased blood pressure (systolic and diastolic)
	Pallor
	Vasodilation
	Profuse sweating
	Subjective report of feeling excessively warm
	Flushed appearance of skin

GASTROINTESTINAL PATHOPHYSIOLOGY

Gastrointestinal Organ Symptoms (Alphin-Tollison, 1981; Cain, 1987; Given and Simmons, 1979; Way, 1983)

It is very important for the physical therapist to carefully assess the patient's complaints because GI tract symptoms can sometimes imitate musculoskeletal dysfunction. Symptoms, including pain, can be related to various GI organ disturbances and differ in character depending on the affected organ. The most clinically meaningful GI symptoms reported in a physical therapy practice include:

- Dysphagia
- Odynophagia
- Melena
- Epigastric pain with radiation to the back
- Symptoms associated with meals
- Early satiety with weight loss
- Bloody diarrhea
- Fecal incontinence
- Referred shoulder pain
- Tenderness over McBurney's point

Dysphagia

Dysphagia is the sensation of food catching or sticking in the esophagus. Initially, this sensation may just occur with coarse, dry foods and may eventually progress to include anything swallowed, even thin liquids and saliva. Achalasia is a process by which the circular and longitudinal muscular fibers of the lower esophageal sphincter do not relax. This disorder contributes to esophageal stricture. Closure *(achalasia)* of the esophageal sphincter may also create an obstruction of the esophagus. Other possible causes of dysphagia include peptic esophagitis (inflammation of the esophagus) with stricture (narrowing) and neoplasm. The presence of dysphagia requires prompt attention by a physician. Treatment is based on a subsequent endoscopic examination.

Odynophagia

Odynophagia or pain during swallowing can be caused by esophagitis or esophageal spasm. Esophagitis may occur secondary to the herpes simplex virus or fungus caused by the prolonged use of strong antibiotics. Pain after eating may occur with esophagitis or may be associated with coronary ischemia. To differentiate esophagitis from coronary ischemia: *esophageal pain* is relieved by upright positioning and is intensified by supine positioning, whereas *cardiac pain* is relieved by nitroglycerin or by supine positioning. Both conditions require medical attention.

Melena

Melena or black, tarry stool occurs as a result of large quantities of blood in the stool. When asked about changes in bowel function, patients may describe black, tarry stools that have an unusual odor. The odor is caused by the presence of blood, and the black color arises as the digestive acids in the bowel oxidize red blood cells. Melena is very sticky and does not clean well. Patients may describe bowel smears on their undergarments.

Upper GI tract (e.g., esophageal, stomach, or duodenal) lesions produce melena. The lesion may be caused by a bleeding ulcer, esophageal varices, or vascular abnormalities of the stomach that break open and bleed easily. *Esophageal varices* are dilated blood vessels usually secondary to cirrhosis of the liver. Blood that would normally be pumped back to the heart must bypass the damaged liver. The blood then "backs up" through the esophagus. Vascular abnormalities of the stomach causing bleeding may include ulcers.

The patient should be asked about the presence of any blood in the stool to determine whether it is melenotic (from the upper GI tract) or bright red (from the distal colon or rectum). Bleeding from internal or external *hemorrhoids* (enlarged veins inside or outside the rectum) is a common cause of bright red blood in the stools.

Epigastric Pain with Radiation

Epigastric pain with radiation posteriorly to the back may occur secondary to long-standing ulcers. For example, the patient may be aware of an ulcer, but does not relate the back pain to the ulcer. Close questioning related to GI symptomatology can provide the physical therapist with knowledge of underlying systemic disease processes. Diagnostic interviewing is especially helpful when patients have neglected medical treatment for so long that back pain caused by an ulcer may in turn create biomechanical changes in muscular contractions and spinal movement. These changes eventually create pain of a biomechanical nature (Rose and Rothstein, 1982). The patient then presents with enough true musculoskeletal findings that a diagnosis of back dysfunction can be supported. However, the symptoms may be associated with a systemic problem. A good medical history can be a very valuable tool in revealing the actual cause of the back pain.

Symptoms Associated with Meals

Patients may or may not be able to relate pain to meals. Pain associated with gastric ulcers (located more proximally in the GI tract) may begin within 30 to 90 minutes after eating, whereas pain associated with duodenal or pyloric ulcers (located distally beyond the stomach) may occur 2 to 4 hours after meals (i.e., between meals). Alternately stated, food is less likely to relieve the pain of a gastric ulcer, but may relieve the symptoms of a duodenal ulcer. The patient with a duodenal ulcer may report pain during the night between 12:00 P.M. and 3:00 A.M. This pain should be differentiated from the nocturnal pain associated with cancer by its intensity and duration. More specifically, the *gnawing pain* of an *ulcer* may be relieved by eating, but the *intense, boring pain* associated with *cancer* is not relieved by any measures.

Early Satiety

Early satiety occurs when the patient feels hungry, takes one or two bites of food, and feels full. The sensation of being full is out of proportion with the time of the previous meal and the initial degree of hunger experienced.

Bloody Diarrhea

Bloody diarrhea is usually associated with a sense of urgency (the patient senses that he or she must find a bathroom immediately and cannot wait), frequency, and cramping pain. There are many potential causes of bloody diarrhea including ulcerative colitis, Crohn's disease, colitis (secondary to overgrowth of bacteria after a long course of antibiotics), benign or malignant colonic obstruction (stools must be liquid to pass by the obstruction), amoebic colitis (patient has a recent history of travel outside of the United States), and angiodysplasia, a vascular lesion in which clusters of vessels (capillaries) break open and bleed. Medical diagnosis is made by fiberoptic endoscopy (visual examination of the interior structures of the intestines with an instrument) and by barium enema.

Fecal Incontinence

Fecal incontinence may be described as an inability to control evacuation of stool and is associated with a sense of urgency, diarrhea, and abdominal cramping. Causes include partial obstruction of the rectum (cancer), colitis, and radiation therapy, especially in the case of women treated for cervical or uterine cancer. The radiation may cause trauma to the rectum resulting in incontinence and diarrhea. Anal distortion secondary to traumatic childbirth, hemorrhoids, and hemorrhoidal surgery may also cause fecal incontinence.

Pain in the Left Shoulder

Pain in the left shoulder (Kehr's sign) can occur as a result of free air or blood in the abdominal cavity, such as ruptured spleen causing distention. The core interview may help the patient to recall any precipitating trauma or injury such as a sharp blow during an athletic event, a fall, or perhaps an automobile accident. The patient may not connect these seemingly unrelated events with the present shoulder pain.

McBurney's Point

Parietal pain caused by inflammation of the peritoneum in acute appendicitis or peritonitis is localized at McBurney's point (see Fig. 6–10). McBurney's point is located by palpation with the patient in a supine position. Isolate the anterior superior iliac spine (ASIS) and the umbilicus: palpate for tenderness halfway between these two surface landmarks. This method differs from palpation of the iliopsoas muscle because the position used to locate the iliopsoas muscle is with the patient in a supine position, with hips and knees flexed and fully supported in a 90-degree position. Palpate one third of the distance between the ASIS and the umbilicus. You may ask the patient to gently flex the hip to assist you in isolating the iliopsoas muscle. Palpate both McBurney's point and the iliopsoas muscle for reproduction of symptoms to rule out iliopsoas abscess associated with appendicitis or peritonitis.

INFLAMMATORY/IRRITABLE BOWEL CONDITIONS

Any disruption of the digestive system can create symptoms, such as pain, diarrhea, and constipation. The bowel is susceptible to altered patterns of normal motility caused by food, alcohol, tobacco, caffeine, drugs, physical and emotional stress, and life style (e.g., lack of regular exercise). During the course of evaluation and treatment with physical therapy, the conversation with the patient may be directed toward the patient's daily life. Physical therapists are often aware of daily stresses affecting a patient—stresses that may aggravate the patient's emotional perception of pain.

Use of the *McGill Pain Questionnaire* provided in Chapter 2, along with a knowledge of underlying types and causes of abdominal pain, can be very helpful in understanding the basis for a patient's subjective report of pain. This knowledge can help the physical therapist to recognize musculoskeletal complaints of a systemic origin that require referral to a physician.

Inflammatory Bowel Disease

(Banks et al, 1983; Cain, 1987; Donaldson, 1983; Kodner and Fry, 1982)

Inflammatory bowel disease (IBD) refers to two inflammatory conditions:

- Ulcerative colitis
- Crohn's disease (also referred to as regional enteritis or ileitus)

By definition, ulcerative colitis is an inflammation and ulceration of the inner lining of the large intestine (colon) and rectum. When inflammation is confined to the rectum only, the condition is known as ulcerative proctitis. Ulcerative colitis is not the same as irritable bowel syndrome (IBS) or spastic colitis (another term for IBS).

Crohn's disease is an inflammatory disease that attacks the terminal end (or distal portion) of the small intestine (ileum), the colon, or both small intestine and colon. This inflammation is patchy and skips over areas of healthy bowel (Banks et al, 1983).

Ulcerative Colitis and Crohn's Disease (Regional Enteritis) (Banks et al, 1983)

Stress-related bowel conditions are considered to be autoimmune diseases in which either the antibodies or other defense mechanisms are directed against the body. These chronic bowel conditions may occur suddenly or gradually and have no known etiology. A possible correlation of the onset of disease with life stresses and poor adaptation to those stresses is cited in the majority of the literature referenced in this section, but this has not been proved conclusively.

Twenty-five per cent of patients with ulcerative colitis and Crohn's disease may present with arthritis or migratory arthralgias (joint pain). The patient may present with monoarthritis (i.e., asymmetric pattern affecting one joint at a time), usually involving an ankle or knee although elbows and wrists can be included. Polyarthritis (involving more than one joint) or sacroiliitis (arthritis of the lower spine and pelvis) is common and may lead to ankylosing spondylitis in rare cases. Whether monoarthritic or polyarthritic, this condition comes and goes with the disease process and may precede repeat episodes of bowel symptoms by 1 to 2 weeks. With proper medical treatment, there is no permanent joint deformity.

Medical testing and diagnosis are required to differentiate between these inflammatory conditions. Most often, the physical therapist is faced with patients presenting complaints of pain located in the shoulder, back, or groin that may have a GI origin and not true musculoskeletal dysfunction at all.

CLINICAL SIGNS AND SYMPTOMS OF ULCERATIVE COLITIS AND REGIONAL ENTERITIS

- Diarrhea
- Constipation
- Fever
- Abdominal pain
- Rectal bleeding
- Night sweats
- Decreased appetite, nausea, weight loss
- Skin lesions
- Uveitis (inflammation of the eye)

The patient may have nonspecific symptoms common to chronic systemic disease

- Depression
- Decreased appetite and resultant fatigue
- Overall muscular weakness from inactivity
- Irritability

Skin lesions may occur as either erythema nodosum (red bumps/purple knots over the ankles and shins) or pyoderma (deep ulcers or canker sores) of the shins, ankles, and calves. Uveitis may cause red and painful eyes, which are sensitive to light but without affecting the patient's vision.

Nutritional Aspects of Inflammatory Bowel Disease

(Banks et al, 1983)

Inflammation alone along with the decrease in functioning surface area of the small intestine increases food requirements causing poor absorption. The disease may progress to the point that the GI tract is no longer able to absorb enough nutrients to sustain life (Table 6–2). Intravenous nutritional support is then required by the patient. This method of intravenous feeding is known as hyperalimentation or total parenteral nutrition (TPN). Nutritional problems may occur associated with the medical treatment of IBD. The use of prednisone decreases vitamin D metabolism, impairs calcium absorption, decreases potassium supplies, and increases the nutritional requirement for protein and calories. Decreased vitamin D metabolism and impaired calcium absorption subsequently result in bone demineralization and osteoporosis.

Irritable Bowel Syndrome

(Donaldson, 1983)

IBS has been called the "common cold" of the stomach and occurs as a result of the digestive tract's reaction to the stresses of daily life as well as to dietary patterns. There are no structural lesions and no progressive organic diseases in process.

CLINICAL SYMPTOMS OF IRRITABLE BOWEL SYNDROME

- Painful abdominal cramps
- Constipation
- Diarrhea

These primary symptoms occur when the natural motility of the bowel (rhythmic peristalsis) is disrupted by tension, smoking, eating, and alcohol consumption. Rapid alterations in the speed of bowel movement create an obstruction to the natural flow of stool and gas. The resultant pressure build-up in the bowel produces pain and spasm.

Medical follow-up is essential and should be augmented by a regular program of exer-

Table 6–2. SYMPTOMS ASSOCIATED WITH NUTRITIONAL DEFICIENCIES*

Symptoms	Nutritional Deficit
Generalized malnutrition, as shown by muscle wasting and growth retardation	Malabsorption of proteins, fats, carbohydrates; insufficient calories
Diarrhea, bloating, gas	Impaired absorption of salt and water caused by carbohydrate and fat malabsorption
Weakness	Anemia; electrolyte (sodium, potassium, bicarbonate, chloride, calcium, magnesium) imbalance
Anemia	Impaired absorption of iron, vitamin B_{12}, folic acid
Sore mouth and lips	Deficiency of iron and B vitamins
Numbness and tingling	Deficiency of vitamin B_{12} or other B vitamins; electrolyte imbalance
Swelling	Protein depletion
Absent menstrual periods	Protein and calorie depletion; rapid loss of weight
Bone pain	Protein depletion; vitamin D and calcium deficiency
Muscle spasms	Electrolyte imbalance (especially low calcium); pregnancy
Easy bleeding or bruising	Vitamin K deficiency

* Adapted from Banks, P.A., Present, D.H., and Steiner, P.: The Crohn's Disease and Ulcerative Colitis Fact Book. National Foundation for Ileitis and Colitis. New York, Scribner & Sons, 1983.

cise and stress management. Physical therapists must be alert to patients with IBS who have developed breath-holding patterns or hyperventilation in response to stress. Teaching proper breathing techniques during exercise and daily relaxation techniques is important.

Constipation (DeVroede, 1983; Peterson, 1983)

Constipation is defined clinically as being a condition of prolonged retention of fecal content in the GI tract resulting from decreased motility of the colon or difficulty in expelling stool. It is a secondary response to many other factors, such as diet, drugs, disease, personality, or lack of exercise (Table 6–3).

The group of associated problems that comprise constipation may be interpreted in a different manner by each individual. Common manifestations of this problem are hard stools, stools that are difficult to expel, infrequent stools, or a feeling of incomplete evacuation after defecation and general discomfort. Intractable constipation is called *obstipation* and can result in a fecal impaction that must be removed.

Diets that are high in refined sugars and low in fiber discourage bowel activity. Transit time of the alimentary bolus from the mouth to the anus is influenced mainly by dietary fiber and is decreased with increased fiber intake. Additionally, motility can be decreased by emotional stress that has been correlated with personality. Constipation associated with severe depression can be improved by exercise (Tucker et al, 1981).

Pressure from stored fecal content on sacral nerves may cause an *aching discomfort in the sacrum, buttocks, or thighs.* Some risks are associated with prolonged constipation including increased urinary tract infections, perforation of the bowel with prolonged storage of feces in one bowel segment, and a possible link between cancer of the colon in women and constipation (Bjelke, 1974; Wynder and Shigematsu, 1967).

Diarrhea (Krejs and Fortran, 1983; Peterson, 1983)

Diarrhea, by definition, is an abnormal increase in stool liquidity and daily stool weight associated with increased stool frequency (i.e., more than three times per day). This may be accompanied by urgency, perianal discomfort, and fecal incontinence. The causes of diarrhea vary widely from one patient to another, but food, alcohol, use of laxatives and other

Table 6–3. CAUSES OF CONSTIPATION*

Neurogenic Causes	Muscular Causes	Mechanical Causes	Rectal Lesions	Drugs
Cortical, voluntary, or involuntary of evacuation	Atony	Bowel obstruction	Thrombosed hemorrhoids	Anesthetic agents (recent general surgery)
Central nervous system lesions	Severe malnutrition	Neoplasm	Perirectal abscess	Antacids (containing aluminum or calcium)
Multiple sclerosis	Metabolic defects	Volvulus (intestinal twisting)		Anticholinergics
Cord tumors	Hypothyroidism	Diverticulitis		Anticonvulsants
Tabes dorsalis	Hypercalcemia	Extra-alimentary tumors (including pregnancy)		Antidepressants
Traumatic spinal cord lesions	Potassium depletion			Antihistamines
	Hyperparathyroidism			Antipsychotics
				Barium sulfate
				Diuretics
				Iron compounds
				Narcotics

* Adapted from Blackow, R.S. (ed): MacBryde's Signs and Symptoms, 6th ed. Philadelphia, J.B. Lippincott, 1983.

Table 6–4. CAUSES OF DIARRHEA*

Malabsorption	Neuromuscular Causes	Mechanical Causes	Nonspecific Causes
Pancreatitis	Irritable bowel syndrome	Incomplete obstruction	Crohn's disease
Carcinoma of the pancreas	Diabetic enteropathy	Neoplasm	Ulcerative colitis
Crohn's disease (regional enteritis)		Adhesions	Diverticulitis
		Stenosis	
		Fecal impaction	
		Muscular incompetency	
		Scleroderma	
		Postsurgical effect	
		Ileal bypass	

* Adapted from Blackow, R.S. (ed): MacBryde's Signs and Symptoms, 6th ed. Philadelphia, J.B. Lippincott, 1983.

drugs, and travel may contribute to the development of diarrhea (Table 6–4).

In normal bowel physiology, there are 9 liters of fluid present in the intestine: 2 liters are from ingested foods and liquids, and the rest are from digestive secretions. It is well known that the first 3 to 5 lb of weight loss for most people starting a diet occurs as a result of water loss from the intestines. The volume of chyme in the small bowel depends on the type of food eaten. Chyme increases with sugar intake and decreases with protein ingestion. Ingestion of alcohol (sugar) can produce diarrhea secondary to a decrease in enzymes and vitamins and hypermobility of the intestines.

Laxative abuse contributes to the production of diarrhea and begins a vicious cycle as chronic laxative users experience excessive secretion of aldosterone and resultant edema when they attempt to stop using laxatives. This edema and increased weight forces the person to continue to rely on laxatives. The use of laxatives in the American population is substantiated by more than 225 million dollars spent on laxatives annually (Darlington, 1966; Product Management, 1975). The abuse of laxatives is common in the anorexic (loss of appetite due to emotional state) and bulemic (eating disorder) population who may ingest up to 100 laxatives at a time.

For the patient describing chronic diarrhea, it may be necessary to probe further about the use of laxatives as a possible contributor to this condition. These questions can be asked tactfully during the core interview when asking about medications, including over-the-counter drugs such as laxatives. Encourage the patient to discuss bowel management without drugs at the next appointment with the physician. A referral to a nutritionist may be appropriate when the physician determines that the patient's diet is contributing to symptoms of diarrhea or constipation. The physical therapist may make the suggestion for patient referral to a nutritionist directly to the patient, by report to the physician, or both.

OVERVIEW OF GASTROINTESTINAL PAIN PATTERNS

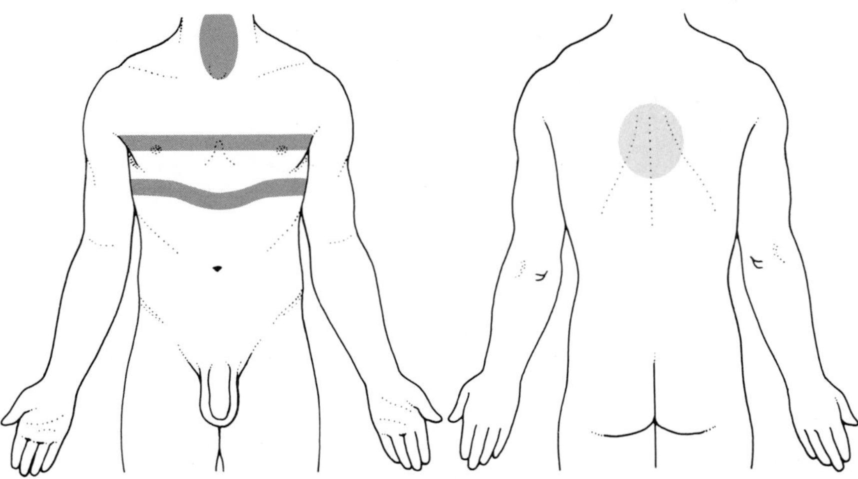

Figure 6–5. Esophagus: Esophageal pain may be projected around the chest at any level corresponding with the esophageal lesion. Only two of the possible bands of pain around the chest are shown here.

Esophagus

Pain

Location (Fig. 6–5):	Substernal discomfort at the level of the lesion Lesion of upper esophagus: pain in the (anterior) neck Lesion of lower esophagus: pain originating from the xyphoid process, radiating around the thorax
Referral:	Severe esophageal pain: pain referred to the middle of the back Back pain may be the only symptom or may be the earliest symptom of esophageal cancer
Description:	Sharp, sticking, knifelike, stabbing Strong burning pain (esophagitis)
Intensity:	Varies from mild discomfort to severe pain
Duration:	May be constant; associated with meals
Associated Signs and Symptoms:	Dysphagia, odynophagia, melena
Possible Etiology:	Obstruction of the esophagus (neoplasm)

Esophageal stricture secondary to acid reflux (peptic esophagitis)
Esophageal stricture of unknown cause
Achalasia
Esophagitis or esophageal spasm
Esophageal varices (usually asymptomatic except bleeding)

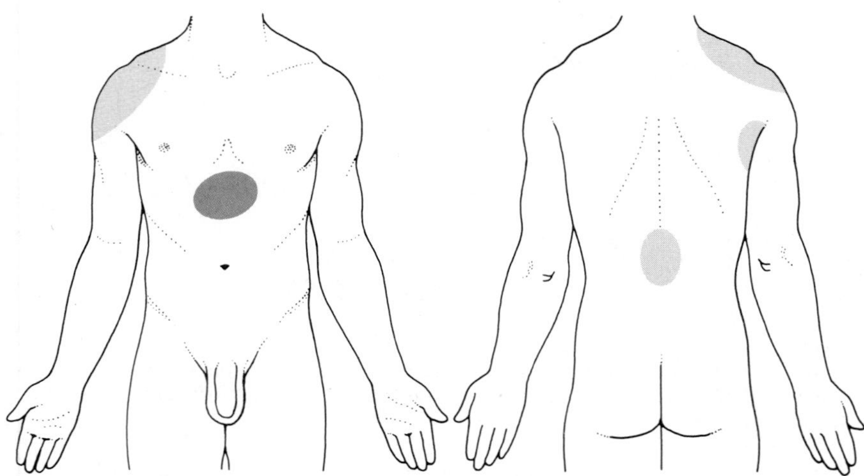

Figure 6–6. Stomach or duodenal pain *(dark red)* may occur anteriorly in the midline of the epigastrium or upper abdomen just below the xyphoid process. Referred pain *(light red)* to the back may occur at the level of the abdominal lesion (T6–T10). Other patterns of referred pain *(light red)* may include the right shoulder and upper trapezius or the lateral border of the right scapula.

Stomach and Duodenum

Pain

Location (Fig. 6–6):	Pain in the midline of epigastrium Upper abdomen just below the xyphoid process
Referral:	Common referral pattern to the back at the level of the lesion (T_6–T_{10}) Right shoulder/upper trapezius Lateral border of the right scapula
Description:	Aching, burning, gnawing, cramplike pain (true visceral pain)
Intensity:	Can be mild or severe
Duration:	Comes in waves

Associated Signs and Symptoms:	Early satiety
	Melena
	Symptoms may be associated with meals
Possible Etiology:	Peptic ulcers: gastric, pyloric, duodenal
	Stomach carcinoma
	Kaposi's sarcoma (most common malignancy associated with acquired immunodeficiency syndrome [AIDS])

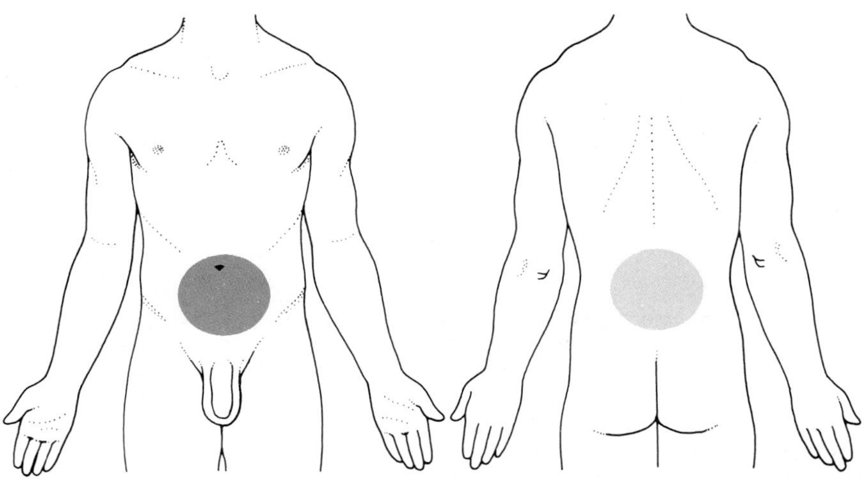

Figure 6–7. Midabdominal pain *(dark red)* caused by disturbances of the small intestine is centered around the umbilicus and may be referred *(light red)* to the low back area.

Small Intestine

Pain

Location (Fig. 6–7):	Midabdominal pain (about the umbilicus)
Referral:	Pain referred to the back if the stimulus is sufficiently intense or if the individual's pain threshold is low
Description:	Cramping pain
Intensity:	Moderate to severe
Duration:	Intermittent (pain comes and goes)
Associated Signs and Symptoms:	Nausea, fever, diarrhea
	Pain relief may not occur after passing stool or gas

Possible Etiology:	Obstruction (neoplasm) Increased bowel motility Crohn's disease (regional enteritis)

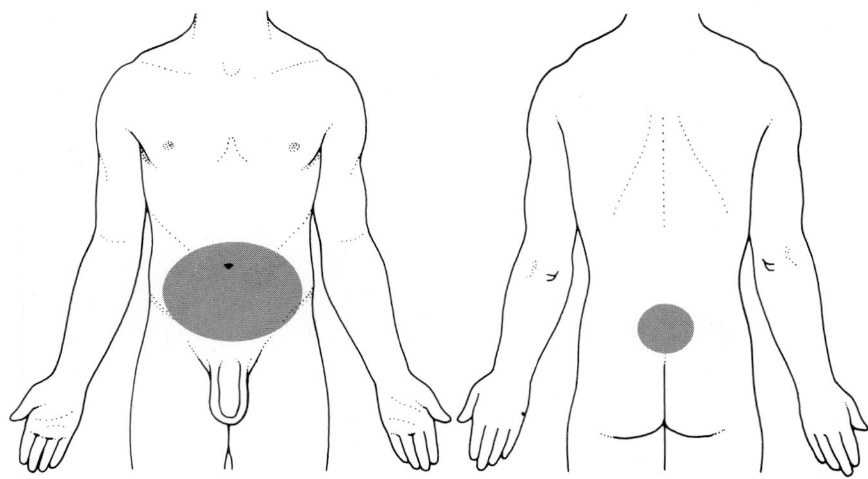

Figure 6–8. Pain associated with the large intestine and colon *(dark red)* may occur in the lower midabdomen across either or both abdominal quadrants. Pain may be referred to the sacrum *(light red)* when the rectum is stimulated.

Large Intestine and Colon

Pain

Location (Fig. 6–8):	Lower midabdomen (across either or both quadrants) Poorly localized
Referral:	Pain may be referred to the sacrum when the rectum is stimulated
Description:	Cramping
Intensity:	Dull
Duration:	Steady
Associated Signs and Symptoms:	Bloody diarrhea, urgency Constipation Pain relief may occur after defecation or passing gas
Possible Etiology:	Ulcerative colitis Crohn's disease (regional enteritis) Carcinoma of the colon Long-term use of antibiotics IBS

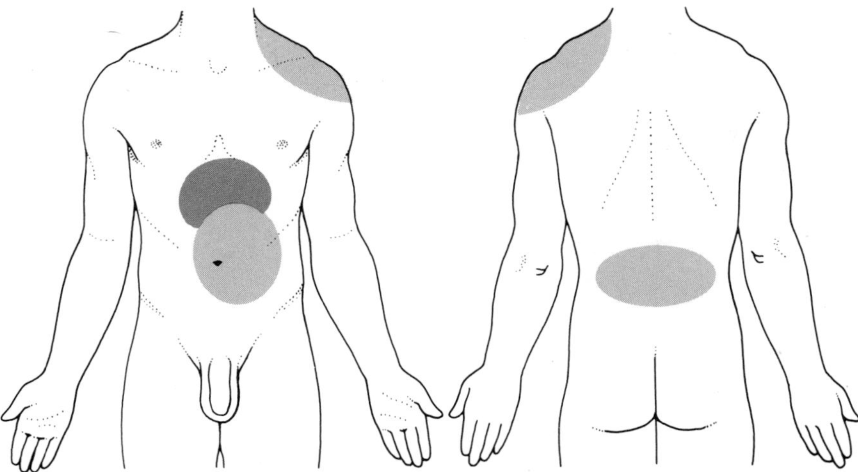

Figure 6–9. Pancreatic pain *(dark red)* occurs in the midline or left of the epigastrium, just below the xiphoid process, but may be referred *(light red)* to the left shoulder or to the middle or low back.

Pancreas

Pain

Location (Fig. 6–9):	Midline or to the left of the epigastrium, just below the xyphoid process
Referral:	Referred pain in the middle or lower back is typical with pancreatic disease
	Somatic pain felt in the left shoulder may result from activation of pain fibers in the left diaphragm by an adjacent inflammatory process in the tail of the pancreas (Way, 1983)
Description:	Terrifying, burning, or gnawing abdominal pain
Intensity:	Severe
Duration:	Constant pain, sudden onset
Associated Signs and Symptoms:	Sudden weight loss
	Jaundice
	Vomiting
	Symptoms may be unrelated to digestive activities (carcinoma)
	Symptoms may be related to digestive activities (pancreatitis)
Possible Etiology:	Pancreatitis
	Pancreatic carcinoma (primarily disease of men, occurs during the 6th to 7th decade)

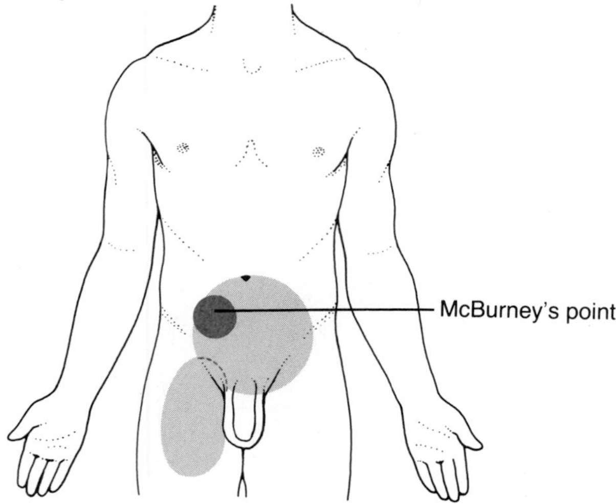

Figure 6–10. Appendix.

Appendix

Pain

Location (Fig. 6–10):	Right lower quardrant pain
	Well localized
Referral:	First referred to epigastric or periumbilical areas
	Referred pain pattern to the right hip
Description:	Aching
Intensity:	Moderate to severe
Duration:	Steadily progresses over time (usually 12 hours with acute appendicitis)
Associated Signs and Symptoms:	Positive McBurney's point for tenderness
	Anorexia, nausea, vomiting, low-grade fever
	Iliopsoas abscess may occur; pain on movement and palpation of muscle

SUMMARY

In this chapter on GI disorders that can refer pain to the musculoskeletal system, we have attempted to discuss the most common GI organ symptoms encountered by the physical therapist in a clinical practice. In the course of this discussion, we have attempted to provide an overview of:

- GI physiology
- Abdominal pain
- GI pathophysiology
    - GI organ symptoms

- Inflammatory/irritable bowel conditions
- GI pain patterns

Systemic Signs and Symptoms Requiring Physician Referral

Bloody diarrhea
Boring, stabbing pain
Chills
Constant pain
Cutting, knifelike pain
Dark urine
Dysphagia
Early satiety
Fecal incontinence
Fever
Gnawing, burning pain
Jaundice
Kehr's sign (positive)
Light stools
McBurney's point
Melena
Migratory arthralgias
Night pain
Night sweats
Odynophagia
Skin lesions
Sudden weight loss
Uveitis
Vomiting

The patient may not associate gastrointestinal symptoms or already diagnosed GI disease with his or her musculoskeletal pain, which makes it necessary for the physical therapist to initiate questions to determine the presence of such GI involvement.

Taking the patient's temperature and vital signs during the initial evaluation is recommended for any patient who has musculoskeletal pain of unknown origin. Fever, low-grade fever over a long period (even if cyclic), or night sweats is indicative of systemic disease.

SUBJECTIVE EXAMINATION

Special Questions to Ask

After completing the initial intake interview, if there is cause to suspect GI involvement, include the following additional questions:

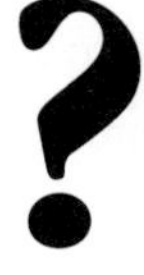

□ Do you have any problems chewing or swallowing food? Do you have any pain when swallowing food or liquids? **(Dysphagia, odynophagia)**

□ Do you vomit frequently? **(Esophageal varices, ulcers)**

If so, how often?

Describe the vomitus.

Have you ever vomited blood?

Is your vomitus ever dark brown or black?

Do you ever take any medication for vomiting? If so, what?

Do you ever spit up blood?

Subjective Exam

Special Questions to Ask

□ Have you ever been x-rayed for an ulcer?

If so, when?

Have you ever been treated for an ulcer? If so, when?

Do you still have any pain from your ulcer?

□ Does eating relieve your pain? **(Duodenal or pyloric ulcer)**

How soon after eating?

Does eating aggravate your pain? **(Gastric ulcer, gallbladder inflammation)**

□ Does your pain occur 1 to 3 hours after eating or between meals? **(Duodenal or pyloric ulcers, gallstones)**

Have you ever had gallstones?

□ Are you ever awakened at night with pain? **(Duodenal ulcer, cancer)**

Approximately what time does this occur? **(12:00 A.M. to 3:00 A.M.: ulcer)**

Can you relieve the pain in any way and get back to sleep? If yes, how? **(Ulcer: eating relieves/Cancer: nothing relieves)**

□ Do you have a feeling of fullness after only one or two bites of food? **(Early satiety: stomach and duodenum or gallbladder)**

□ Have you had a sudden weight loss in the last month (i.e., 10 to 15 lb in 2 weeks without trying)? **(Cancer)**

□ How often do you have a bowel movement? **(Constipation/bowel obstruction: normal frequency varies from 3 times a day to once every 3 days)**

□ Do you take laxatives?

If so, how frequently?

□ Do you have diarrhea? **(Ulcerative colitis, Crohn's disease, long-term use of antibiotics, colonic obstruction, amoebic colitis, angiodysplasia)**

Do you have more than two loose stools a day? If so, do you take medication for this problem? What kind of medication do you use?

Do you have a sense of urgency: Do you have to find a bathroom immediately without waiting?

Have you traveled outside of the United States within the last 6 months to 1 year? **(Amoebic colitis associated with bloody diarrhea)**

□ Do you ever have any blood in your stool?

If so, how often?

Is the blood mixed in with the stool or does it coat the surface? **(Distal colon or rectum versus melena)**

Subjective Exam

Special Questions to Ask

Is the blood bright red or are your stools black or tarry? **(Distal colon or rectum versus melena)**

- □ Do you have hemorrhoids?

  If yes, have you ever had surgery for your hemorrhoids? **(Most common cause of bright red blood coating stools/check for fecal incontinence)**

- □ Do you ever have bowel smears on your undergarments? **(Fecal incontinence)**
- □ Do you ever have gray (clay)-colored stools? **(Lack of bile or biliary obstruction: hepatitis, gallstones, cirrhosis, pancreatic carcinoma, hepatotoxic drugs)**
- □ Are your stools ever pencil thin? **(Indicates bowel obstruction)**
- □ Is your pain relieved after passing stool or gas? **(Yes: large intestine and colon; No: small intestine)**
- □ Have you ever had your colon x-rayed?

  If so, when?

  Have you ever undergone a colonoscopy or proctoscopy? If so, why and how long ago?

- □ Have you ever had abdominal surgery?

  If so, when? What type was it?

- □ When was the last time that you went to a doctor because you had abdominal or intestinal problems?
- □ Have you sustained any injuries in the last week during a sports activity, fall, automobile accident, etc.? **(Ruptured spleen associated with pain in the left shoulder: positive Kehr's sign)**
- □ Do you ever have episodes of fever and night sweats? **(Hallmark sign of systemic disease)**
- □ Medications: Follow the usual line of questions provided in the subjective examination: Look for long-term use of antibiotics or hepatotoxic drugs. See Table 6–3 for a list of medications that cause constipation.
- □ Do you have any other medical or health-related problems?

PHYSICIAN REFERRAL

A 67-year-old man is seeing you through home health care for a home program after discharge from the hospital 2 weeks ago for a total hip replacement. His recovery has been slowed down by chronic diarrhea. A 25-year-old woman who is diagnosed as having a sacroiliac pain and joint dysfunction asks you what exercises she can do for constipation. A 44-year-old man with biceps tendinitis reports several episodes of fever and chills, diarrhea, and abdominal pain, which he contributes to "the stress of meeting deadlines on the job."

When to Refer a Patient to a Physician

These are common examples of symptoms of a GI nature that are described by patients

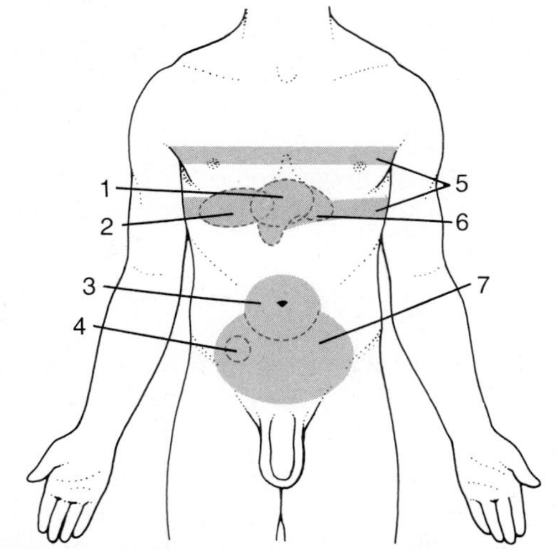

Figure 6–11. Full figure pain pattern: (1) stomach/duodenum; (2) liver/gallbladder/common bile duct; (3) small intestine; (4) appendix; (5) esophagus; (6) pancreas; and (7) large intestine/colon.

and are unrelated to current physical therapy treatment. These patients may be seeking the physical therapist's advice as being the only medical personnel with whom they have contact. Knowing the pain patterns associated with GI involvement and which follow-up questions to ask can assist the physical therapist in deciding when to suggest that the patient return to a physician for a medical examination and treatment.

On the other hand, the physical therapist may be evaluating a patient who presents with shoulder, back, or groin pain and limitations that are not true musculoskeletal lesions, but rather, the result of GI involvement. The presence of associated GI symptoms in the absence of conclusive musculoskeletal findings will alert the physical therapist to the possible need for medical referral. Correlate the *history* with *pain patterns* and any *unusual findings* that may indicate systemic disease. Figures 6–11 and 6–12 provide a summary of all the pain patterns described including the referred pain of systemic origin that can mimic pain and dysfunction associated with musculoskeletal lesions.

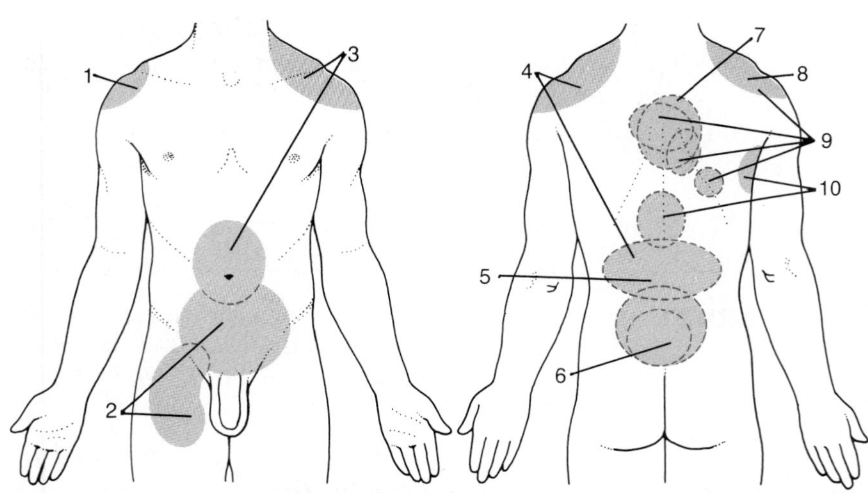

Figure 6–12. Referred pain patterns: Full figure: (1) liver/gallbladder/common bile duct; (2) appendix; (3) pancreas; (4) pancreas; (5) small intestine; (6) colon; (7) esophagus; (8) stomach/duodenum; (9) liver/gallbladder/common bile duct; and (10) stomach/duodenum.

CASE STUDY

Referral

A 21-year-old woman comes to you with complaints of pain on hip flexion when she lifts her right foot off the brake in the car. There are no other aggravating factors, and she is unaware of any way to relieve the pain when she is driving her car. Before the onset of symptoms, she jogged 5 to 6 miles/day, but could not recall any injury or trauma that might contribute to this pain. The *Family/Personal History* form has no indication of personal illness, but a complex list of positive family history for heart disease, diabetes, ulcerative colitis, stomach ulcers, stomach cancer, and alcoholism.

Additional Questions To Ask

It is suggested that the physical therapist use the physical therapy interview to assess the patient's complaints today and follow-up with appropriate additional questions, such as those noted here.

Lead-in Comments to the Patient. From your family history form, I notice that a number of your family members have reportedly been diagnosed with various diseases.

Do you have any other medical or health-related problems?

Have you sustained any injuries to the lower back, side, or abdomen in the last week, for example, during a sports activity, fall, or automobile accident?

Although the symptoms that you have described appear to be a musculoskeletal problem, I would like to investigate the possibility of a urologic, abdominal, or gynecologic source of this irritation. I will ask you some additional questions that may seem to be unrelated to the problem with your hip, but which will help me to assimilate the whole picture of the history, symptoms, and actual physical results from my examination today.

General Systemic

What other symptoms have you had with this problem if any? For example, have you had any:

- Numbness
- Fatigue
- Legs giving out from under you
- Burning, tingling
- Weakness

Gastrointestinal

Have you had any:

- Nausea
- Diarrhea
- Loss of appetite

CASE STUDY

- Feeling of fullness after only 2 to 3 bites of a meal
- Unexpected weight gain or loss (10 to 15 lb without trying)
- Vomiting
- Constipation
- Blood in your stool

If yes to any of these, follow-up with *Special Questions to Ask* from this chapter.

Have you noticed any association between when you eat and your symptoms?

After allowing the patient to respond you may want to prompt her by asking if eating relieves the pain or aggravates the pain.

Is your pain relieved or aggravated during or after you have a bowel movement?

Gynecologic

Since your hip/groin/thigh symptoms started, have you been examined by a gynecologist to rule out any gynecologic causes of this problem?

If no:

- Have you ever been told that you have ovarian cysts, uterine fibroids, retroverted uterus, endometriosis, an ectopic pregnancy, or any other gynecologic problem?
- Are you pregnant or have you recently terminated a pregnancy either by miscarriage or abortion?
- Are you using an intrauterine (IUD) device?
- Are you having any unusual vaginal discharge?

If yes to any of these questions, see the follow-up questions for women in Chapter 12.

Urologic

Have you had any problems with your kidneys or bladder?

If yes, please describe.

Have you noticed any changes in your ability to urinate since your pain or symptoms started?

If no, it may be necessary to provide examples of what changes you are referring to; for example, difficulty in starting or stopping the flow of urine, numbness, or tingling in the groin or pelvis, painful urination, urinary incontinence.

Have you had burning with urination during the last 1 to 3 weeks?

Have you noticed any blood in your urine?

Objective Examination

Your objective examination reveals tenderness on palpation over the right anterior, upper thigh muscles into the groin with reproduction of the pain on resisted trunk flexion only. This woman attends daily ballet classes, stretches daily, and seems to be very active physically. All tests for flexibility were negative

CASE STUDY

for tightness, including the Thomes test for tight hip flexors. Other special tests for hip and a neurologic screen had negative results. The patient's temperature was normal when it was taken today during the intake screen of vital signs, but during the physical therapy interview, when specifically asked about fevers and night sweats, she indicated several recurrent episodes of night sweats during the last 3 months.

Results

Although the patient's complaints are primarily musculoskeletal, the absence of trauma, positive family history for systemic disease, limited musculoskeletal findings, and the patient's remark concerning the presence of night sweats will alert the physical therapist to the need for a medical referral to rule out the systemic origin of symptoms.

The patient's condition gradually worsened during a 3-week period and a repeat blood test and re-examination by the physician led to an eventual diagnosis of Crohn's disease (regional gastroenteritis). The patient was treated with medications that reduced abdominal inflammation and eliminated subjective reports of pain on active hip flexion.

References

Alphin-Tollinson, A.: *In* Nursing 81 Books: Performing GI procedures. Horsham, PA, Intermed Communications, 1981, pp. 138–155.

Banks, P.A., Present, D.H., and Steiner, P.: National Foundation for Ileitis and Colitis. The Crohn's Disease and Ulcerative Colitis Fact Book. New York, Charles Scribner's Sons, 1983.

Bauwens, D.B., and Paine, R.: Thoracic pain. *In* Blacklow, R.S. (ed): MacBryde's Signs and Symptoms, 6th ed. New York, J.B. Lippincott, 1983, pp. 139–164.

Bjelke, E.: Epidemiologic studies of cancer of the stomach, colon and rectum. Scand. J. Gastroenterol., *9*(Suppl. 31), 1974.

Cain, J.A.: Lecture material presented to senior physical therapy students in "Clinical Medicine" course. Missoula, MT, University of Montana, 1987.

Darlington, R.C.: O.T.C. laxatives. J. Am. Pharm. Assoc. *6*:470, 1966.

DeVroede, G.: Constipation: Mechanism and management. *In* Sleisenger, M.H., and Fortran, J.S. (eds): Gastrointestinal Disease, 2nd ed. Philadelphia, W.B. Saunders Company, 1983, pp. 288–303.

Donaldson, R.M., Jr.: Crohn's disease. *In* Sleisenger, M.H., and Fortran, J.S. (eds): Gastrointestinal Disease, 2nd ed. Philadelphia, W.B. Saunders Company, 1983, pp. 1088–1118.

Given, B.A., and Simmons, S.J.: Gastroenterology in Clinical Nursing. Baltimore, C.V. Mosby, 1979.

Kodner, I.J., and Fry, R.D.: Inflammatory bowel disease. Clinical Symposia. Summit, NJ, CIBA Pharmaceutical Company, *34*:1, 1982.

Krejs, G.J., and Fortran, J.S.: Diarrhea. *In* Sleisenger, M.H., and Fortran, J.S. (eds): Gastrointestinal Disease, 2nd ed. Philadelphia, W.B. Saunders Company, 1983, pp. 257–277.

Long, B.C.: Assessment of the gastrointestinal system. *In* Phipps, W.J., Long, B.C., and Woods, N.: Medical-Surgical Nursing: Concepts and Clinical Practice. St. Louis, C.V. Mosby, 1987, pp. 1453–1470.

Peterson, M.L.: Constipation and diarrhea. *In* Blacklow, R.S. (ed): MacBryde's Signs and Symptoms, 6th ed. New York, J.B. Lippincott, 1983, pp. 375–392.

Product Management Drugs Cosmet.: What the public spent for drugs, cosmetics, toiletries in 1974. Product Management Drugs Cosmet., *4*:37, 1975.

Rose, S.J., and Rothstein, J.M.: Muscle mutability: General concepts and adaptations to altered patterns of use. Phys. Ther. *62*:1773, 1982.

Travell, J.G., and Simons, D.G.: Myofascial Pain and Dysfunction: The Trigger Point Manual. Baltimore, Williams & Wilkins, 1983.

Tucker, D.M., Sandstead, H.H., Logan, G.M., Jr., et al: Dietary fiber and personality factors ad determinants of stool output. Gastroenterology, *81*:879, 1981.

Way, L.W.: Abdominal pain. *In* Sleisenger, M.H., and Fortran, J.S. (eds): Gastrointestinal Disease, 2nd ed. Philadelphia, W.B. Saunders Company, 1983, pp. 207–221.

Wynder, E.L., and Shigematsu, T.: Environmental factors of cancer of the colon and rectum. Cancer, *20*:1520, 1967.

Bibliography

Kirsner, J.B., and Shorter, R.G., (eds): Diseases of the Colon, Rectum and Anal Canal. Baltimore, Williams & Wilkins, 1988.

Chapter 7

Overview of Renal and Urologic Signs and Symptoms

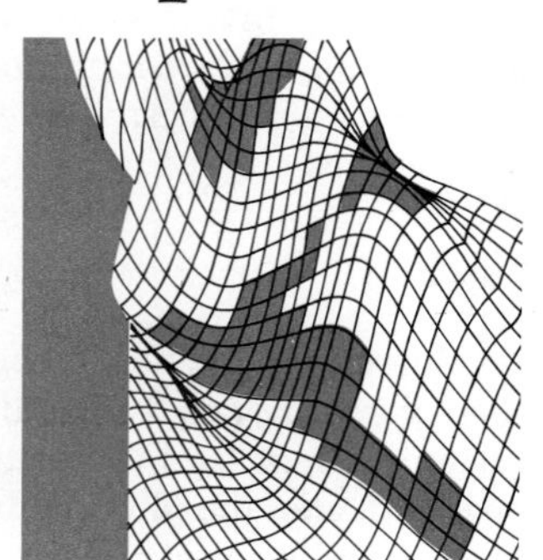

☐ ***Clinical Signs and Symptoms of:***

- Urinary Tract Problems
- Renal Impairment
- Cystitis and Urethritis
- Obstruction of the Upper Urinary Tract
- Obstruction of the Lower Urinary Tract
- Prostatitis

A 40-year-old athletic man comes to your clinic for an evaluation of back pain that he attributes to a very hard fall on his back while he was alpine skiing 3 days ago. His chief complaint is a dull, aching costovertebral pain on the left side, which is unrelieved by a change in position or by treatment with ice, heat, or aspirin. He stated that "even the skin on my back hurts." He has no previous history of any medical problems. After further questioning the patient reveals that inspiratory movements do not aggravate the pain, and he has not noticed any change in color, odor, or volume of urine output. However, percussion of the costovertebral angle results in the reproduction of the symptoms. This type of symptomatology may suggest renal involvement even without obvious changes in urine. Whether secondary to trauma or of insidious onset, a patient's complaints of flank pain, low back pain, or pelvic pain may be of renal or urologic origin and should be screened carefully through the subjective and objective examinations. Medical referral may be necessary.

The urinary tract, consisting of kidney, ureters, bladder, and urethra, is an integral component of human functioning that disposes of the body's toxic waste products and unnecessary fluid and expertly regulates extremely complicated metabolic processes. Disruption within this system can result in severe dysfunction of physiologic homeostasis. An understanding of the basic anatomy, physiology, and pathophysiology of the urinary tract will help the therapist to determine more clearly if the patient's symptoms are musculoskeletal in origin or are related to disorders of this system.

This chapter is intended to guide the physical therapist in understanding the origins and relationships of renal, ureteral, bladder, and urethral symptoms. It includes basic urinary tract anatomy and physiology and focuses on the major categories of urinary tract disease, related diagnostic procedures, and resultant clinical signs and symptoms, including pain patterns. In addition, a general discussion of renal failure and its related symptoms, medical consequences, and treatment options are presented.

UPPER URINARY TRACT

Structure

The upper urinary tract consists of the kidneys and ureters. The kidneys are located in the posterior upper abdominal cavity in a space behind the peritoneum (retroperitoneal space) (Fig. 7–1). Their position is in front of and on both sides of the vertebral column at the level of T12 to L2. The upper portion of the kidney is in contact with the diaphragm and moves with respiration. The kidneys are protected by the rib cage and abdominal organs anteriorly and by large back muscles and ribs posteriorly. The lower portions of the kidney and the ureters extend below the ribs and are separated from the abdominal cavity by the peritoneal membrane.

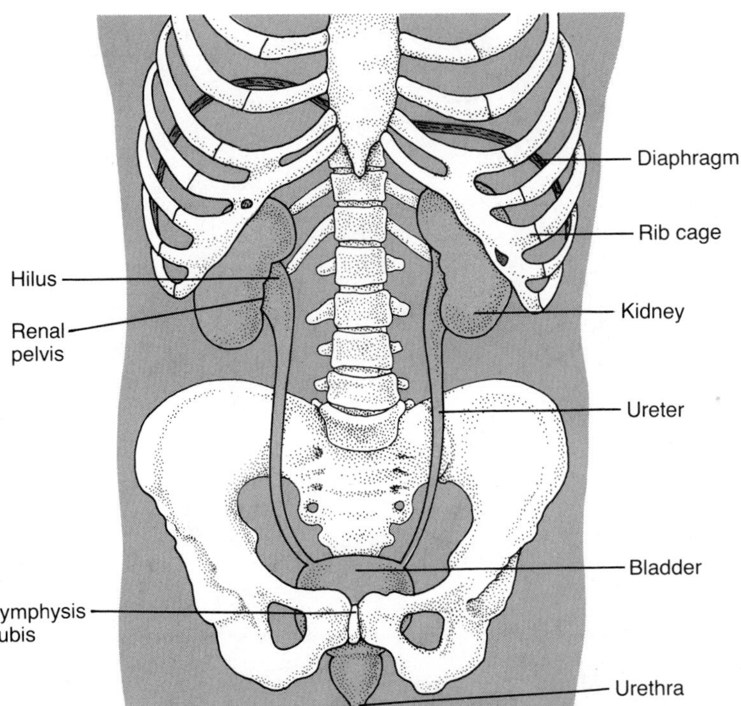

Figure 7–1. Schematic representation of urinary tract structures. The upper portion of each kidney is protected by the rib cage, and the bladder is partially protected by the symphysis pubis.

Each kidney is approximately 4 to 6 oz (180 g); approximately 5 inches in length (11.5 cm); 3 inches wide (7.5 cm); and 1 inch (2.5 cm) thick. The central notch or hilus of each kidney supplies the organ with blood and nerves and contains the renal pelvis, which is the opening into the ureter (see Fig. 7–1). From the ureter, urine flows into the bladder where it is stored until it is excreted through the urethra (i.e., a tubular structure connected to the bladder).

Function

The functional unit of the kidney is the nephron. Each kidney contains about one million nephrons. The nephron consists of several structures that form urine and maintain critical physiologic functions. The glomerulus, which is a cluster of capillaries, and Bowman's capsule, are the structures that filter blood. The proximal convoluted tubule, the loop of Henle, and the distal convoluted tubule are the urine formation structures, which reabsorb the substances that the body needs and excretes the waste materials. Urine is collected in and transported out of the body through the collecting ducts (Fig. 7–2).

Formation and excretion of urine by the nephrons is the major activity of the kidney. Through this process, the kidney is able to maintain a homeostatic environment in the body. Besides the excretory function of the kidney, which includes formation of urine and removal of wastes and excessive fluid, the kid-

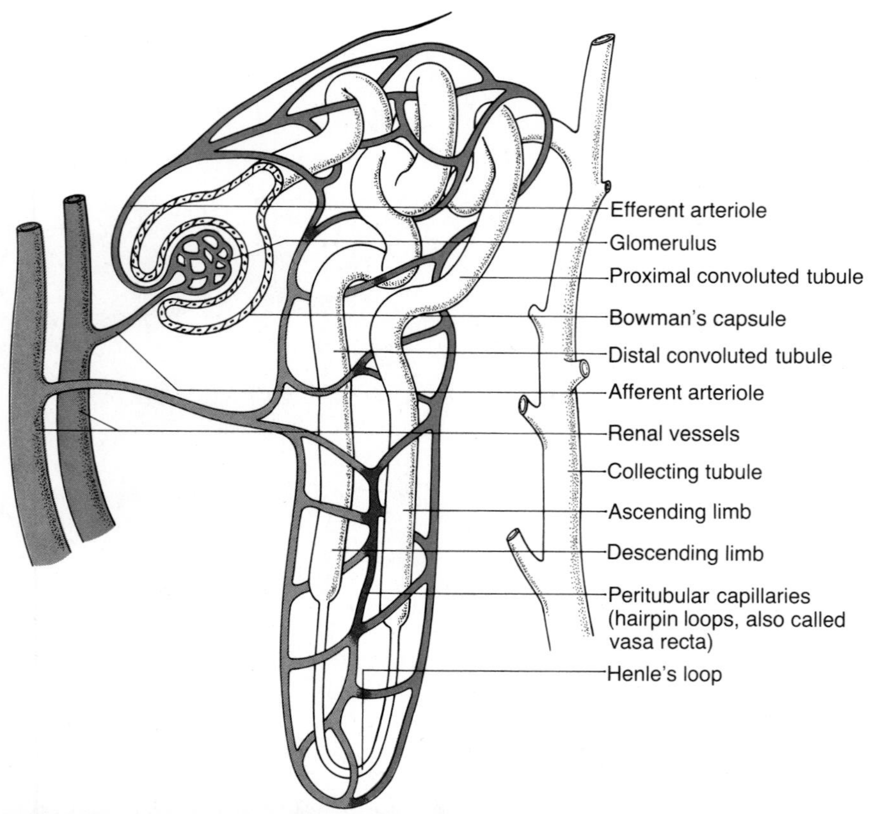

Figure 7–2. Components of the nephron. The afferent arteriole carries blood to the glomerulus for filtration through Bowman's capsule and the renal tubular system. (From Foster, R.L., Hunsberger, M.M., and Anderson, J.J.: Family-Centered Nursing Care of Children. Philadelphia, W.B. Saunders Company, 1989.)

ney also plays an integral role in the balance of various essential body functions including:

- Acid-base balance
- Electrolyte balance
- Control of blood pressure with renin
- Formation of red blood cells (RBCs)
- Activation of vitamin D and calcium balance

The failure of the kidney to perform any of these functions results in severe alteration and disruption of the body's homeostasis.

LOWER URINARY TRACT

Structure and Function

The lower urinary tract consists of the bladder and urethra. From the renal pelvis, urine is moved by peristalsis to the ureters and into the bladder. The bladder, which is a muscular, membranous sac, is located directly behind the symphysis pubis and is used for storage and excretion of urine. The urethra is connected to the bladder and serves as a channel through which urine is passed from the bladder to the outside of the body.

Voluntary control of urinary excretion is based on learned inhibition of reflex pathways from the walls of the bladder. Release of urine from the bladder occurs under voluntary control of the urethral sphincter (Farley and Miller, 1987a).

Urine Formation

Urine is a very complex body fluid that consists of 95% water and approximately 5% solids. It represents many biologic functions and is the end-product of vast numbers of metabolizing cells. There is a great quantity of blood flow through the kidneys, because about 20 to 25% of the blood from each heart beat flows through the kidney (Fischbach, 1988). Blood enters the glomerulus of each nephron through the afferent arteriole. Urine formation begins in the glomerular capillaries with dissolved substances and fluid passing into the tubular system of the nephron. As this "filtrate" (water and dissolved substances) passes along the tubular system, more solutes may be added to the filtrate from the blood of capillaries that surround the tubular system and renal tubular tissue. Some solutes that were originally filtered and some water are then reabsorbed back into the blood from the tubules. This process depends on the needs of the body and the influence of hormones, such as aldosterone and antidiuretic hormone (ADH). For example, ADH increases the permeability of water-absorbing structures, such as tubule and renal duct walls, as part of urine formation. Fluid regulation, sodium regulation, blood chemistry, blood pressure, and nutrient intake also influence the character of urine formation (Guyton, 1986).

Elements of Urine (Table 7-1)

The primary elements contained in large quantities in the urine are urea, creatinine, metabolic acids, and sodium chloride. Many other dissolved substances are also present, and the composition of urine depends mainly on the amount and type of waste material produced by the body. Certain chemical elements of the blood, such as glucose, have a threshold level—a certain level of the substance must be reached in the blood before it is excreted by the kidney into the urine. All substances excreted in the urine are also present in some amount in the blood. By monitoring both urine and blood components of these elements, a description of renal function or "clearance" can be calculated and is a very valuable indicator of normal or abnormal renal function.

Protein and cellular components of the blood, such as RBCs and white blood cells (WBCs) should not usually be present in the urine. These cells are typically too large to pass through the glomerular capillary membrane and, if present in the urine, may indicate renal damage or other problems within the urinary tract.

Normal urine does, however, contain small numbers of cells and other components from

Table 7–1. URINE ANALYSIS (URINALYSIS)*

	Test	Normal Result
General Measurements	Color	Yellow-amber
	Turbidity	Clear
	pH	4.6–8.0
	Specific gravity	1.01–1.025
Other Components	Glucose	Negative
	Ketones	Negative
	Blood	Negative
	Protein	Negative
	Bilirubin	Negative
Sediment	RBCs	Negative
	WBCs	Negative
	Casts	Occasional
	Mucous threads	Occasional
	Crystals	Occasional

* Normal values are taken from Kee, J.: Laboratory and Diagnostic Tests with Nursing Implications. Norwalk, CT, Appleton & Lange, 1987.

the entire length of the urinary tract. These elements include casts (substances formed in the renal tubules by precipitation and jelling of urinary mucoproteins), crystals (vary with the pH of urine, but usually normal even in large quantity), and mucous threads (mixture of mucus, pus, and epithelial cells). Along with bacteria, these elements are examined through the use of a microscope (Fischbach, 1988). Abnormalities exist with the presence of certain types of casts (e.g., those formed from the presence of RBCs, WBCs, or protein in the urinary tract) and specific types of crystals (those formed from abnormal body metabolism, such as gout, not just urinary pH-related). Mucous threads in large quantities can indicate urinary tract irritation.

RENAL AND URINARY TRACT PROBLEMS

Pathologies of the upper and lower urinary tract can be categorized according to primary causative factors. Three general categories—inflammatory/infectious, obstructive, and mechanical (neuromuscular)—are used for discussion and classification of clinical symptoms in this text.

Inflammatory/Infectious

Inflammatory disorders of the kidney and urinary tract can be caused by bacterial infection, by changes in immune response, and by toxic agents such as drugs and radiation. Common infections of the urinary tract develop in either the upper or lower urinary tract (Table 7–2). Lower urinary tract infections (UTIs) include cystitis (bladder infection) or urethritis (urethra). Symptoms of UTI depend on the location of the infection in either the upper or lower urinary tract (although rarely, both could occur simultaneously).

Disorders of the Upper Urinary Tract

Infections or inflammations of the upper urinary tract (kidney and ureters) are considered to be more serious because these lesions can be a direct threat to renal tissue itself.

Pyelonephritis. Pyelonephritis, or inflammation of the renal parenchyma, is a relatively common renal infection and is associated directly with bacteria that enter through the urethra and ascend through the bladder, ureter, and to the kidney. It is usually sudden in onset and is associated with chills, fever,

Table 7–2. URINARY TRACT INFECTIONS

Upper Urinary Tract Infection	Lower Urinary Tract Infection
Renal infections, such as pyelonephritis (renal parenchyma, i.e., kidney tissue)	Cystitis (bladder infection)
Acute or chronic glomerulonephritis (glomeruli)	Urethritis (urethra infection)
Renal papillary necrosis	
Renal tuberculosis	

and dull pain in the flank over one or both kidneys. Palpation of the kidney elicits pain or tenderness. In many cases, there are also signs of bladder or urethral infection, such as urgency, burning, and frequency of urination. It is most commonly associated with pregnancy, obstruction, or trauma of the urinary tract and chronic health problems (e.g., diabetes mellitus).

Glomerulonephritis. Glomerulonephritis is an inflammatory problem of the glomeruli of both kidneys. Many causative factors are related to this pathology, which include immunologic reactions, streptococcal infections, vascular injuries, and diabetes mellitus (Farley and Miller, 1987b). Glomerulonephritis can be *acute* (2 to 3 weeks after skin or strep throat infection), with school-aged children at highest risk, or *chronic* (slow, progressive destruction of glomeruli with gradual loss of renal function). There may be little or no evidence of renal infection or predisposing infection with chronic glomerulonephritis.

Renal Papillary Necrosis. This condition characterized by the destruction (necrosis) of tissue in the renal medulla (inner portion of kidney containing collecting structures). It usually affects both kidneys and is associated with various underlying problems, such as pyelonephritis, diabetes mellitus, urinary tract obstruction, sickle cell disease, and analgesic abuse. The cause of this problem is thought to involve an alteration in renal blood flow, which results in ischemia to the renal medullary tissue and subsequent necrosis.

Patients with renal papillary necrosis become ill rapidly and suddenly and are not likely to seek medical attention from a physical therapist. However, because of its association with other problems such as diabetes, the physical therapist may be treating a patient who develops papillary necrosis.

The condition is characterized by high fever, chills, kidney tenderness, severe abdominal tenderness, and rebound abdominal pain (pain felt on release of pressure). The urine contains RBCs, WBCs without bacteria, and occasional fragments of medullary tissue. This sloughing of tissue produces ureteral obstruction and destruction of nephrons, leading to renal failure (LaValle, 1986).

Renal Tuberculosis. This condition is caused by the organism responsible for pulmonary tuberculosis *(Mycobacterium tuberculosis)* and is a blood-borne infection secondary to an infection in another site (pulmonary tuberculosis). It is most common in men between 20 and 40 years of age. Signs and symptoms are usually mild and include loss of appetite, weight loss, and intermittent fever. RBCs may also be present in the urine and *M. tuberculosis* is also present in urine (Farley and Miller, 1987b).

CLINICAL SIGNS AND SYMPTOMS OF UPPER URINARY TRACT INFECTIONS (Table 7–3)

Symptoms of upper urinary tract infection, particularly renal infection, can be categorized according to urinary tract manifestations or systemic manifestations due to renal impairment. Clinical signs and symptoms of urinary tract involvement can include:

- Unilateral costovertebral tenderness
- Flank pain
- Fever and chills
- Skin hypersensitivity
- Hematuria (blood in urine)
- Pyuria (pus in urine)
- Bacteriuria (presence of bacteria in urine)

CLINICAL SIGNS AND SYMPTOMS OF RENAL IMPAIRMENT (see Table 7–3)

- Hypertension
- Decreased urinary output
- Dependent edema
- Weakness
- Anorexia (loss of appetite)
- Dyspnea
- Mild headache
- Proteinuria (protein in urine, urine may be foamy)
- Abnormal blood serum level, such as elevated blood urea nitrogen (BUN) and creatinine

Whether symptoms are systemic or involve the urinary tract, or both, renal and ureteral infections are extremely serious conditions, which, if not treated promptly and properly, can result in permanent kidney damage.

Disorders of the Lower Urinary Tract

The bladder and urine both include a number of defenses against bacterial invasion. These defenses are mechanisms such as voiding, urine acidity, and osmolality, and the bladder mucosa itself, which is thought to have antibacterial properties (LaValle, 1986). Urine in the bladder and kidney is normally sterile, but urine itself is a good medium for bacterial growth. Interferences in the defense mechanisms of the bladder, such as the presence of residual or stagnated urine, changes in urinary pH or concentration, or obstruction of urinary excretion, can promote bacterial growth.

Routes of entrance of bacteria to the urinary tract can be *ascending* (most commonly up the urethra into the bladder and then into the ureters and kidney), *blood-borne* (bacterial invasion through the bloodstream), and *lymphatic* (bacterial invasion through the lymph system, the least common route).

A lower UTI occurs most commonly in women because of the short female urethra and the proximity of the urethra to the vagina and rectum. The rate of occurrence increases with age and sexual activity. Chronic health problems, such as diabetes mellitus, gout, hypertension, and obstructive urinary tract problems, are also predisposing risk factors for the development of these infections.

Cystitis, or inflammation of the bladder, occurs usually due to ascending UTIs. This condition may be acute or chronic. Structural and functional abnormalities of the lower uri-

Table 7–3. CLINICAL SYMPTOMS OF INFECTIOUS/INFLAMMATORY URINARY TRACT PROBLEMS

Upper Urinary Tract	Lower Urinary Tract	Renal Impairment
Costovertebral tenderness	Urinary frequency	Decreased urinary output
Flank pain	Urinary urgency	Hypertension
Fever and chills	Dysuria	Dependent edema
Hyperesthesia of dermatomes	Hematuria	Weakness
Hematuria	Pyuria	Anorexia
Pyuria	Bacteriuria	Shortness of breath
Bacteriuria	Low back pain	Mild headache
		Proteinuria
		Abnormal blood serum values

nary tract, obstruction of urine flow, and impaired bladder innervation all promote this problem.

Urethritis is an inflammation of the urethra that can be due to several different organisms, including those that are sexually transmitted (gonococcus, *Chlamydia trachomatis*). Inflammation of the urethra occurs most commonly along its anterior portion, although posterior and external meatal involvement is possible.

CLINICAL SIGNS AND SYMPTOMS OF CYSTITIS AND URETHRITIS (see Table 7–3)

Lower urinary tract symptoms are directly related to irritation of the bladder and urethra. The intensity of symptoms depends on the severity of the infection. These symptoms include:

- Urinary frequency
- Urinary urgency
- Dysuria (discomfort, such as pain or burning during urination)
- Hematuria (presence of RBCs in the urine: may be gross to slight)
- Pyuria (presence of WBCs in the urine)
- Low back pain

Patients presenting with any of these symptoms should be referred promptly to a physician for further diagnostic work-up and possible treatment. Infections of the lower urinary tract are potentially very dangerous due to the capability of upward spread and resultant damage to renal tissue. Some patients, however, are asymptomatic and routine urine culture and microscopic examination are the most reliable methods of detection and diagnosis.

Obstructive

Urinary tract obstruction can occur at any point in the urinary tract and can be the result of *primary* urinary tract obstructions (obstructions occurring within the urinary tract) or *secondary* urinary tract obstructions (obstructions resulting from disease processes outside of the urinary tract). A primary obstruction might include problems such as acquired or congenital malformations, strictures, renal or ureteral calculi (stones), polycystic kidney disease, or neoplasms of the urinary tract (e.g., bladder, kidney).

Secondary obstructions produce pressure on the urinary tract from outside and might be related to conditions such as prostatic enlargement (benign or malignant), abdominal aortic aneurysm, gynecologic conditions, such as pregnancy, pelvic inflammatory disease, and endometriosis, or neoplasms of the pelvic or abdominal structures.

Obstruction of any portion of the urinary tract results in a back-up or collection of urine behind the obstruction. The result is dilatation or stretching of the urinary tract structures also positioned behind the point of blockage. Muscles near the affected area contract in an attempt to push urine around the obstruction. Pressure accumulates above the point of obstruction and can result eventually in severe dilatation of the renal collecting system (hydronephrosis) and renal failure. The greater the intensity and duration of the pressure, the greater is the destruction to renal tissue.

Because urine flow is decreased with obstruction, urinary stagnation and infection or stone formation can result. Stones are formed because urine stasis permits clumping or precipitation of organic matter and minerals. Lower urinary tract obstruction can also result in constant bladder distention, hypertrophy of bladder muscle fibers, and formation of herniated sacs of bladder mucosa. These herniated sacs result in a large, flaccid bladder that cannot empty completely. In addition, these sacs retain stagnant urine that cause infection and stone formation.

Disorders of the Upper Urinary Tract

Obstruction of the upper urinary tract may be sudden (acute) or slow in development. Tumors of the kidney or ureters may develop slowly enough that symptoms are totally absent or very mild initially with eventual progression to pain and signs of impairment. *Acute* ureteral or renal blockage by a stone (calculus consisting of mineral salts), for example, may result in excruciating, spasmodic, and radiating pain accompanied by severe nausea and vomiting.

Renal tumors may also be detected as a flank mass combined with unexplained weight loss, fever, pain and hematuria. The presence of any amount of blood in the urine must always result in referral to a physician for further diagnostic evaluation, because this is a primary symptom of urinary tract neoplasm.

CLINICAL SIGNS AND SYMPTOMS OF OBSTRUCTION OF THE UPPER URINARY TRACT

- Pain (depends on the rapidity of onset and on the location)
    - Acute, spasmodic, radiating
    - Mild and dull flank pain
    - Lumbar discomfort with some renal diseases or renal back pain with ureteral obstruction
- Hyperesthesia of dermatomes (T10-L1)
- Nausea and vomiting
- Palpable flank mass
- Hematuria
- Fever and chills
- Abdominal muscle spasms
- Renal impairment indicators (Table 7–4; see also Table 7–3)

Disorders of the Lower Urinary Tract

Common conditions of obstruction of the lower urinary tract are bladder tumors (bladder cancer is the most common site of urinary tract cancer) and prostatic enlargement, either benign (benign prostatic hypertrophy [BPH]) or malignant (cancer of the prostate). An enlarged prostate gland can occlude the urethra partially or completely.

Benign prostatic hypertrophy is a common complaint in men over 50 years of age. Because of its position around the urethra, enlargement of the prostate quickly interferes

Table 7–4. RENAL BLOOD STUDIES*

Test	Normal Result	Renal Impairment
Creatinine	0.6–1.2 mg/dl†	Increased
BUN	8.0–25.0 mg/dl	Increased
Uric acid	2.8–7.8 mg/dl	Increased
Potassium	3.5–5.0 meq/l‡	Increased
Sodium	135–145 meq/l	Depends on the type of impairment
Calcium	9.0–10.6 mg/dl	Decreased
Phosphorus	2.5–4.5 mg/dl	Increased
RBCs	Male: 4.6–6.0 (ml/mm³)§ Female: 4.0–5.0	Decreased
Hematocrit	Male: 40–54% Female: 36–46%	Decreased
Hemoglobin	Male: 13.5–18 g/dl Female: 12–16 g/dl	Decreased

* Normal values are taken from Kee, J.: Laboratory and Diagnostic Tests with Nursing Implications. Norwalk, CT, Appleton & Lange, 1987.

† mg/dl = milligrams per 100 milliliters.

‡ meq/l = milliequivalent per liter.

§ ml/mm³ = million per cubic millimeter.

Reference values for laboratory tests vary from one laboratory to another. Always refer to the normal values used in each hospital or laboratory as being the appropriate reference for normal.

with the normal passage of urine from the bladder. Urination becomes increasingly difficult, and the bladder never feels completely empty. If left untreated, continued enlargement of the prostate eventually obstructs the bladder completely and emergency measures become necessary to empty the bladder. If the prostate is greatly enlarged, chronic constipation may result. The usual remedy is prostatectomy. Cancer of the prostate may occur in men over 60 years of age. Prostatitis is a relatively common inflammation of the prostate and may be acute or chronic (Miller and Keane, 1987). (See the case study at the end of this chapter.)

Cancer of the prostate is the second most common site of cancer among men and is often diagnosed when the man seeks medical assistance because of symptoms of urinary obstruction or sciatica. The sciatic (low back, hip, and leg) pain is caused by metastasis of the cancer to the bones of the pelvis, lumbar spine, or femur.

CLINICAL SIGNS AND SYMPTOMS OF OBSTRUCTION OF THE LOWER URINARY TRACT

Lower urinary tract symptoms of blockage are related most commonly to bladder or urethral pressure. This pressure results in bladder distention and subsequent pain. Common symptoms of lower urinary tract obstruction include:

- Bladder palpable above the symphysis pubis
- Suprapubic or pelvic pain
- Difficulty in voiding
- Hesitancy: difficulty in initiating urination or an interrupted flow of urine
- Small amounts of urine with voiding
- Lower abdominal discomfort with a feeling of the need to void
- Nocturia (unusual voiding during the night)
- Hematuria (RBCs in the urine)

CLINICAL SIGNS AND SYMPTOMS ASSOCIATED WITH PROSTATITIS

- Sudden moderate-to-high fever
- Chills
- Low back and perineal pain
- Urinary frequency and urgency
- Nocturia
- Dysuria
- General malaise
- Arthralgia
- Myalgia

Mechanical (Neuromuscular)

Mechanical problems of the urinary tract relate specifically to difficulty with emptying of urine from the bladder. Improper emptying of the bladder results in urinary retention and impairment of voluntary bladder control (incontinence). Several possible causes of mechanical bladder dysfunction include mechanical stress (e.g., exercise, coughing), spinal cord injury, central nervous system disease (e.g., multiple sclerosis and Guillain-Barré syndrome), UTI, partial urethral obstruction, trauma, and removal of the prostate gland (Farley et al, 1987c).

Many of these mechanical problems are neurogenic and may require bladder retraining or artificial drainage, such as urinary catheterization. There are three primary categories of neurogenic bladder dysfunction—flaccid (hypotonic), spastic (hypertonic), and uninhibited (Tanagho, 1984).

Flaccid Bladder

Flaccid bladder can be the consequence of smooth muscle denervation of the bladder wall. This is a lower motor neuron dysfunction of the spinal cord involving the region of the cord where the spinal reflex for micturition is located (parasympathetic nervous system via S2, S3, and S4) (Perkash, 1982). Most spinal cord lesions are both sensory and motor lesions and result in a limp, flaccid bladder with a greatly increased capacity. The patient has no urgency to void and must empty the bladder mechanically by using some form of massage or internal pressure, such as the Valsalva or Credé maneuver. This type of bladder dysfunction can result in a urinary back-up, ureteral and renal parenchymal dilatation, and eventual impairment.

Spastic Bladder

A spastic bladder preserves reflex bladder activity, but the detrusor muscle contracts with very small amounts of urine present (20 to 50 ml). This is considered to be an upper motor neuron problem with the presence of a lesion above the spinal reflex centers and results in urinary incontinence. A high pressure system occurs due to the continual spastic activity as the bladder and sphincter alternately spasm resulting in a high rate of bladder destruction. This condition of noncongruent bladder/sphincter spasming is known as the *detruser sphincter dysynergism.* The spastic bladder can respond to minimal stimuli, such as touching or stroking the genitalia or thighs. UTI causes further, more severe spasm (Perkash, 1982).

Treatment may include the use of anticholinergic drugs to decrease the bladder spasm, intermittent urinary catheterization, and possible surgical destruction of the sphincter muscles (McGuire, 1986).

Uninhibited Bladder

The uninhibited bladder is one that is neither flaccid nor spastic. The patient has a lack of control or sensation of bladder activity and becomes incontinent. This problem most commonly originates from a cerebral lesion, such as a stroke, head injury, or impaired cerebral function. Control can sometimes be established through the use of a persistent retraining schedule. However, if loss of control is a result of unconsciousness, treatment may be limited to external or indwelling urinary drainage or to use of waterproof or absorbent pads.

Mechanical bladder dysfunctions of any kind predispose the patient to various additional urinary tract problems, including infection, obstruction, or kidney damage. These patients need to be assessed carefully for any symptoms relating to further urinary tract impairment and need immediate referral if a problem is suspected.

Renal Failure

A patient is unlikely to seek treatment for renal problems from the physical therapist. However, renal patients may receive treatment for primary musculoskeletal lesions in both inpatient and outpatient clinics. An understanding of the basic physiologic problems associated with end-stage renal disease (chronic renal failure) is necessary to appropriately evaluate the patient's complaints and to treat musculoskeletal conditions in these individuals.

Etiologies

Renal failure exists when the kidneys can no longer maintain the homeostatic balances within the body that are necessary for life. Three primary categories help to define the possible etiologies of renal failure: prerenal, renal, and postrenal.

The *prerenal* classification includes disorders that primarily affect blood supply to the kidney. Renal impairment results from renal tissue ischemia caused by conditions such as hypertension, heart failure, or hypovolemic shock. The *renal* category is specific to problems that involve direct damage to the renal tissue itself, such as infection, diabetes mellitus, collagen diseases (e.g., systemic lupus erythematosus [SLE]), and chemical or radiation toxicity. *Postrenal* problems are related to conditions that block or obstruct the flow of urine. These problems occur anywhere from the renal pelvis to the distal portion of the urinary tract or urethra. Tumors or blockages of the urethra (e.g., calculi), bladder, ureters, or renal pelvis cause a back-up of urine, dilatation of urinary tract structures, and eventual renal damage (Hahn, 1987).

Treatment of renal failure involves several

elements that are designed to replace the lost excretory and metabolic functions of this organ. Treatment options include:

- Dialysis (removal of wastes and fluid; and balance of electrolytes through the use of an artificial kidney or the patient's peritoneal membrane)
- Diet (restricted in sodium, potassium, fluid, and some protein)
- Drug therapy (used to assist in regulation of lost metabolic processes)
  - Antihypertensives
  - RBC production stimulants, such as testosterone derivatives
  - Vitamin replacements, especially active vitamin D
  - Phosphate binders (usually antacids) used to remove phosphate through the gastrointestinal (GI) tract
- Renal transplantation (completely *replaces* lost functions; patients need immunosuppressants and antirejection drugs for a period of time)

The choice of treatment options, such as dialysis, transplantation, or no treatment, depends on many factors including the patient's age, underlying physical problems, and availability of compatible organs for transplantation. Untreated or chronic renal failure results eventually in death.

Clinical Symptoms

Failure of the filtering and regulating mechanisms of the kidney can be either acute (sudden in onset and potentially reversible) or chronic (called uremia, which develops gradually and is usually irreversible). Patients with either type of renal failure develop symptoms characteristic of impaired fluid and waste excretion and altered renal regulation of other body metabolic processes, such as pH regulation, RBC production, and calcium phosphorus balance.

Blood serum abnormalities typical of the failing kidney include elevated BUN, creatinine, and uric acid levels, elevated phosphorus levels combined with decreased calcium levels (imbalance results in bone deterioration), and decreased bicarbonate levels (imbalance results in metabolic acidosis). Normal blood serum results are shown in Table 7–4.

Urine volume is frequently decreased (oliguria) or is totally absent (anuria). This insufficiency in the excretion of urine causes an accumulation of fluid in both the vascular system and in body tissues which, in turn, causes hypertension and edema. Some patients with renal failure have a normal output of urine, but the urine is greatly decreased in waste products and may contain abnormal constituents, such as glucose, protein, and blood cells.

Due to the limited ability of the impaired kidney to produce erythropoietin (hormone essential for RBC production in the bone marrow), many renal patients are severely anemic. The anemia is usually associated with extreme fatigue and intolerance to even normal daily activities. A pale skin color is also characteristic of the decrease in RBCs.

In addition, the continuous presence of toxic waste products in the bloodstream (urea, creatinine, uric acid) results in damage to many other body systems, including the central nervous system, peripheral nervous system, eyes, GI tract, integumentary system, endocrine system, and cardiopulmonary systems (Table 7–5).

RENAL AND UROLOGIC PAIN

Upper Urinary Tract (Renal/Ureteral)

The kidneys and ureters are innervated by both sympathetic and parasympathetic fibers. The kidneys receive sympathetic innervation from the lesser splanchnic nerves through the renal plexus, which is located next to the renal arteries. Renal vasoconstriction and increased renin release are associated with sympathetic stimulation. Parasympathetic innervation is derived from the vagus nerve, and the function of this innervation is not known (Perlmutter and Blacklow, 1983).

Renal sensory innervation is not completely understood even though the capsule (cover-

Table 7–5. SYSTEMIC MANIFESTATIONS OF RENAL FAILURE

Systemic Symptoms	Probable Causes
Urinary System	
Decreased urinary output	Damaged renal tissue
Abnormal urinary constituents (blood cells, protein, casts)	
Cardiopulmonary	
Hypertension	Fluid overload
Congestive heart failure	
Pulmonary edema	
Pericarditis	Uremic toxins irritate pericordial sac
Gastrointestinal Tract	
Bleeding	Irritation of gastric mucosa by uremic toxins combined with platelet changes
Nausea and vomiting	
Uremic breath	Uremic toxins change saliva
Anorexia	
Nervous System	
Central (CNS)	
Irritability	Effect of uremic toxins on brain cells (usually resolve with dialysis treatment)
Impaired judgment	
Inability to concentrate	
Seizures	
Lethargy/coma	
Sleep disturbances	
Peripheral (PNS)	
Loss of vibratory sense and deep tendon reflexes	Effect of uremic toxins on peripheral nerves
Impairment of motor nerve conduction velocity	
Burning, tingling, paresthesias	
Tremors	Electrolyte imbalances (calcium, sodium, potassium)
Muscle cramps, muscle twitching	
Foot drop	
Weakness	
Integumentary (Skin)	
Pruritus (itching)/excoriation (scratching)	Skin calcifications related to calcium/phosphorus imbalances
Hyperpigmentation	Retained uremic pigments
Pallor	Anemia
Bruising	Platelet dysfunction
Eyes	
Band keratopathy	Corneal calcifications related to calcium/phosphorus imbalance
Visual blurring	
Red eyes	Conjunctival calcifications related to calcium/phosphorus imbalance
Endocrine	
Fertility and sexual dysfunction	Effect of uremic toxins on menstrual cycles, ovulation, and sperm production
Hyperparathyroidism	Result of calcium/phosphorus imbalance

Table 7–5. SYSTEMIC MANIFESTATIONS OF RENAL FAILURE Continued

Systemic Symptoms	Probable Causes
Hematopoietic	
Anemia	Decreased production of erythropoietin by kidney Destruction of RBCs by dialysis
Platelet dysfunction	Uremic toxins interfere with platelet aggregation
Skeletal	
Renal osteodystrophy (demineralization of bones)	Related to decreased calcium absorption and resultant calcium/phosphorus imbalance
Joint pain	Joint calcifications

ing of the kidney) and lower portions of the collecting system seem to respond with pain to stretching (distention) or puncture. Information transmitted by renal and ureteral pain receptors are transmitted by sympathetic nerves that enter the spinal cord at T10 to L1 (Richard, 1986).

Because visceral and cutaneous sensory fibers enter the spinal cord in close proximity and actually converge on some of the *same* neurons, when visceral pain fibers are stimulated, concurrent stimulation of cutaneous fibers also occurs. The visceral pain is then felt as though it is skin pain (hyperesthesia), similar to the occasion when the alpine skiier stated that "even the skin on my back hurts." Renal and urethral pain can be felt throughout the T10 to L1 dermatomes.

Renal pain is felt typically in the posterior subcostal and costovertebral regions, whereas ureteral pain is felt in the groin and genital area (see Fig. 7–3). Radiation forward around the flank into the lower abdominal quadrant and abdominal muscle spasm with rebound tenderness can occur on the same side as the source of pain. The pain can also be generalized throughout the abdomen. Nausea, vomiting, and impaired intestinal motility (progressing to intestinal paralysis) can occur with severe, acute pain (Perlmutter and Blacklow, 1983). Nerve fibers from the renal plexus are also in direct communication with the spermatic plexus and, due to this close relationship, testicular pain may also accompany renal pain (Richard, 1986). Neither renal nor ureteral pain is altered by changing body position.

Typical renal pain sensation is aching and dull in nature, but can occasionally be a severe, boring type of pain. The constant dull and aching pain usually accompanies distention or stretching of the renal capsule, pelvis, or collecting system. This stretching can result from intrarenal fluid accumulation, such as inflammatory edema, inflamed or bleeding cysts, and bleeding or neoplastic growths. Whenever the renal capsule is punctured, a dull pain can also be felt by the patient. Ischemia of renal tissue due to blockage of blood flow to the kidneys results in a *constant* dull or a *constant* sharp pain.

Pseudorenal pain (Smith, 1984) may occur secondary to radiculitis or irritation of the costal nerves caused by mechanical derangements of the costovertebral or costotransverse joints. Disorders of this sort are common in the cervical and thoracic areas, but the most common sites are T10 to T12 (Smith and Raney, 1976). Irritation of these nerves causes costovertebral pain that often radiates into the ipsilateral lower abdominal quadrant. The onset is usually acute with some type of traumatic history, such as lifting a heavy object, sustaining a blow to the costovertebral area, or falling from a height onto the buttocks. The pain is affected by body position, and although the patient may be awakened at night when assuming a certain position (e.g., sidelying on the affected side), it is usually absent on awakening and increases gradually during the day. The pain is also aggravated by prolonged periods of sitting, especially when driving on rough roads in the car, and again is relieved by changing to another position. Radiculitis may mimic ureteral colic or renal pain, but true renal pain is seldom affected by movements of the spine.

Ureteral obstruction (e.g., from a urinary calculus or "stone" consisting of mineral salts) results in distention of the ureter and causes intermittent or constant severe pain until the stone is passed. Pain of this origin usually starts in the costovertebral angle and radiates to the ipsilateral lower abdomen, upper thigh, testis, or labium (see Fig. 7–4). Movement of a stone down a ureter can cause *renal colic,* an excruciating pain that radiates to the region just described and usually increases in intensity in waves of colic or spasm.

Chronic ureteral and renal pain tend to be vague, poorly localized, and easily confused with many other problems of abdominal or pelvic origin. There are also areas of *referred pain* related to renal or ureteral lesions. For example, if the diaphragm becomes irritated due to pressure from a renal lesion, shoulder pain may be felt. If a lesion of the ureter occurs *outside* the ureter, pain may occur on movement of the adjacent iliopsoas muscle. Abdominal rebound tenderness results when the adjacent peritoneum becomes inflamed (Perlmutter and Blacklow, 1983). Active trigger points along the upper rim of the pubis and the lateral half of the inguinal ligament may lie in the lower internal oblique muscle and possibly in the lower rectus abdominis. These trigger points can cause increased irritation and spasm of the detrusor and urinary sphincter muscles, producing urinary frequency, retention of urine, and groin pain (Travell and Simons, 1983).

Lower Urinary Tract (Bladder/Urethra)

Bladder innervation occurs through sympathetic, parasympathetic, and sensory nerve pathways. Sympathetic bladder innervation assists in the closure of the bladder neck during seminal emission. Afferent sympathetic fibers also assist in providing awareness of bladder distention, pain, and abdominal distention due to bladder distention. This input reaches the cord at T9 or higher. Parasympathetic bladder innervation is at S2, S3, and S4 and provides motor coordination for the act of voiding. Afferent parasympathetic fibers assist in sensation of the desire to void, proprioception (position sensation), and perception of pain (Perlmutter and Blacklow, 1983).

Sensory receptors are present in the mucosa of the bladder and in the muscular bladder walls. These fibers are more plentiful near the bladder neck and the junctional area between the ureters and bladder.

Urethral innervation, also at the S2, S3, and S4 level, occurs through the pudendal nerve. This is a mixed innervation of both sensory and motor nerve fibers. This innervation controls the opening of the external urethral sphincter (motor) and an awareness of the imminence of voiding and heat (thermal) sensation in the urethra (McGuire, 1986).

Bladder or urethral pain is felt above the pubis (suprapubic) or low in the abdomen. The sensation is usually characterized as one of urinary urgency, a sensation to void, and dysuria (painful urination). Irritation of the neck of the bladder or of the urethra can result in a burning sensation localized to these areas, probably due to the urethral thermal receptors (see Fig. 7–5).

Other causes of pain similar to upper or lower urinary tract pain of either an acute or chronic nature may include:

Perforated viscus (any large internal organ)

Intestinal obstruction

Cholecystitis (inflammation of the gallbladder)

Pelvic inflammatory disease

Tubo-ovarian abscess

Ruptured ectopic pregnancy

Twisted ovarian cyst

OVERVIEW OF RENAL AND UROLOGIC PAIN PATTERNS

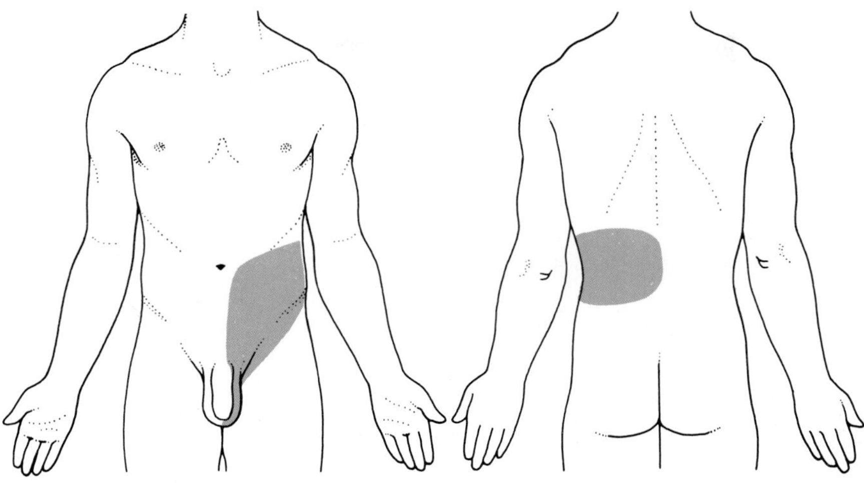

Figure 7–3. Renal pain is felt typically in the posterior subcostal and costovertebral region *(dark red)*. It can radiate forward around the flank into the lower abdominal quadrant. Testicular pain may also accompany renal pain.

Kidney

Location (Fig. 7–3)	Posterior subcostal and costovertebral region
	Usually unilateral
Referral:	Radiates forward, around the flank or the side into lower abdominal quadrant (T11 to T12)
	Pressure from the kidney on the diaphragm may cause ipsilateral shoulder pain
Description:	Dull aching, boring
Intensity:	Acute: severe, intense
	Chronic: vague and poorly localized
Duration:	Constant
Associated Signs and Symptoms:	Hyperesthesia of associated dermatomes (T9 to T10)
	Ipsilateral or generalized abdominal pain
	Spasm of abdominal muscles
	Nausea and vomiting when severely acute
	Testicular pain may occur in men
	Unrelieved by a change in position

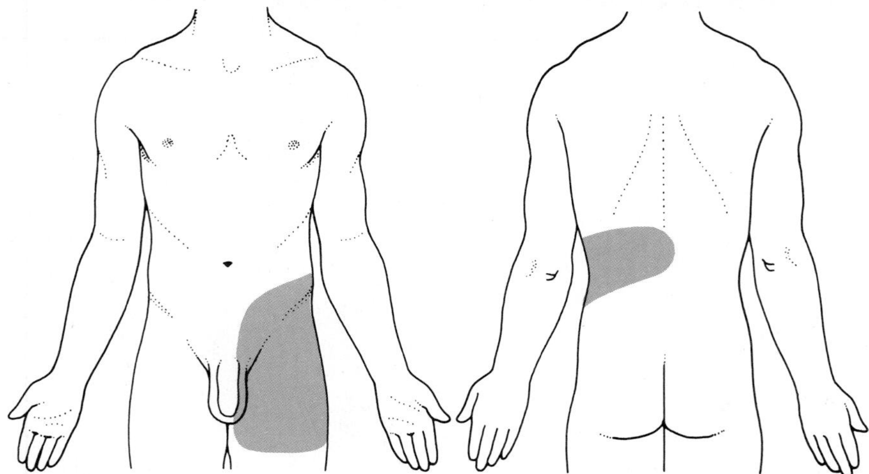

Figure 7–4. Ureteral pain *(dark red)* may begin posteriorly in the costovertebral angle and may then radiate arteriorly *(dark red)* to the ipsilateral lower abdomen, upper thigh, testes, or labium.

Ureter

Location (Fig. 7–4)	Costovertebral angle Unilateral or bilateral
Referral:	Radiates to the lower abdomen, upper thigh, testis, or labium on the same side (groin and genital area)
Description:	Described as crescendo waves of colic
Intensity:	Excruciating, severe
Duration:	Intermittent or constant without relief until treated or until the calculus (kidney stone) is passed
Associated Signs and Symptoms:	Rectal tenesmus (painful spasm of anal sphincter with urgent desire to evacuate the bowel/bladder; involuntary straining with little passage of urine or feces) Nausea, abdominal distention, vomiting Hyperesthesia of associated dermatomes (T10 and L1) Tenderness over the kidney or ureter Unrelieved by a change in position Movement of iliopsoas may aggravate symptoms associated with a lesion outside the ureter

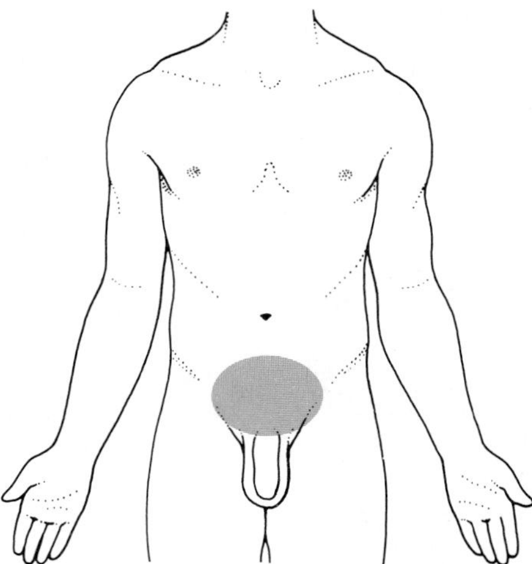

Figure 7–5. Bladder or urethral pain *(dark red)* is usually felt suprapubically or in the lower abdomen.

Bladder/Urethra

Location (Fig. 7–5)	Suprapubic or low abdomen
Referral:	Pelvis
	Can be confused with gas
Description:	Sharp, localized
Intensity:	Moderate to severe
Duration:	Intermittent; may be relieved by emptying the bladder
Associated Signs and Symptoms:	Great urinary urgency
	Tenesmus
	Dysuria
	Hot or burning sensation during urination

DIAGNOSTIC TESTING

Urinalysis

Routine screening of urine composition is called urinalysis (UA) and is the commonly used method of determining various properties of urine. This analysis is actually a series of several tests of urinary components and is a very valuable aid in the diagnosis of urinary tract or metabolic disorders. Normal urinary constituents are shown in Table 7–1. A more detailed examination of the chemical, electrolyte, and cellular composition of urine can also be done to assist in the identification of disease processes. Urine cultures are also very important studies in the diagnosis of UTIs.

Blood Studies

A blood sample can be separated (by centrifuge) into two primary constituents: serum (plasma) and cellular elements (RBCs, WBCs, and platelets). Studies of the serum portion of the blood are usually labeled "blood chemistry" or "serum panel" evaluations. These studies measure many of the chemicals that are present in the blood serum. The examination and description of the cellular elements of the blood are called hematology and include counting of various cellular types as well as defining important cellular characteristics (e.g., size, shape, and amount of hemoglobin).

Various blood studies can be done to assess renal function (see Table 7–4). These studies examine both the serum and cellular components of the blood for specific changes characteristic of renal performance. Substances that must be examined in the serum are those that are a *direct* reflection of renal function, such as creatinine and others that are more *indirect* in renal evaluation (e.g., BUN, pH-related substances, uric acid, various ions, and electrolytes and cellular components [RBCs]).

Creatinine is a byproduct of normal muscle metabolism and is regulated and excreted almost solely by the kidney. There are very few factors other than renal function changes that will affect or influence the presence of creatinine in the blood serum. Creatinine is present in very small amounts in the blood serum and in very large amounts in the urine. It can rise in the serum with only mild renal impairment.

Urea is formed in the liver and consists of the primary nonprotein nitrogenous endproduct of dietary protein breakdown in the body. It is excreted in the urine as a waste product. A rise in the BUN level usually indicates an impairment of excretion by the renal tubules, but other metabolic factors, such as shock, dehydration, GI hemorrhage, or excessive protein intake can cause an increase in this value. Another component affected by metabolic processes, but reflective of renal function, is *uric acid* (increases also occur in gout, malignancies, starvation, and shock). PH-related substances, such as bicarbonate, certain ions, and electrolytes, are also measured to assist in the determination of renal performance, but these substances are influenced greatly by other body processes (Richard, 1986). Potassium, a critical ion that is very plentiful within body cells, must be balanced meticulously by the kidney because its accumulation in the bloodstream can result in abnormalities of cardiac muscle contraction and can potentially lead to lethal arrhythmias.

RBCs (erythrocytes) also need to be assessed carefully because erythropoiesis (RBC production) is influenced greatly by the functioning kidney. The total RBC count and hematocrit (percentage of RBCs per plasma) are valuable indicators of the kidney's ability to produce erythropoietin.

SUMMARY

Most renal and urologic conditions present with a combination of systemic signs and symptoms accompanied by either pelvic, flank, or low back pain. The patient may have a history of recent trauma or previous medical history of UTIs to alert the clinician to possible systemic origin of symptoms.

To assist the physical therapist with appropriate questioning and possible patient referral, in this chapter we have emphasized:

- Urinary tract structure and physiology
- Renal and urinary tract problems, including inflammatory, obstructive, and mechanical disorders
- Discussion of chronic renal failure and the medical consequences of this condition
- An overview and discussion of renal and urinary tract pain patterns
- A discussion of common pertinent diagnostic testing and laboratory studies

Signs and Symptoms Requiring Physician Referral

The physical therapist is advised to question the patient further whenever any of the following signs and symptoms are reported or observed because they may indicate systemic disease, and the patient should therefore be referred to a physician for further evaluation.

Abdominal muscle spasms
Anorexia
Anuria (totally absent urine)
Decreased urinary output
Dependent edema
Dyspnea
Dysuria
Fever and chills
Flank pain
Foul odor to urine
Headache
Hematuria (change in color: black, brown, gray, or red)
Hesitancy
Hypertension
Incontinence
Low back and perineal pain
Nausea and vomiting
Proteinuria
Pyuria (cloudy)
Shoulder pain (result of pressure from the kidney on the diaphragm)
Skin hyperesthesia (T10–L1)
Small amounts of urine with voiding
Spasmodic, radiating pain to the testis, labia, thigh, suprapubic or pelvic area
Unilateral costovertebral tenderness
Unusual nocturia
Urinary frequency
Urinary urgency
Weakness

SUBJECTIVE EXAMINATION

Special Questions to Ask

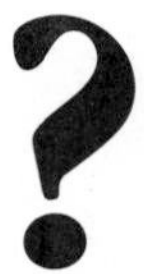

Patients may be reluctant to answer the physical therapist's questions concerning bladder and urinary function. The physical therapist is advised to explain the need to rule out possible causes of pain related to the kidneys and bladder and to give the patient time to respond if answers seem to be uncertain. For example, the physical therapist may ask the patient to observe urinary function over the next 2 days and he or she may inform the patient that these questions will be reviewed again at the next appointment.

- □ Do you have any problems with your kidneys or bladder? If so, can you describe them?
- □ Have you ever had kidney or bladder stones? If so, how were these stones treated?

Subjective Exam

Special Questions to Ask

- □ Have you ever had an injury to your bladder or to your kidneys? If so, how was this injury treated?
- □ Have you had any infections of the bladder? How were these infections treated?

  Were they related to any specific circumstances (e.g., pregnancy, intercourse)?
- □ Have you had any kidney infections? How were these infections treated?

  Were they related to any specific circumstances (e.g., pregnancy, after bladder infections, after strep throat or strep skin infections)?
- □ Have you ever had surgery on your bladder or kidneys? If so, what kind of surgery and how long ago did it occur?
- □ Have you ever had flank (kidney or ureter) or suprapubic (bladder or urethra) pain?

  If so, what relieves this pain?

  Does a change of position affect it? (Inflammatory pain may be relieved by a change in position. Renal colic remains unchanged by a change in position.)

  For women: Have you noticed any unusual vaginal discharge during the time that you had pain just above the pubic area (suprapubic pain)? (Infection)

  For men: Have you noticed any unusual discharge from your penis during the time you had pain above the pubic area (suprapubic pain)? (Infection)
- □ Have you noticed a change in the amount or number of times that you urinate in the last 2 to 3 weeks? (Infection)
- □ How much fluid do you usually drink on an average day (excluding alcohol)?
- □ When you urinate, do you ever have trouble starting the flow of urine? (Urethral obstruction)
- □ Do you urinate in a steady stream or do you start and stop the flow of urination? (Urethral obstruction)
- □ Has your urine stream changed in size? If so, please describe. (Urethral obstruction)
- □ When you are finished urinating, do you feel like your bladder is completely empty? (Bladder dysfunction)
- □ Do you ever have a pain or a burning sensation when you urinate? (Lower urinary tract irritation)
- □ Have you ever had or been treated for a venereal disease? (May cause a burning sensation on urination or urgency)
- □ Have you had a need to urinate during the night that is unusual for you during the last 2 to 3 weeks?

Subjective Exam

Special Questions to Ask

Does this happen every night or just when you drink a large amount of fluid before bedtime? (Diminished bladder capacity, inability to empty the bladder completely)

□ Do you ever have urinary dribbling or incontinence? If so, describe this experience.

Is it related to coughing, laughing, exercise, or having a bowel movement? (Stress incontinence; may be caused by medications, such as antihistamines, antispasmodics, sedatives, diuretics, and psychotropic drugs) (Nursing, 1984)

□ Does your urine ever look brown, red, or black? (Hematuria or may be normal with some medications and foods such as beets or rhubarb)

□ Is your urine clear? If not, please describe how it looks. How frequently does this happen? (Could indicate upper or lower UTI)

□ Have you ever noticed a foul or unusual odor coming from your urine? (Infection, secondary to medication)

For men: Have you ever been treated for a prostate problem? If so, how long ago did it occur and what was the treatment?

PHYSICIAN REFERRAL

Pain related to urinary tract pathology is often similar to pain felt from an injury to the back, flank, abdomen, or upper thigh. Further diagnostic testing and medical examination must be performed by the physician to differentiate urinary tract conditions from musculoskeletal problems. The proximity of the kidneys, ureters, bladder, and urethra to the ribs, vertebrae, diaphragm, and accompanying muscles and tendinous insertions can often make it difficult to accurately identify the patient's problems.

The physical therapist must be able to recognize the systemic origin of urinary tract symptoms that mimic musculoskeletal pain. Many conditions that produce urinary tract pain also include an elevation in temperature and abnormal urinary constituents, such as change in color, odor, or amount of urine. The presence of any amount of blood in the urine always requires a referral to a physician. However, the presence of abnormalities in the urine may not be obvious, and thus a thorough diagnostic analysis of the urine may need to be done. Careful questioning of the patient regarding urinary tract history, urinary patterns, urinary characteristics, and pain patterns elicit valuable information relating to potential urinary tract symptoms.

Referral by the physical therapist to the physician is recommended when the patient presents with any combination of systemic signs and symptoms presented in this chapter. Damage to urinary tract structures can occur concurrently with trauma and damage to musculoskeletal structures, which are located in the same anatomic location. For example, the alpine skiier discussed at the beginning of the chapter had a dull, aching costovertebral pain on the left side, which was unrelieved by a change of position or by ice, heat, or aspirin. His pain is related directly to a traumatic episode, and musculoskeletal injury is a definite possibility in his case. He has no medical history of urinary tract problems and denies any urine changes. Because the pain is constant and is unrelieved by usual measures, and the location of the pain is approximate to the renal structures, a medical follow-up and urinalysis would be recommended.

The physical therapist should review the signs and symptoms listed earlier in this chapter when making a medical referral and also the findings of the objective examination combined with the medical history and present symptomatology.

CASE STUDY

Referral

The patient is self-referred and states that he has been to your hospital-based outpatient clinic in the past. He has a very extensive chart containing his entire medical history for the last 20 years.

Background Information

He is a 44-year-old man who describes his current occupation as "errand boy/gopher," which requires minimal lifting, bending, or strenuous physical activity. His chief complaint today is pain in the lower back, which comes and goes and seems to be aggravated by sitting. The pain is poorly described, and the patient is unable to specify any kind of descriptive words for the type of pain, intensity, or duration.

Special Questions to Ask

See Chapter 12 for Special Questions to Ask about the back. The patient's answer to any questions related to bowel and bladder functions is either "I don't know" or "Well, you know," which makes a complete interview impossible.

Subjective/Objective Findings

There are radiating symptoms of numbness down the left leg to the foot. The patient denies any saddle anesthesia. Deep tendon reflexes are intact bilaterally, and the patient stands with an obvious scoliotic list to one side. The patient is unable to tell you whether his symptoms are relieved or alleviated on performing a lateral shift to correct the curve. There are no other positive neuromuscular findings or associated systemic symptoms.

Result

After 3 days of treatment over the course of 1 week, the patient has had no subjective improvement in symptoms. Objectively, the scoliotic shift has not changed. A second opinion is sought from two other staff members, and the consensus of agreement is to refer the patient to his physician. The physician performs a rectal examination and confirms a positive diagnosis of prostatitis based on the results of laboratory tests. These test results were consistent with the patient's physical findings and previous history of prostate problems 1 year ago. The patient was reluctant to discuss bowel or bladder function with the female therapist, but readily suggested to his physician that his current symptoms mimicked an earlier episode of prostatitis.

It is not always possible to elicit thorough responses from patients concerning matters of genitourinary function. If the patient hesitates or is unable to answer questions satisfactorily, it may be necessary to present the questions again at a later time (e.g., next treatment session), to ask a colleague of the same sex to confer with the patient, or to refer the patient to his or her physician for further evaluation. Occasionally, the patient will answer negatively to any questions regarding observed changes in urinary function and will then report back at the next session that there was some pathology that was not noted earlier.

In this case, a close review of the extensive medical records may have alerted the physical therapist to the patient's previous treatment for the same problem, which he was reluctant to discuss.

CASE STUDY

References

Farley, F., and Miller, P.: Assessment of urinary function. *In* Phipps, W., Long, B., and Woods, N. (eds): Medical-Surgical Nursing: Concepts and Clinical Practice, 3rd ed. St. Louis, C.V. Mosby, 1987a, pp. 1577–1593.

Farley F., and Miller, P.: Interventions for persons with problems of the urinary tract. *In* Phipps, W., Long, B., and Woods, N. (eds): Medical-Surgical Nursing: Concepts and Clinical Practice. St. Louis, C.V. Mosby, 1987b, pp. 1595–1625.

Farley, F., Miller, P., Roberts, R., and Broadwell, D.: Interventions for persons with urinary disorders. *In* Phipps. W., Long, B., and Woods, N. (eds): Medical-Surgical Nursing: Concepts and Clinical Practice, 3rd ed. St. Louis, C.V. Mosby, 1987c, pp. 1627–1654.

Fischbach, F.: A Manual of Laboratory Diagnostic Tests, 2nd ed. Philadelphia, J.B. Lippincott, 1988.

Guyton, A.: Textbook of Medical Physiology, 7th ed. Philadelphia, W.B. Saunders Company, 1986.

Hahn, K: The many signs of renal failure. Nursing 87, *17*:34, 1987.

LaValle, S.: Infections and obstructive diseases of the kidney. *In* Richard, C. (ed): Comprehensive Nephrology Nursing. Boston, Little Brown, 1986, pp. 86–97.

McGuire, E.: Neuromuscular dysfunction of the lower urinary tract. *In* Walsh, P., Perlmutter, A., Gittes, T., and Stamey, T. (eds): Campbell's Urology, 5th ed. Philadelphia, W.B. Saunders Company, 1986, pp. 616–638.

Miller, B.F., and Keane, C.B.: Encyclopedia and Dictionary of Medicine, Nursing, and Allied Health, 4th ed. Philadelphia, W.B. Saunders Company, 1987.

Nursing 84 Books: Renal and urologic disorders. Springhouse, PA, Springhouse Corporation, 1984.

Perkash, I.: Management of neurogenic dysfunction of the bladder and bowel. *In* Kottke, G., Stillwell, K., and Lehmann, J. (eds): Krusen's Handbook of Physical Medicine and Rehabilitation, 3rd ed. Philadelphia, W.B. Saunders Company, 1982, pp. 724–745.

Perlmutter, A., and Blacklow, R.: Urinary tract pain, hematuria and pyuria. *In* Blacklow, R.S. (ed): MacBryde's Signs and Symptoms. Philadelphia, J.B. Lippincott, 1983, pp. 181–192.

Richard, C.: Renal assessment with nursing implications. *In* Richard, C. (ed): Comprehensive Nephrology Nursing. Boston, Little Brown, 1986.

Smith, D.R.: Symptoms of disorders of the genitourinary tract. *In* Smith, D.R. (ed): General Urology, 11th ed. Los Altos, CA, Lange Medical Publications, 1984, pp. 27–35.

Smith, D.R., and Raney, F.L., Jr.: Radiculitis distress as a mimic of renal pain. J Urol., *116*:269, 1976.

Tanagho, E.: Neuropathic bladder disorders. *In* Smith, D. (ed): General Urology, 11th ed. Los Altos, CA, Lange Medical Publications, 1984, pp. 405–443.

Travell, J.G., and Simons, D.G.: Myofascial Pain and Dysfunction. The Trigger Point Manual. Baltimore, Williams & Wilkins, 1983.

Chapter 8

Overview of Hepatic and Biliary Signs and Symptoms

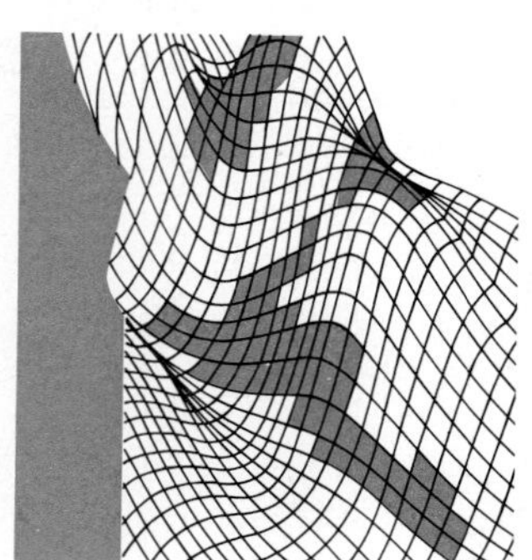

☐ ***Clinical Signs and Symptoms of:***

Liver Disease
Gallbladder Disease
Hepatitis A
Hepatitis B
Chronic Active Hepatitis
Chronic Persistent Hepatitis
Toxic and Drug-Induced Hepatitis
Cirrhosis
Portal Hypertension
Hepatic Encephalopathy
Liver Abscess
Liver Neoplasm
Acute Cholecystitis
Chronic Cholecystitis
Primary Biliary Cirrhosis

According to the American Liver Foundation, 27,000 Americans die each year from one of more than 100 varieties of liver diseases. Medical understanding of these diseases has increased in the last decade owing to the advances in diagnostic techniques, including ultrasonography and computed tomography. The increased knowledge in the field of viral hepatitis and advances made in the basic sciences that pertain to liver structure and function have also contributed to a better understanding of the pathogenesis and, therefore, treatment of liver diseases.

As with many of the organ systems in the human body, the hepatic and biliary organs (liver, gallbladder, and common bile duct) can develop diseases that mimic primary musculoskeletal lesions. The musculoskeletal symptoms associated with hepatic and biliary pathology are generally confined to the midback, scapular, and right shoulder regions. These musculoskeletal symptoms can occur alone (as the only presenting symptom) or in combination with other systemic signs and symptoms discussed in this chapter.

LIVER AND BILIARY PHYSIOLOGY

Liver (Nursing 81, 1981)

Structure

The liver is the largest internal organ in the human body, weighing slightly more than 3 lb (1200 to 1600 g) in the average adult. It performs more than 100 separate functions including the formation and secretion of bile; detoxification of harmful substances; production of clotting factors; storage of vitamins; and metabolism of carbohydrates, fats, and proteins. Located above the right kidney, stomach, pancreas, and intestines and immediately below the diaphragm, the liver divides into a left and right lobe (the right lobe is six times larger than the left), which are separated by the falciform ligament. Glisson's capsule, a network of connective tissue, covers the entire organ and extends into the parenchyma along blood vessels and bile ducts (Fig. 8–1).

Within the parenchyma, cylindrical lobules comprise the basic functional units of the liver, consisting of cellular plates that radiate from a central vein—like spokes in a wheel (Fig. 8–2). Small bile canaliculi (an extremely narrow tubular passage or channel) fit between the cells in the plates and empty into terminal bile ducts. These ducts join two larger ones, which merge into a single hepatic duct after leaving the liver. The hepatic duct then joins the cystic duct to form the common bile duct (see Fig. 8–1).

Functions

The liver receives blood from two major sources: the hepatic artery and the portal vein (see Fig. 8–2). These two vessels carry approximately 1500 ml/min of blood to the liver, almost 75% of which is supplied by the portal vein. Sinusoids (offshoots of both the hepatic artery and the portal vein) run between each row of hepatic cells. Phagocytic Kupffer's cells

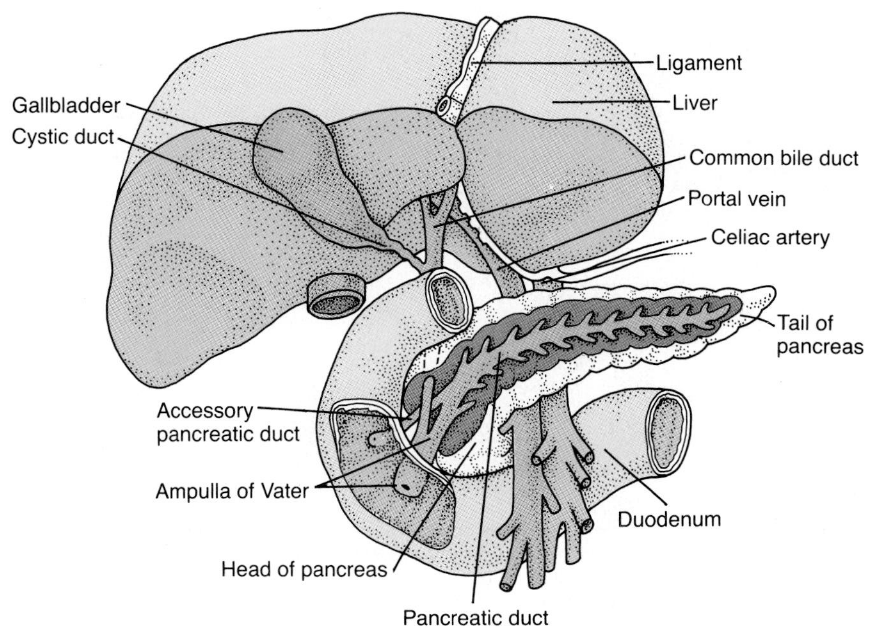

Figure 8–1. Anatomy of the liver, gallbladder, common bile duct, and pancreas.

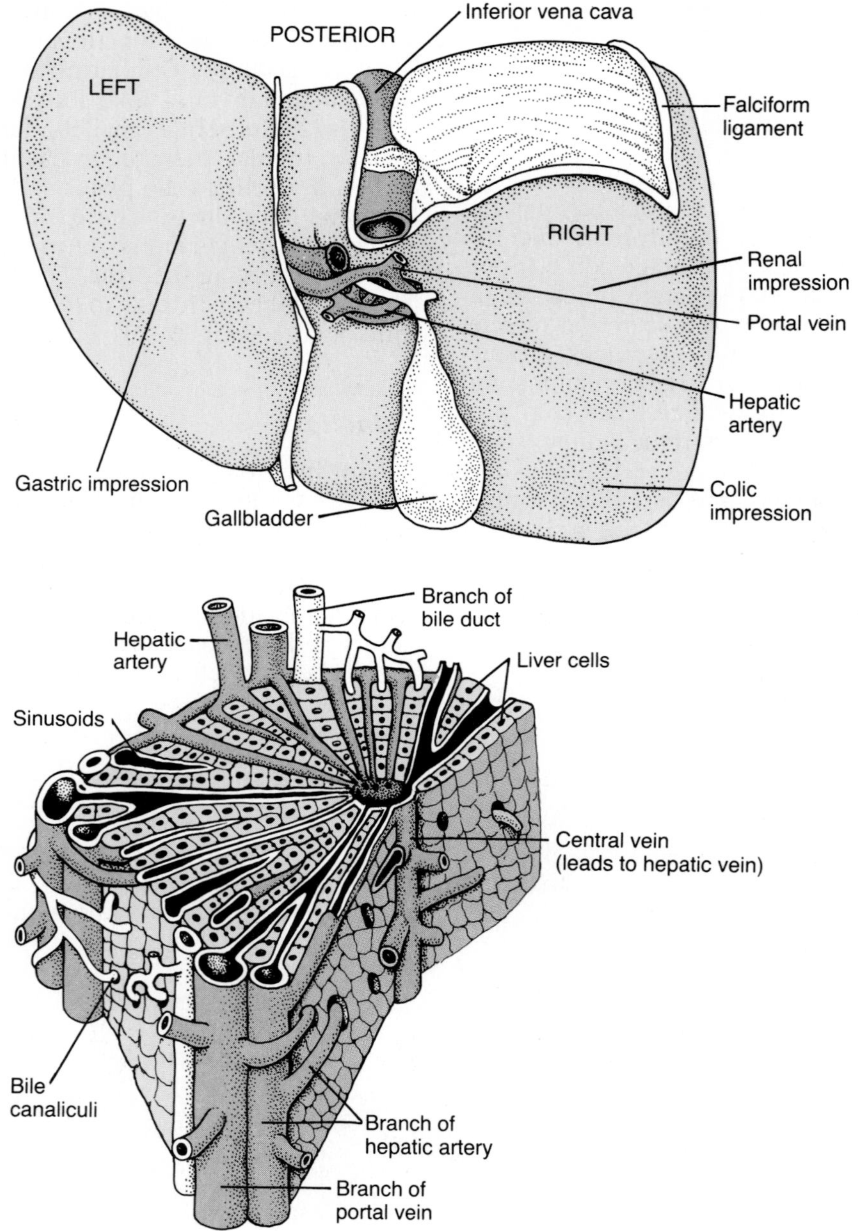

Figure 8–2. The liver receives blood from the hepatic artery and the portal vein. Most of the blood supply arriving in the portal vein has already passed through the intestine. The cylindrical plates radiating from the central vein are visualized. (From Jackson, G: Digestion: Fueling the system. New York: Torstar Books, 1984, p. 101.)

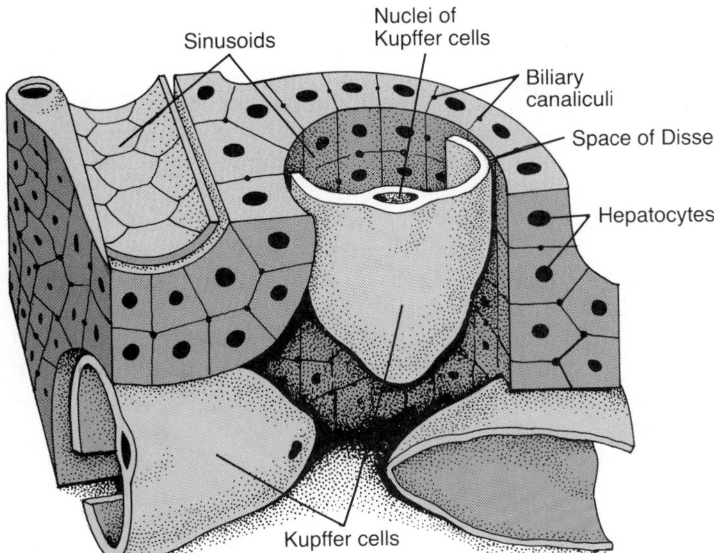

Figure 8–3. Kupffer cells lining the hepatic sinusoid.

(Fig. 8–3), part of the reticuloendothelial system, line the sinusoids, destroying old or defective red blood cells (RBCs) and detoxifying harmful substances, including the metabolism and inactivation of many drugs. The liver has a large lymphatic supply, and consequently, cancer frequently metastasizes to the liver.

Bilirubin Metabolism. One of the liver's most important functions is the conversion of bilirubin into bile. Bilirubin (red bile pigment) is the end-product of RBCs (heme) and comes from hemoglobin, myoglobin, and respiratory enzymes. When hemoglobin (an oxygen-carrying blood protein) breaks down, it produces a compound called biliverdin. This substance then converts to bilirubin, which is taken up by the liver and excreted into bile. Six grams of hemoglobin are broken down daily forming 250 to 350 mg of bilirubin. The liver is capable of excreting two or three times this amount, which occurs, for example, after a blood transfusion or in the case of a patient with anemia. This excessive capacity of the liver explains why these patients are not jaundiced (yellow skin and yellow mucous membranes due to a build-up of bilirubin and deposition of bile pigments).

Eighty per cent of this bilirubin metabolism takes place in the reticuloendothelial* cells in the liver and spleen. Twenty per cent of this process occurs within RBCs in the spleen and bone marrow. The enzyme, microsomal heme oxygenase, actually converts the heme to bilirubin. The bilirubin is then transported in the plasma tightly bound to albumin, a transport protein carrying large organic anions, such as fatty acids, bilirubin, hormones such as cortisol and thyroxine, and many drugs and antibiotics. The bilirubin must compete with these other substances for albumin.

During the albumin-bound transport time, the bilirubin is not water-soluble and is called *unconjugated bilirubin.* The subsequent excretion of bilirubin depends on its transfer from the blood plasma to the liver cell, its conjugation (joining) to the acid glucoronide, and its secretion into the bile channels as water-soluble conjugated bilirubin. After being secreted into the bile channels, the conjugated bilirubin is then secreted into the duodenum. In the gastrointestinal tract, the conjugated bilirubin is then metabolized to urobilinogen,

* The reticuloendothelial cells are a system of macrophages within the network of cells in the liver and spleen.

which is excreted in the feces or is reabsorbed. Reabsorbed urobilinogen is either recycled by the liver and re-excreted in bile or excreted in the urine (Luckmann and Sorenson, 1987).

Bilirubin is readily bound to elastic tissue (skin, blood vessels, sclerae, synovium), which in turn becomes easily icteric (jaundiced or yellow).

Gallbladder (Nursing 81, 1981)

Structure

The gallbladder is a pear-shaped organ that lies in the fossa on the underside of the liver (see Fig. 8–2) and is capable of holding 50 ml (2 oz) of bile. Attached to the liver above, to the peritoneum, and to blood vessels, the gallbladder is divided into four parts: the fundus (broad inferior end), the body (funnel-shaped and bound to the duodenum), the neck (which empties into the cystic duct), and the infundibulum, which lies between the body and the neck and sags to form Hartmann's pouch (Fig. 8–4). The hepatic artery supplies both the cystic and hepatic ducts with blood; the blood then drains out of the gallbladder through the cystic vein. Lymph vessels in the submucosal layer also drain the gallbladder and the head of the pancreas.

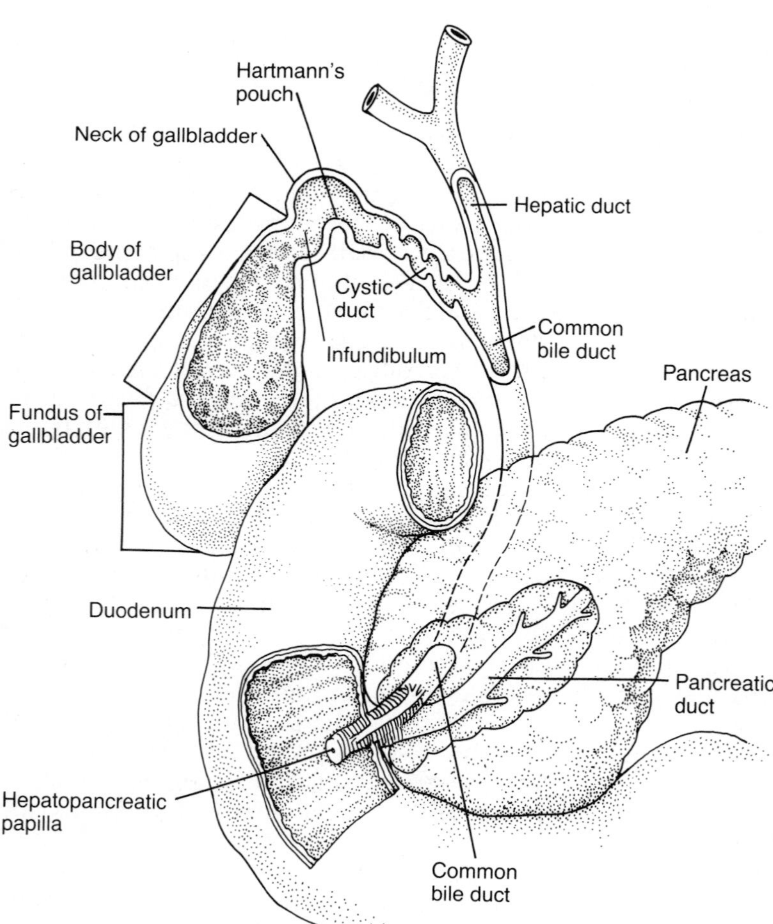

Figure 8–4. The gallbladder and its divisions: fundus, body, infundibulum, and neck. Obstruction of either the hepatic or common bile duct by stone or spasm blocks the exit of bile from the liver, where it is formed, and prevents bile from ejecting into the duodenum.

Function

The biliary duct system provides a passage for bile from the liver to the intestine and regulates the bile flow. The gallbladder itself collects, concentrates, and stores bile. After the ingestion of fats, the gallbladder contracts and empties its contents into the common bile duct that leads into the duodenum. The normally functioning gallbladder also removes water and electrolytes from hepatic bile, increases the concentration of the larger solutes, and lowers bile pH below 7.0.

Bile helps by alkalinizing the intestinal contents and plays a role in the emulsification, absorption, and digestion of fat. Its chief constituents are conjugated bile salts, cholesterol, phospholipid, bilirubin, and electrolytes. The bile salts emulsify fats by breaking up large fat globules into smaller ones so that they can be acted on by the fat-splitting enzymes of the intestine and pancreas. A healthy liver produces bile according to the body's needs and does not require stimulation by drugs. Infection or disease of the liver, inflammation of the gallbladder, or any obstruction such as the presence of gallstones can interfere with the flow of bile into the duodenum (Miller and Keane, 1987).

In gallbladder disease, bile becomes more alkaline, altering bile salts and cholesterol and predisposing the organ to stone formation. With liver damage, normal bile formation is compromised and affects the digestion and absorption of fats. The patient often has an intolerance to fatty foods, anorexia, nausea, vomiting, flatulence (excess gas in the stomach or intestines), and diarrhea or constipation (Alyn, 1982).

PRIMARY SIGNS AND SYMPTOMS OF LIVER DISEASE (Nursing 81, 1981)

- Sense of fullness of the abdomen
- Anorexia, nausea, and vomiting
- Jaundice (a result of increased serum bilirubin levels)
- Ascites (abnormal accumulation of serous fluid in the peritoneal cavity)
- Edema and oliguria (reduced urine secretion in relation to fluid intake)
- Right upper quadrant (RUQ) abdominal pain
- Right shoulder pain
- Neurologic symptoms
    - Confusion
    - Muscle tremors
    - Asterixis (motor disturbance resembling body or extremity flapping)*
- Pallor (often linked to cirrhosis or carcinoma)
- Bleeding disorders
    - Purpura (blood under the skin and through the mucous membranes that appears deep red or purple)
    - Ecchymosis (bruises)
- Spider angiomas (branched dilatation of the superficial capillaries resembling a spider)†
- Palmar erythema (redness of the skin over the palms)
- Light-colored or clay-colored feces

LIVER AND BILIARY PATHOPHYSIOLOGY

Taking a careful patient history and making close observations of the patient's physical condition can detect telltale signs of hepatic disease.

---

* To test for asterixis (flapping tremor), ask the patient to raise both arms, with wrists flexed and fingers extended. Watch for quick, irregular extensions and flexions of the wrists and fingers when the wrists are held out straight and the hands are flexed upward (Nursing 81, 1981).

† Both spider angiomas and palmar erythema occur as a result of increased estrogen levels normally detoxified by the liver.

PRIMARY SIGNS AND SYMPTOMS OF GALLBLADDER DISEASE

- Right upper abdominal and epigastric pain
- Jaundice (result of blockage of the common bile duct)
- Fever, chills
- Indigestion
- Nausea
- Intolerance of fatty foods

Referred Shoulder Pain

Referred shoulder pain may be the only presenting symptom of hepatic or biliary disease. Sympathetic fibers from the biliary system are connected through the celiac and splanchnic plexuses to the hepatic fibers in the region of the dorsal spine. These connections account for the intercostal and radiating interscapular pain that accompanies gallbladder disease (see Fig. 8–5, page 204). Although the innervation is bilateral, most of the biliary fibers reach the cord through the right splanchnic nerves producing pain in the right shoulder (Given and Simmons, 1979; Way, 1983).

Diagnosis of liver or gallbladder disease is made by x-ray or ultrasonic scan of the gallbladder and CT scan of the abdomen including the liver. Gallstones (cholelith) located in the gallbladder or in the bile ducts consist of cholesterol crystals, fragments of bacteria, and calcium and can be related to an increased serum cholesterol and high dietary fat intake.

Jaundice (Miller and Keane, 1987)

Jaundice (icterus) is not a disease. It is a symptom of a number of different diseases and disorders of the liver and gallbladder that causes yellowness of skin, sclerae, mucous membranes, and excretions. The change in color is due to staining by the bile pigment, bilirubin (hyperbilirubinemia). Normally, the liver cells absorb the bilirubin and secrete it along with other bile constituents. If the liver is diseased, or if the flow of bile is obstructed, or if destruction of erythrocytes is excessive, the bilirubin accumulates in the blood and eventually produces jaundice.

It may be the first, and sometimes the only, manifestation of disease (Schiff, 1983). It is usually first noticeable in the eyes when the concentration of serum bilirubin exceeds 2 mg/100 ml, although it may come on so gradually that it is not immediately noticed by those in daily contact with the jaundiced person.

Dark urine and light stools associated with jaundice occurs when the bilirubin level increases from a normal value of less than 1 milligram per deciliter (mg/dl: deciliter = 100 ml) to a value of 2 or 3 mg/dl. When bilirubin reaches this level, the sclera of the eye takes on a yellow hue. When the bilirubin level reaches 5 to 6 mg/dl, the skin becomes yellow. The liver's function to metabolize bilirubin from the blood is impaired by any damage to the liver. Impairment of liver function caused by cirrhosis (chronic disease of the liver), liver cancer, or infection/inflammation of the liver results in jaundice. Normally, bile causes the stool to assume a brown color. Light-colored stools (almost white) and urine the color of tea or cola indicate an inability of the liver or biliary system to properly excrete bilirubin. These changes in urine, stool, or skin color may be caused by hepatitis, gallstones, or pancreatic cancer blocking the bile duct, cirrhosis, or hepatotoxic medications.

Causes of Jaundice

The causes of jaundice are numerous including:

- Hereditary forms
- Drug-induced hepatitis
- Alcoholic hepatitis
- Acute or chronic hepatitis
- Viral hepatitis
- Cirrhosis
- Biliary tract obstruction
  - Common duct stone
  - Neoplasm
  - Common duct stricture (previous gallbladder surgery)

Classifications of Jaundice

Jaundice may be caused by a wide range of disorders that result in the excessive accumulation of bilirubin in the blood serum. Jaundice can be classified broadly according to where the pathologic events that cause the jaundice take place.

Prehepatic. In the prehepatic state, bilirubin increases before it reaches the liver as a result of overproduction of bilirubin secondary to hemolysis (destruction of RBCs) (Luckmann and Sorenson, 1987).

Intrahepatic. In the *intrahepatic* state, bilirubin increases as a result of pathology within the liver itself. This pathology may include hepatocellular diseases (e.g., viral or drug-induced hepatitis), metabolic and infiltrative disorders (e.g., anorexia or metastatic tumors), immaturity of the liver conjugating system (e.g., neonatal jaundice), or disorders of the intrahepatic biliary system (e.g., primary biliary cirrhosis) (Ockner, 1988).

Extrahepatic. Extrahepatic jaundice occurs when bilirubin increases due to a problem occurring after the bilirubin leaves the liver. This may occur with large bile duct obstruction, such as bile duct strictures, gallstones, pancreatitis, and tumors, that affects the ducts themselves or important adjacent structures (Ockner, 1988).

Conjugated or Unconjugated. In addition, jaundice can also be categorized according to whether the bilirubin is primarily conjugated or unconjugated. Those pathologies that develop due to excessive bilirubin or to defective conjugation of bilirubin in the liver result in *unconjugated hyperbilirubinemia.* The pathologies related to improper excretion of bilirubin from the liver or to obstructed flow of bile from outside the liver result in *conjugated hyperbilirubinemia.* Thus, a logical first step in the physician's diagnosis of a jaundiced patient is to determine whether the bilirubin is predominantly conjugated or unconjugated. This determination can be done by both urine and blood serum testing (Andreoli et al, 1986). It is interesting to note that there are situations in which more than one mechanism may be responsible for jaundice in the same patient.

Clinical History and Observations

A careful history and close observation of the patient are important in determining whether a person may need a medical referral for possible jaundice. Jaundice in the postoperative patient is not uncommon, but may be a potentially serious complication of surgery and anesthesia. Clinical management of jaundice is complicated by anything capable of damaging the liver including stress, hypoxemia, blood loss, infection, and administration of multiple drugs. The following factors are considered when evaluating the clinical history and observations (Sherlock, 1985):

- *Occupation:* employment involving alcoholic consumption; contact with rats carrying Weil's disease, (a type of Mediterranean jaundice)
- *Place of origin:* Mediterranean, Africa, Far East (may suggest carriage of hepatitis B antigen)
- *Personal/family history:* history of jaundice, hepatitis, anemia, splenectomy, cholecystectomy
- *Contact with jaundiced persons:* dialysis patients, drug abusers, homosexuals, prostitutes
- *Injections* within the last 6 months: blood tests, drug abuse, tuberculosis testing, dental treatment, tatoo (receiving or removal), blood or plasma transfusion
- *Consumption of shellfish*
- *Previous travel* to areas where hepatitis is endemic (present in a community at all times)
- *Onset* is important in determining the type
  - Viral hepatitis
    - Nausea
    - Anorexia
    - Aversion to smoking for smokers
    - Sudden onset (develops in a matter of hours)
  - Cholestatic
    - Slow onset
    - Persistent pruritus (itching)
    - Dark urine and light stools preceding illness

- *Age and sex:*
  Incidence of type A hepatitis decreases with age (most commonly seen in children)
  No age is exempt from type B hepatitis and non-A, non-B hepatitis
  Probability of cancerous biliary obstruction occurring increases with age
- *Skin color:*
  Mild yellow—hemolytic jaundice (rupture of RBCs with the release of hemoglobin into the blood plasma)
  Orange—hepatocellular jaundice (involving liver directly)
  Green hue—Prolonged biliary obstruction
- *Mental state:* hepatocellular jaundice
  Slight intellectual deterioration
  Mild personality change
  Flapping tremor may indicate developing hepatic coma

Kernicterus (Van Dyke et al, 1982)

Kernicterus (hyperbilirubinemia in the newborn) or physiologic jaundice of the newborn occurs as a result of increased bilirubin in the system. Maximum serum bilirubin concentration (mean 6 to 8 mg/dl) occurs at 3 to 4 days of age, at which time a mild condition of jaundice may occur in approximately 50% of all healthy full-term newborns. The incidence of jaundice is higher with premature newborns.

The cause of this condition is multifactorial. The liver is one of the last organs to mature and function fully. During the first few days of life, the liver cannot conjugate (the joining of a toxic substance with some natural substance of the body to form a detoxified product for elimination from the body) bilirubin efficiently due to the deficiency of the required liver enzyme. The unconjugated bilirubin cannot be excreted into the intestine, thus build-up of bilirubin in the bloodstream causes the characteristic yellow skin of jaundice. This is especially true with premature infants who have an even more undeveloped liver.

Other factors include accelerated RBC breakdown, impaired hepatic uptake, increased conjugation with excretion of bilirubin by the neonatal liver, and enhanced circulation of bilirubin. Kernicterus may occur in the case of mother/infant blood group incompatibility. For example, if the mother has A+ blood type and the neonate has O+, the baby carries the mother's antibodies to the infant's O+ blood. These antibodies break down the infant's RBCs (hemolysis), releasing large amounts of bilirubin into the blood that the immature liver of the newborn cannot handle. Exchange transfusion (mechanical removal of the baby's blood and replacement with fresh blood) is the treatment for blood group incompatibility.

Finally, it is generally accepted that the use of oxytocin approximately doubles the incidence of neonatal hyperbilirubinemia and increases its severity in a dose-related manner. Studies have shown that infants born after oxytocin-induced labor exhibit enhanced osmotic fragility of RBCs (Singhi and Singh, 1979). The antidiuretic effects of oxytocin, along with the large amounts of electrolyte-free dextrose solutions used to administer it, cause osmotic swelling of RBCs and thus, more rapid destruction of the cells with resultant hyperbilirubinemia (Buchan, 1979).

Physiologic jaundice does not require treatment, but at 13 mg/dl of bilirubin, the effect of too much bilirubin in the bloodstream can cause irreversible brain damage called *kernicterus.*

Phototherapy will be initiated for the newborn. This exposure to prolonged irradiation with visible blue light modifies bilirubin into a water-soluble form, helps the reabsorption process, and facilitates excretion of bilirubin. At 20 mg/dl, a partial or complete exchange via a blood transfusion may be required to prevent potential brain damage; even with the exchange, subsequent neurologic involvement including motor delays are not uncommon (Ross Laboratories, 1983).

Liver Diseases

Viral Hepatitis (Alyn, 1982; Miller and Keane, 1987; Nursing 81, 1981)

Hepatitis is an inflammation of the liver. Viral hepatitis is an acute infectious inflammation caused by one of three different forms of hepatitis: hepatitis A virus (infectious hepatitis), hepatitis B virus (serum or long-incubation hepatitis), and non-A, non-B (NANB) hepatitis. These three forms of hepatitis are caused by different viruses, have different incubation periods, and have different modes of transmission. However, they manifest similar symptoms and pathologic changes within the hepatic tissue.

Hepatitis is a major uncontrolled public health problem for several reasons: All the causative agents have not been identified, there are no specific therapeutic drugs for its treatment, its incidence has increased in relation to illicit drug use, and it can be communicated before the appearance of observable clinical symptoms. It is spread easily to others and usually results in an extended period of convalescence with loss of time from school or work.

There is a vaccine available that is used to provide active immunity against type B hepatitis for people considered to be at high risk (e.g., physicians, dentists, nurses, aides, laboratory technicians, immunocompromised patients, dialysis patients, household members in close contact with a patient with hepatitis, homosexually active men, prostitutes, and drug addicts). A vaccine for hepatitis A is under investigation. Immune serum globulin (ISG), referred to as gamma globulin, has been found to be 80 to 90% effective in producing passive immunity (i.e., by transferring antibodies) for 3 to 4 months to type A hepatitis when administered promptly (as soon as possible after exposure, but within 2 weeks after the onset of jaundice).

Hepatitis affects patients in three stages: the initial or preicteric stage, the icteric or jaundiced stage, and the recovery period. During the *initial stage,* which lasts for 1 to 3 weeks, the patient experiences vague gastrointestinal (GI) and general body symptoms. Fatigue, malaise, lassitude, weight loss, and anorexia are common. Many people develop an aversion to food, alcohol, and cigarettes. Nausea, vomiting, diarrhea, arthralgias, and influenza-like symptoms may occur. The liver becomes enlarged and tender, and intermittent pruritus may develop. One to 4 days before the icteric stage, the urine darkens and the stool lightens as less bilirubin is conjugated and excreted.

The *icteric stage* is characterized by the appearance of jaundice, which peaks in 1 to 2 weeks and persists for 6 to 8 weeks. During this stage, the acuteness of the inflammation subsides. The GI symptoms begin to disappear, and after 1 to 2 weeks of jaundice, the liver decreases in size and becomes less tender. During the icteric stage, the postcervical lymph nodes and spleen are enlarged. Persons who have been treated with human ISG may not develop jaundice.

The *recovery stage* lasts for 3 to 4 months, during which time the patient generally feels well, but fatigues easily.

Acute: Hepatitis A Virus (HAV). HAV primarily affects children and young adults and is highly contagious through close personal contact (Table 8–1). It is commonly found in environments in which there is poor sanitation and overcrowding, such as in day-care centers, schools, and similar institutions. The most common cause is ingestion of contaminated food, water, or milk. Outbreaks of HAV often occur after people have eaten seafood from polluted water.

HAV is highly contagious, and infection depends on exposure to viruses from an infected person; the primary mode of transmission is the oral-fecal route.* The peak viral excretion occurs during the 2-week period before the onset of jaundice and before the infected person becomes clinically ill. Thus, the greatest danger of infection is during the incubation period when the person is probably unaware that the virus is present.

CLINICAL SIGNS AND SYMPTOMS OF HEPATITIS A

Hepatitis A is often acquired in childhood as a mild infection with symptoms similar to the "flu" and may be

---

* The oral-fecal route of transmission occurs primarily due to poor or improper handwashing and personal hygiene, particularly after using the lavatory and then handling food for public consumption. This route of transmission may also occur through the shared use of oral utensils, such as straws, silverware, and toothbrushes.

misdiagnosed or ignored. It does not usually cause lasting damage to the liver, although the following symptoms may persist for weeks:

- Extreme fatigue
- Anorexia
- Fever
- Arthragias and myalgias (generalized aching)
- Right upper abdominal pain
- Clay-colored stools
- Dark urine
- Icterus (jaundice)
- Headache
- Pharyngitis
- Alterations in the senses of taste and smell
- Loss of desire to smoke or drink alcohol

Table 8–1. HEPATITIS

Type	Source	Incubation Period	Course	Signs and Symptoms
A (hepatitis A virus)	Raw shellfish contaminated by sewage	20–37 days* (15–49 days)	Does not progress to chronic liver disease	Mental and physical fatigue Nausea and vomiting Diarrhea RUQ pain Headache Arthralgias
	Oral contact with fecal material			
	Water			Influenza-like symptoms: fever, cough, sore throat Hives or skin rash Clay-colored stools Dark-colored urine Jaundice Pain over the liver, especially after exercise
B (hepatitis B virus)	Blood products†	60–110 days (25–160)	10% develop chronic liver disease	Low-grade fever Mental and physical fatigue Nausea, anorexia, vomiting Diarrhea RUQ pain Headache Arthralgias Symptoms worse than type A Hives or skin rash Pain over liver especially after exercise
	Syringes and needles‡			
	Vaginal or anal intercourse			
	Saliva			
	Breast milk			
	Vertical transmission: perinatal			
Non-A	Blood transfusions	35–70 days (21–84)	10–40% develop chronic liver diseae	Mental and physical fatigue Nausea, anorexia, vomiting
	Syringes and needles			
Non-B (virus other than hepatitis A or B)	Vertical transmission: perinatal			RUQ pain Headache Arthralgias Hives or skin rash

* Usual range with outside limits given in parentheses.
† Including inoculation with contaminated syringe or contaminated blood products.
‡ Including sharing of needles among drug addicts, scarification in primitive tribes, acupuncture.

Studies have been conducted dealing with the natural history of acute hepatitis and have provided perspective on the frequency of skin and joint manifestations in these infections (Stewart et al, 1978). More than one third of the adults studied had joint pains during the course of their illness. There was no difference in the incidence of these symptoms between hepatitis B surface antigen (HBsAg)-positive and HBsAg-negative patients, although the duration of joint symptoms was slightly longer (more than 2 weeks) in patients who were HBsAg-positive.* Examination of the HBsAg-negative patients showed a strong association between arthralgia and the age of the patient (Table 8–2), the frequency of this symptom increasing with age. Joint pains affected only 18% of children compared with 45% of adults over 30 years of age (Gocke, 1982).

Treatment is primarily symptomatic, and bedrest is recommended for patients who are jaundiced in order to avoid complications from liver damage. Hospitalization may be required for anyone who has excessive vomiting and subsequent fluid and electrolyte imbalance. In most patients, there is total recovery with lifelong immunity to type A hepatitis thereafter.

Acute: Hepatitis B Virus (HBV). HBV is generally transmitted parenterally or, in other words, by some method other than through the intestine, such as by subcutaneous, intramuscular, or intravenous means. This can occur for example, when the blood of an infected human comes in contact with the blood or mucous membrane of another person. Posttransfusion hepatitis may occur after the transfusion of blood or blood products (e.g., commercially prepared plasma). HBV can also be spread through contact with human secretions (e.g., tears, saliva, semen, feces, urine, menstrual secretions) which qualifies it as being a sexually transmitted disease passed along to others either by heterosexual or homosexual intercourse. A third method of transmission is called *vertical transmission* by which an infant is infected by its mother either during pregnancy or after birth (see Table 8–1).

Whereas type A has usually been eliminated from the body by the time jaundice appears, the body is not always able to rid itself of HBV and the virus can persist in body fluids indefinitely. Nurses, physicians, laboratory technicians, blood-bank workers, and dentists are frequent victims of HBV, often as a result of wearing defective gloves while working. Persons who are carriers of the disease are not only a threat to others, but also they themselves are at risk for chronic hepatitis, cirrhosis of the liver, and primary hepatocellular carcinoma. Approximately 10% of infected persons become carriers, but the greater risk for spread of the disease comes from commercially prepared clotting concentrates derived from plasma of commercial donors. Widespread use of screening tests of donor blood has reduced this problem, but not eliminated it.

Type B viral hepatitis follows a course similar to that of type A. The onset, however, is usually insidious, whereas type A has an abrupt

* Serologic profiles reflecting the presence or absence of characteristic markers for HAV and HBV in serum are now well standardized and practical for diagnosing and monitoring viral hepatitis. HBsAg-positive and HBsAg-negative are two of those markers (Overby, 1982).

Table 8–2. ASSOCIATION OF ARTHRALGIA WITH AGE IN HBsAg NEGATIVE PATIENTS

Age (yrs)	No Arthralgia	Arthralgia	Total	% Suffering From Arthralgia
0–14	95	21	116	18
15–29	96	41	137	30
>30	56	45	101	45
Total	247	107	354	30

* From Stewart, J.S., Farrow, L.J., Clifford, R.E., et al: A three-year survey of viral hepatitis in West London. Q. J. Medicine, *187*:365, 1978.

onset. Type B differs from type A in the degree of sickness and number of symptoms. Type B occurs less frequently and has a higher mortality rate than type A.

> **CLINICAL SIGNS AND SYMPTOMS OF HEPATITIS B**
>
> Hepatitis B may be asymptomatic but can include:
>
> - Jaundice
> - Arthralgias
> - Rash

Acute: Non-A, Non-B Hepatitis. About 85% of all cases of viral hepatitis can be traced to either HAV or HBV. The remaining 10 to 15% are caused by at least one and possibly several other types of viruses classified together under the term NANB hepatitis. Clinically, NANB hepatitis is similar to type B hepatitis (see Table 8–1). It can develop into chronic hepatitis and is often associated with blood transfusions. NANB hepatitis accounts for 60 to 90% of post-transfusion hepatitis in the United States and usually results from commercial blood donations rather than from a volunteer donor.

Chronic Hepatitis (Miller and Keane, 1987). Chronic hepatitis is used to describe an illness associated with prolonged inflammation of the liver after unresolved viral hepatitis or *chronic active hepatitis* (CAH) of unknown etiology. "Chronic" is defined as inflammation of the liver for 6 months or more. The symptoms and biochemical abnormalities may continue for months or years. It is divided by findings on liver biopsy into CAH and *chronic persistent hepatitis* (CPH).

Chronic Active Hepatitis. This type of hepatitis refers to seriously destructive liver disease that can result in cirrhosis. CAH is often a result of viral infection (HBV or NANB but not due to HAV), but can also be secondary to drug sensitivity (e.g., methyldopa [Aldomet], an antihypertensive medication and isoniazid [INH], an antitubercular drug). Steroid therapy is sometimes recommended for patients with evidence of aggressive liver inflammation and necrosis (identified by liver biopsy) as a result of these drugs.

If left untreated, the course of patients with CAH is unpredictable and may range from progressive deterioration of liver function to spontaneous remissions and exacerbations (Boyer and Miller, 1982). In untreated cases, the mortality from CAH can be as high as 50% within 3 to 5 years.

> **CLINICAL SIGNS AND SYMPTOMS OF CHRONIC ACTIVE HEPATITIS**
>
> The clinical signs and symptoms of chronic active hepatitis may range from asymptomatic to the patient who is bedridden with cirrhosis and advanced hepatocellular failure. In the latter, the prominent signs and symptoms may reflect multisystem involvement including:
>
> - Fatigue
> - Jaundice
> - Abdominal pain
> - Anorexia
> - Arthralgia
> - Fever
> - Splenomegaly and hepatomegaly
> - Weakness
> - Ascites
> - Hepatic encephalopathy

Chronic Persistent Hepatitis. This type of hepatitis occurs most commonly secondary to a viral infection (usually hepatitis B or NANB hepatitis). Many patients with CPH are asymptomatic and appear to be healthy or have only minor complaints. Episodes of acute illness are infrequent, and the prognosis for recovery is good (Koff and Galambos, 1982). No treatment is necessary because the condition slowly resolves on its own. CPH is generally considered benign, usually asymptomatic, anicteric (without jaundice), and without progression to cirrhosis.

CLINICAL SIGNS AND SYMPTOMS OF CHRONIC PERSISTENT HEPATITIS

- RUQ pain
- Anorexia
- Mild fatigue
- Malaise

Nonviral Hepatitis (Nursing 81, 1981; Zimmerman and Maddrey, 1982)

Nonviral hepatitis is a form of liver inflammation that occurs secondary to exposure to certain chemicals or drugs. It is considered to be a toxic or drug-induced hepatitis from which most patients recover without serious complications. Specific chemical hepatotoxins may include carbon tetrachloride, trichloroethylene, poisonous mushrooms (*Amanita phalloides* and related species, rare in the United States but more common in Europe), alcohol (most common in the United States) and vinyl chloride. Careful questioning of patients regarding occupational exposure to these toxins is important.

Drug-induced hepatitis occurs after the administration of one of various drugs to patients who demonstrate a hypersensitivity reaction. Whereas toxic hepatitis appears to affect all people indiscriminately, drug-induced hepatitis occurs only in a small number of people. The drugs that may cause hepatitis include (Overby, 1982):

- Acetaminophen (suicide attempts)
- Thiazide diuretics (rare)
- Halothane (anesthetic)
- Sulfonamides (antibiotic)
- Isoniazid (a tuberculosis chemotherapeutic)
- Chlorpromazine (psychotropic)
- Oral contraceptives
- Methyldopa (antihypertensive)
- Diphenylhydantoin (anticonvulsant)

A number of other anti-inflammatory and minor analgesic agents have caused hepatic injury (Table 8–3). Again, the mechanism by which these agents induce overt injury is clearly unusual susceptibility of individual patients (i.e., the adverse effects are idiosyncratic reactions) (Zimmerman, 1978). Some drugs (e.g., oral contraceptives) may impair liver function and produce jaundice without causing necrosis, fatty infiltration of liver cells, or a hypersensitive reaction.

Table 8–3. COMMON HEPATOTOXIC DRUGS

Drug or Drug Type	Clinical Uses
Tetracyclines	Antibiotic
Cytotoxic drugs	Antineoplastic
Acetaminophen	Analgesic/antipyretic
Tannic acid	Astringent
Aspirin	Anti-inflammatory/analgesic/antipyretic
Monoamine oxidase inhibitors	Antidepressant
Chlorpromazine and other phenothiazines	Antipsychotic
Oxacillin sodium	Antibiotic
Halothane	Gas anesthetic
Isoniazid	Antitubercular
Aminosalicylic acid	Antitubercular
Rifampin	Antibiotic
Erythromycin estolate	Antibiotic
Oral contraceptives	Contraceptive
Anabolic steroids	Anticatabolic/increase hemoglobin
Novobiocin	Antibiotic
Chloramphenicol	Antibiotic
Radiographic contrast agents	Diagnostic testing

CLINICAL SIGNS AND SYMPTOMS OF TOXIC AND DRUG-INDUCED HEPATITIS

Clinical signs and symptoms of toxic and drug-induced hepatitis vary with the severity of liver damage and causative agent. In most patients, symptoms resemble those of acute viral hepatitis:

- Anorexia, nausea, vomiting
- Fatigue and malaise
- Jaundice
- Dark urine
- Clay-colored stools
- Headache, dizziness, drowsiness (carbon tetrachloride poisoning)
- Fever, rash, arthralgias, epigastric or RUQ pain (halothane anesthetic)

Cirrhosis

Cirrhosis is a chronic hepatic disease characterized by the destruction of liver cells and by the replacement of connective tissue by fibrous bands. As the liver becomes more and more scarred (fibrosed), blood and lymph flow becomes impaired and causes hepatic insufficiency and increased clinical manifestations. The causes of cirrhosis can be varied, although alcohol is the most common cause of liver disease in the United States. The following list describes the primary causes of cirrhosis:

- Alcoholic cirrhosis (Laennec's cirrhosis)
- Biliary cirrhosis (caused by any bile duct disease that suppresses bile flow)
- Posthepatic cirrhosis
- Cardiac cirrhosis (rare form resulting from right ventricular failure)
- Pigment cirrhosis (as a result of hemochromatosis, a disorder of iron metabolism)
- Idiopathic cirrhosis (unknown causes account for approximately 10% of patients)

EARLY CLINICAL SIGNS AND SYMPTOMS OF CIRRHOSIS

- Mild RUQ pain (progressive)
- GI symptoms
  - Anorexia
  - Indigestion
  - Weight loss
  - Nausea and vomiting
  - Diarrhea or constipation
- Dull abdominal ache
- Ease of fatigue (with mild exertion)
- Weakness
- Fever

The activity level of the patient with cirrhosis is determined by the symptoms. Because hepatic blood flow diminishes with moderate exercise, rest periods are advised and are adjusted according to the level of fatigue experienced by the patient both during the exercise and afterwards at home. The person may return to work with medical approval, but is advised to avoid straining, such as lifting heavy objects, if portal hypertension and esophageal varices are a problem. Because stress decreases hepatic blood flow, any reduction of stress at home, at work, or during treatment is therapeutic (Alyn, 1982).

Portal Hypertension. As the cirrhosis progresses and hepatic insufficiency and portal hypertension occur, late symptoms that affect the entire body develop (Table 8–4). Portal hypertension is the elevated pressure in the portal vein (through which blood passes from the GI tract and spleen to the liver). As the blood meets increased resistance from fibrotic tissue, portal pressure rises and the blood backs up into the spleen. The blood then bypasses the liver through collateral vessels.

SIGNS AND SYMPTOMS OF PORTAL HYPERTENSION

- Ascites (abnormal collection of fluid in the peritoneal cavity)
- Dilated collateral veins
  - Esophageal varices (upper GI)
  - Hemorrhoids (lower GI)
- Splenomegaly (enlargement of the spleen)
- Thrombocytopenia (decreased number of blood platelets for clotting)

Table 8–4. CLINICAL MANIFESTATIONS OF CIRRHOSIS

Body System	Clinical Manifestations
Respiratory	Limited thoracic expansion (due to ascites) Hypoxia Dyspnea Cyanosis Clubbing
Central nervous system (CNS) (progressive to hepatic coma)	Subtle changes in mental acuity (progressive) Mild memory loss Poor reasoning ability Irritability Paranoia and hallucinations Slurred speech Asterixis (tremor of outstretched hands) Peripheral neuritis Peripheral muscle atrophy
Hematologic	Impaired coagulation/bleeding tendencies Nosebleeds Easy bruising Bleeding gums Anemia (usually caused by GI blood loss from esophageal varices)
Endocrine (due to liver's inability to metabolize hormones)	Testicular atrophy Menstrual irregularities Gynecomastia (excessive development of breasts in the man) Loss of chest and axillary hair
Integument (cutaneous and skin)	Severe pruritus (itching) Extreme dryness Poor tissue turgor Abnormal pigmentation Prominent spider angiomas (benign tumor made up of blood vessels) Palmar erythema (redness caused by extensive collection of arteriovenous anastomoses) Jaundice
Hepatic	Hepatomegaly (enlargement of the liver) Ascites Edema of the legs Hepatic encephalopathy
Gastrointestinal (GI)	Anorexia Nausea Vomiting Diarrhea

Ascites. Ascites is an abnormal accumulation of serous (edematous) fluid within the peritoneal cavity. In portal and venous hepatic hypertension, there is increased pressure within the sinusoids and hepatic veins (see Fig. 8–2). As the pressure increases, there is movement of protein-rich plasma filtrate into the hepatic lymphatics. Some fluid enters the thoracic duct, but if the pressure is high enough, the excess fluid will ooze from the surface of the liver into the peritoneal cavity.

The liver is the only organ that synthesizes albumin, a plasma protein. Albumin maintains colloid osmotic pressure in the vasculature. With decreased albumin, the plasma colloid osmotic pressure is decreased, allowing fluid to escape to the interstitial fluid spaces. Likewise, because this fluid has a high colloidal osmotic pressure owing to its high protein content, it is not readily reabsorbed from the peritoneal cavity (Miller and Keane, 1987). This shift of fluid is noticeable as edema in dependent locations, such as the ankles, and fluid accumulates in the abdomen (ascites) (Alyn, 1982).

For the physical therapist, the development of abdominal hernias and lumbar lordosis observed in patients with ascites may present symptoms mimicking musculoskeletal involvement, such as groin or low back pain.

Esophageal Varices. Esophageal varices are dilated veins of the lower esophagus that develop when hepatic fibrosis compresses hepatic veins impeding outflow through the vena cava and increasing portal pressure. These thin-walled vessels accommodate portal circulation poorly and become dilated, causing rupture with subsequent hemorrhaging. The hemorrhage occurs because of two underlying pathophysiologic processes: the diseased liver fails to produce blood clotting factors and the increased portal hypertension predisposes the patient to peptic ulceration and hemorrhage. Additionally, alcohol is toxic to gastric mucosa and can induce hemorrhagic gastritis (Purtilo, 1989). Esophageal varices are, in terms of hospitalization and ultimate mortality, the single most significant complication of cirrhosis (Conn, 1982; Gitnick, 1982). Hemorrhage from esophageal varices almost always occurs in cirrhotic patients with ascites and often occurs when the abdomen is tightly distended.

CLINICAL SIGNS AND SYMPTOMS TO INDICATE HEMORRHAGE ASSOCIATED WITH ESOPHAGEAL VARICES

- Restlessness
- Pallor
- Tachycardia
- Cooling of the skin
- Hypotension

Hepatic Encephalopathy (Hepatic Coma) (Nursing 81, 1981; Popper and Schaffner, 1974)

Hepatic encephalopathy leading to coma is a neurologic condition that occurs secondary to chronic liver disease. Any disease of the liver that becomes destructive of liver parenchyma or results in abnormal shunting of blood around functioning liver tissue may predispose the patient to hepatic encephalopathy (Zieve, 1982). Ammonia from the intestine (produced by protein breakdown) is normally transformed by the liver to urea, glutamine, and asparagine. When portal blood shunts past the liver, ammonia directly enters the systemic circulation and is carried to the brain. The excess of ammonia reaches the brain as a result of reduced hepatic function or of the bypass of blood around the liver parenchyma. Other factors that predispose to rising ammonia levels include:

- Excessive protein intake
- Excessive accumulation of nitrogenous body wastes (constipation, GI hemorrhage)
- Bacterial action on protein and urea to form ammonia
- Fluid and electrolyte abnormalities
- Sedatives, tranquilizers, narcotic analgesics
- Severe infection (bacterial pneumonia, pyelonephritis, septicemia [blood poisoning], spontaneous bacterial peritonitis)

Clinical manifestations of hepatic encephalopathy vary, depending on the severity of neurologic involvement, and develop in four stages as the ammonia level increases in the serum with the following accompanying clinical features:

Prodromal Stage (Stage I) (subtle symptoms that may be overlooked)

- Slight personality changes
    - Disorientation, confusion
    - Euphoria or depression
    - Forgetfulness
    - Slurred speech
- Slight tremor
- Muscular incoordination
- Impaired handwriting

Impending Stage (Stage II)

- Tremor progresses to asterixis
- Resistance to passive movement (increased muscle tone)

- Lethargy
- Aberrant behavior
- Apraxia* (Nursing 88, 1988)
- Ataxia
- Facial grimacing and blinking

Stuporous Stage (Stage III) (patient can still be aroused)

- Hyperventilation
- Marked confusion
- Abusive and violent
- Noisy, incoherent speech
- Asterixis
- Muscle rigidity
- Positive Babinski reflex†
- Hyperactive deep tendon reflexes

Comatose Stage (Stage IV) (patient cannot be aroused, responds only to painful stimuli)

- No asterixis
- Positive Babinski reflex
- Hepatic fetor (musty, sweet odor to the breath due to the liver's inability to metabolize the amino acid, methionine)

For the physical therapist, the inpatient with impending hepatic coma has difficulty in ambulating and is unsteady. Protection from falling and seizure precautions must be taken. Skin breakdown in a patient who is malnourished due to liver disease, immobile, jaundiced, and edematous can occur in less than 24 hours. Careful attention to skin care, passive exercise, and frequent changes in position are required.

Medical treatment involves a variety of possible measures including dietary measures, administration of neomycin, an antibacterial substance administered orally or by enema to eliminate ammonigenic substances from the GI tract. This cleansing produces osmotic diarrhea and prevents accumulation of amniogenic blood proteins (Nursing 84, 1984).

Liver Abscess (Nursing 81, 1981)

A liver abscess occurs when bacteria or protozoa destroy hepatic tissue and produce a cavity that fills with infectious organisms, liquified liver cells, and leukocytes. Necrotic tissue then isolates the cavity from the rest of the liver.

Whereas liver abscess is relatively uncommon, it carries a mortality of 30 to 50%. This rate rises to more than 80% with multiple abscesses and to more than 90% with complications such as rupture into the peritoneum, pleura, or pericardium.

CLINICAL SIGNS AND SYMPTOMS OF LIVER ABSCESS

Clinical signs and symptoms of liver abscess depend on the degree of involvement; some patients are acutely ill, others are asymptomatic. Depending on the type of abscess, the onset may be sudden or insidious. The most common signs include:

- Right abdominal pain
- Right shoulder pain
- Weight loss
- Fever, chills
- Diaphoresis
- Nausea and vomiting
- Anemia

Signs of right pleural effusion, such as dyspnea and pleural pain, develop if the abscess extends through the diaphragm. Extensive damage to the liver may cause jaundice. Treatment consists of long-term antibiotic therapy.

* This type of motor apraxia can be best observed by keeping a record of the patient's handwriting and drawings of simple shapes, such as a circle, square, triangle, rectangle. Check for progressive deterioration (Nursing 88, 1988).

† A reflex action of the toes normal during infancy, but abnormal after 12 to 18 months. It is elicited by a firm stimulus (usually scraping with the handle of a reflex hammer) on the sole of the foot from the heel along the lateral border of the sole to the little toe, across the ball of the foot to the big toe. Normally such a stimulus causes all the toes to flex downward. A positive Babinski reflex occurs when the great toe flexes upward and the smaller toes fan outward (Miller and Keane, 1987).

Liver Cancer

Metastatic tumors occur 20 times more often than primary liver tumors because the liver is one of the most common sites of metastasis from other primary cancers (e.g., colorectal, stomach, pancreas, esophagus, lung, breast). Although various sarcomas as well as lymphomas may originate in the liver, more than 98% of primary cancers of the liver are hepatomas, cholangiocellular carcinomas, or mixed types (Foster, 1982; Moertel, 1982). Persons with occupational exposure to vinyl chloride over a long period may develop liver angiosarcoma, a malignant tumor.

Primary liver tumors (hepatocellularcarcinoma [HCC]) are usually associated with cirrhosis, but can be linked to other predisposing factors (Nursing 84, 1984):

- Fungal infection (common in moldy foods of Africa)
- Viral hepatitis
- Excessive use of anabolic steroids
- Trauma
- Nutritional deficiencies
- Exposure to hepatotoxins

Several types of benign and malignant hepatic neoplasms can result from the administration of chemical agents. For example, adenoma (a benign tumor) can occur in recipients of oral contraceptives. Regression of the tumor occurs after withdrawal of the drug.

Interference with liver function does not occur until approximately 80 to 90% of the liver is replaced by metastatic carcinoma or primary carcinoma. Cholangiocarcinoma is a primary cancer that develops in bile ducts within the liver. Cholangiocarcinoma is not associated with cirrhosis, but both hepatocarcinoma and cholangiocarcinoma are fatal despite treatment with chemotherapy (Purtilo, 1989). Metastatic tumors to the liver originating in some organs (stomach, lung) never give rise to hepatic symptoms, whereas others produce hepatic symptoms or jaundice with less than 60% replacement of the liver. Certain tumors (colon, breast, melanoma) typically replace the 90% of liver mentioned before jaundice develops. Melanomas are associated with such minimal tissue reaction that almost complete hepatic replacement is required before hepatic symptoms develop (Edmondson and Peters, 1982).

About one half of the patients with hepatic metastases die without hepatic signs or symptoms (Edmondson and Peters, 1982).

CLINICAL SIGNS AND SYMPTOMS OF LIVER NEOPLASM

If clinical signs and symptoms of liver neoplasm do occur (whether of primary or metastatic origin), these may include:

- Jaundice (icterus)
- Progressive failure of health
- Anorexia and weight loss
- Overall muscular weakness
- Epigastric fullness and pain or discomfort
- Constant ache in the epigastrium or mid-back
- Early satiety (cystic tumors)

Gallbladder and Duct Disease

Cholelithiasis

Gallstones, or cholelithiasis, are stonelike masses called calculus, which form in the gallbladder possibly as a result of changes in the normal components of bile. The hepatic secretion of an excess quantity of cholesterol relative to bile salt and phospholipids creates a situation in which the gallbladder bile becomes supersaturated with cholesterol precipitating out to form stones. The exact mechanism by which this happens is not understood, but abnormal metabolism of cholesterol and bile salts is a possibility. Although there are two types of stones, pigment and cholesterol stones, most types of gallstone disease in the United States, Europe, and Africa are from cholesterol stones (Tan and Warren, 1982). Most cholesterol stones are not pure cholesterol, but a mixture of cholesterol, calcium salts, bile acids, fatty acids, protein, and phospholipids, with some fraction of bile pigment at the center (Nursing 84, 1984).

Cholelithiasis is the fifth leading cause of hospitalization among adults and accounts for 90% of all gallbladder and duct diseases. The risk factors to look for in a patient's history that correlate with the incidence of gallstones include the following (Tan and Warren, 1982):

- Age: incidence increases with age
- Sex: women affected more than men
- Elevated estrogen levels
    - Pregnancy
    - Oral contraceptives
    - Postmenopausal therapy
    - Multiparity (woman who has had two or more pregnancies resulting in viable offspring)
- Obesity
- Diet: high cholesterol, low fiber
- Diabetes mellitus
- Liver disease

Patients with gallstones may be asymptomatic or may present with symptoms of a gallbladder attack described in the next section. The prognosis is usually good with medical treatment, depending on the severity of disease, presence of infection, and response to antibiotics.

Cholecystitis

Cholecystitis, or inflammation of the gallbladder, may be acute or chronic and occurs as a result of gallstones impacted in the cystic duct (see Fig. 8–1), causing painful distention of the gallbladder. Other causes of acute cholecystitis may be typhoid fever or a malignant tumor obstructing the biliary tract. Whatever the cause of the obstruction, the normal flow of bile is interrupted and the gallbladder becomes distended and ischemic. The acute form is most common during middle age; the chronic form, among the elderly (Nursing 81, 1981).

Gallstones may also cause chronic cholecystitis (persistent gallbladder inflammation) in which the gallbladder atrophies and becomes fibrotic, adhering to adjacent organs. It is not unusual for patients to have repeated episodes before seeking medical attention (Miller and Keane, 1987). Prognosis for both acute and chronic cholecystitis is good with medical intervention, which may include controlling the symptoms with dietary measures (e.g., restrict fat and alcohol intake, eating smaller meals more often) or surgical removal of the gallbladder (cholecystectomy).

CLINICAL SIGNS AND SYMPTOMS OF ACUTE CHOLECYSTITIS

- Chills, low-grade fever
- Jaundice
- GI symptoms
    - Nausea
    - Anorexia
    - Vomiting
- Tenderness over the gallbladder
- Severe pain in the RUQ and epigastrium (increases on inspiration and movement)
- Pain radiating into the right shoulder and between the scapulae

CLINICAL SIGNS AND SYMPTOMS OF CHRONIC CHOLECYSTITIS

Clinical signs and symptoms of chronic cholecystitis may be vague or a sense of indigestion and abdominal discomfort after eating unless a stone leaves the gallbladder and causes obstruction of the common duct (called choledocholithiasis) causing:

- Biliary colic: severe, steady pain for 3 to 4 hours in RUQ
- Pain may radiate to the mid-back between the scapulae (due to splanchnic fibers synapsing with phrenic nerve fibers) (Nursing 84, 1984)
- Nausea (intolerance of fatty foods: decreased bile production results in decreased fat digestion)
- Abdominal fullness
- Heartburn
- Excessive belching
- Constipation and diarrhea

Primary Biliary Cirrhosis (Van Dyke et al, 1982)

Primary biliary cirrhosis (PBC) is a chronic, progressive, inflammatory disease of the liver that involves primarily the intrahepatic bile ducts and results in impairment of bile secretion. The disease, which often affects middle-aged women, begins with pruritus or biochemical evidence of cholestasis and progresses at a variable rate to jaundice, portal hypertension, and liver failure. The cause of PBC is unknown, although various factors are being investigated.

No specific treatment has been established yet for PBC (other than supportive measures) for the clinical symptoms described.

CLINICAL SIGNS AND SYMPTOMS OF PRIMARY BILIARY CIRRHOSIS

- Pruritus
- Jaundice
- GI bleeding
- Ascites
- Fatigue
- RUQ pain (posterior)
- Sensory neuropathy of hands/feet (rare)
- Osteoporosis (decreased bone mass)
- Osteomalacia (softening of the bones)

OVERVIEW OF LIVER/BILIARY PAIN PATTERNS

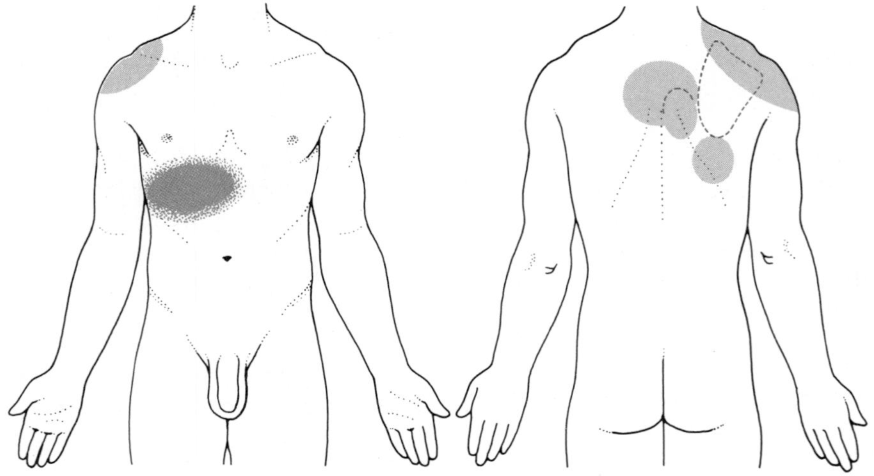

Figure 8–5. Pain from the liver, gallbladder, and common bile duct *(dark red)* occur typically in the midepigastrium or right upper quadrant of the abdomen with referred pain *(light red)* to the right shoulder, interscapular, or subscapular areas.

Liver

Pain

Location (Fig. 8–5):	Pain in the midepigastrium or RUQ of abdomen
	Pain over the liver, especially after exercise (hepatitis)
Referral:	RUQ pain may be associated with right shoulder pain
	Both RUQ and epigastrium pain may be associated with back pain between the scapulae
	Pain may be referred to the right side of the midline in the interscapular or subscapular area
Description:	Dull abdominal aching
	Sense of fullness of the abdomen or epigastrium
Intensity:	Mild at first, then increases steadily
Duration:	Constant
Associated Signs and Symptoms:	Nausea, anorexia (viral hepatitis)
	Early satiety (cystic tumors)
	Aversion to smoking for smokers (viral hepatitis)
	Aversion to alcohol (hepatitis)
	Arthralgias and myalgias (hepatitis A or B)
	Headaches (hepatitis A, drug-induced hepatitis)
	Dizziness/drowsiness (drug-induced hepatitis)
	Low-grade fever (hepatitis A)
	Pharyngitis (hepatitis A)
	Extreme fatigue (hepatitis A, cirrhosis)
	Alterations in the sense of taste and smell (hepatitis A)
	Rash (hepatitis B)
	Jaundice
	Dark urine, light stools
	Ascites
	Edema and oliguria
	Neurologic symptoms (hepatic encephalopathy) Confusion, forgetfulness Muscle tremors Asterixis Slurred speech Impaired handwriting
	Pallor (often linked with cirrhosis or carcinoma)

	Bleeding disorders Purpura Ecchymosis
	Spider angiomas
	Palmar erythema
	Light-colored or clay-colored feces
	Diaphoresis (liver abscess)
	Early satiety (cystic tumors)
	Overall muscular weakness (cirrhosis, liver carcinoma)
	Peripheral neuropathy (chronic liver disease)
Possible Etiology:	Any liver disease Hepatitis Cirrhosis Metastatic tumors
	Pancreatic carcinoma
	Liver abscess
	Medications: use of hepatotoxic drugs

Gallbladder

Pain

Location (see Fig. 8–5):	Pain in the midepigastrium (heartburn)
	RUQ of abdomen
Referral:	RUQ pain may be associated with right shoulder pain
	Both may be associated with back pain between the scapulae
	Pain may be referred to the right side of the midline in the interscapular or subscapular area
Description:	Dull aching
	Deep visceral pain (gallbladder suddenly distends)
	Biliary carcinoma is more persistent and boring
Intensity:	Mild at first, then increases steadily to become severe
Duration:	2 to 3 hours
Aggravating Factors:	Respiratory inspiration
	Upper body movement
	Lying down
Associated Signs and Symptoms:	Dark urine, light stools
	Jaundice

	Skin: green hue (prolonged biliary obstruction)
	Persistent pruritus (cholestatic jaundice)
	Pain and nausea occur 1 to 3 hours after eating (gallstones)
	Pain immediately after eating (gallbladder inflammation)
	Intolerance of fatty foods or heavy meals
	Indigestion, nausea
	Excessive belching
	Flatulence (excessive intestinal gas)
	Anorexia
	Weight loss (gallbladder cancer)
	Bleeding from skin and mucous membranes (late sign of gallbladder cancer)
	Vomiting
	Feeling of fullness
	Low-grade fever, chills
Possible Etiology:	Gallstones (cholelithiasis)
	Gallbladder inflammation (cholecystitis)
	Neoplasm
	Medications: use of hepatotoxic drugs

Common Bile Duct

Pain

Location (see Fig. 8–5):	Pain in midepigastrium or RUQ of abdomen
Referral:	Epigastrium: heartburn (choledocholithiasis)
	RUQ pain may be associated with right shoulder pain
	Both may be associated with back pain between the scapulae
	Pain may be referred to the right side of the midline in the interscapular or subscapular area
Description:	Dull aching
	Vague discomfort (pressure within common bile duct increasing)
	Severe, steady pain in RUQ (choledocholithiasis)
	Biliary carcinoma is more persistent and boring
Intensity:	Mild at first, increases steadily
Duration:	Constant
	3 to 4 hours (choledocholithiasis)

Associated Signs and Symptoms:	Dark urine, light stools
	Jaundice
	Nausea after eating
	Intolerance of fatty foods or heavy meals
	Feeling of abdominal fullness
	Skin: green hue (prolonged biliary obstruction)
	Low-grade fever, chills
	Excessive belching (choledocholithiasis)
	Constipation and diarrhea (choledocholithiasis)
	Sensory neuropathy (primary biliary cirrhosis)
	Osteomalacia (primary biliary cirrhosis)
	Osteoporosis (primary biliary cirrhosis)
Possible Etiology:	Common duct stones
	Common duct stricture (previous gallbladder surgery)
	Pancreatic carcinoma (blocking the bile duct)
	Medications: use of hepatotoxic drugs
	Neoplasm
	Primary biliary cirrhosis
	Choledocholithiasis (obstruction of common duct)

SUMMARY

This chapter on hepatic and biliary signs and symptoms has included diseases of the liver, gallbladder, and common bile duct. In the course of this discussion, we have attempted to provide an overview of:

- Liver and biliary physiology, including bilirubin metabolism
- Liver pathophysiology
  - Jaundice: classifications, kernicterus, and clinical history and observations
  - Viral hepatitis: acute and chronic
  - Nonviral hepatitis
  - Cirrhosis
  - Portal hypertension
  - Ascites
  - Esophageal varices
  - Hepatic encephalopathy
  - Liver abscess
  - Liver cancer
- Gallbladder and duct disease
  - Cholelithiasis
  - Cholecystitis
  - Primary biliary cirrhosis
- Overview of liver/biliary pain patterns
  - Liver
  - Gallbladder
  - Common bile duct

Signs and Symptoms Requiring Physician Referral

A careful history and close clinical observations may elicit indications that the patient is demonstrating signs and symptoms related to the hepatic and biliary systems requiring medical referral. The physical therapist is advised to question the patient further whenever any of the following signs and symptoms are reported or observed:

Anorexia
Alterations in sense of taste/smell
Arthralgias
Ascites
Asterixis
Aversion to cigarettes, alcohol
Changes in skin color (yellow, green)
Constipation
Dark urine
Diaphoresis
Diarrhea
Dizziness
Drowsiness
Early satiety
Ecchymosis
Edema
Excessive belching
Fatigue
Feeling of abdominal fullness
Fever, chills
Flatulence
Headaches
Heartburn
Intolerance to fatty foods
Jaundice
Light stools
Malaise
Mental confusion
Muscle tremors
Myalgias
Nausea, especially after eating
Oliguria
Pallor
Palmar erythema
Pharyngitis
Pruritus
Purpura
Restlessness
Skin rash
Slurred speech
Spider angiomas
Tachycardia
Vomiting
Weakness

SUBJECTIVE EXAMINATION

Special Questions to Ask

- □ Have you ever had jaundice, anemia, or a splenectomy?
- □ Do you have any contact with rodents or exposure to toxins (carbon tetrachloride, beryllium, or vinyl chloride)? (Predispose to hepatic disease)
- □ Do you work in a clinical laboratory or with dialysis patients? **(Hepatitis)**
- □ Have you been out of the country in the last 6 months to a year? (Countries where hepatic disease is endemic)
- □ Have you had any recent contact with hepatitis or with a jaundiced person?
- □ Have you eaten any raw shellfish recently? **(Jaundice)**
- □ Have you had any recent blood or plasma transfusion, blood tests, acupuncture, ear piercing, tattoos, or dental work done? **(Viral hepatitis)**
- □ Have you had any kind of injury or trauma to your abdomen? **(Possible damage to the liver)**
- □ Do you bruise or bleed easily? **(Liver disease)**
- □ Have you noticed a change in the color of your stools or urine? **(Jaundice)**
- □ Has your weight fluctuated 10 to 15 lb or more recently without a change in diet? **(Cancer, cirrhosis, ascites)**

Subjective Exam

Special Questions to Ask

- □ Have you noticed your clothes fitting tighter around the waist from abdominal swelling or bloating? **(Ascites)**
- □ Do you have a feeling of fullness after only one or two bites of food? **(Early satiety: stomach and duodenum, cystic tumors or gallbladder)**
- □ Does eating relieve your pain? **(Duodenal or pyloric ulcer)**

  How soon after eating?
- □ Does eating aggravate your pain? **(Gastric ulcer, gallbladder inflammation)**
- □ Are there any particular foods you have noticed that aggravate your symptoms?

  If yes, which ones? **(Intolerance to fatty foods)**
- □ **For patients with just shoulder or back pain:** Have you noticed any association between when you eat and when your symptoms increase or decrease?
- □ Has anyone in your family ever been diagnosed with Wilson's disease (excessive copper retention) or hemochromatosis (excessive iron absorption)? (Hereditary)
- □ When asking about drug history, keep in mind that oral contraceptives may cause cholestasis (suppression of bile flow) or liver tumors. Some common OTC drugs (e.g., acetaminophen) may have hepatotoxic effects (Nursing 84, 1984).
- □ **For women** Are you currently using oral contraceptives? **(Hepatitis, adenoma)**
- □ Use questions outlined in *The Physical Therapy Interview* to determine possible consumption of alcohol as a hepatotoxin.
- □ Have you noticed any unusual aversion to odors, food, alcohol, or (for patients who smoke) smoking? **(Jaundice)**

PHYSICIAN REFERRAL

A careful history and close observation of the patient are important in determining whether a person may need a medical referral for possible hepatic or biliary involvement. Any patient presenting with midback, scapular, or right shoulder pain without a history of trauma (including forceful movement of the spine, repetitive movements of the shoulder or back, or easy lifting) should be screened for possible systemic origin or symptoms.

For the physical therapist treating the inpatient population, jaundice in the postoperative patient is not uncommon and may be a potentially serious complication of surgery and anesthesia. Clinical management of jaundice is complicated by anything capable of damaging the liver including stress (emotional or physical), hypoxemia, blood loss, infection, and administration of multiple drugs.

When making the referral, it is important to report to the physician the results of your objective findings, especially when there is a lack of physical evidence to support a musculoskeletal lesion. The *Special Questions to Ask* may assist the physical therapist in assessing the patient's overall health status in making the determination whether a medical referral is required. Any time the patient reports accompanying systemic signs or symptoms that have not been evaluated or treated, the physician should be notified.

CASE STUDY

Referral

A 29-year-old male law student has come to you (self-referral) with the following complaints: Status post whiplash injury now with headaches; accident occurred 18 months ago.

The headaches occur two to three times each week, starting at the base of the occiput and progressing up the back of his head to localize in the forehead, bilaterally. The patient has a sedentary life-style with no regular exercise, and he describes his stress level as being "6" on a scale from 0 to 10. The *Family/Personal History* form indicates that he has had hepatitis.

What follow-up questions will you ask this patient related to the hepatitis?

(Introductory remarks: I see from your History form that you have had hepatitis.)

Past Medical History

When did you have hepatitis?

(Remember the three stages when trying to determine whether this person may still be contagious requiring necessary handwashing and hygiene precautions, including avoidance of any body fluids on your part through the use of protective gloves. This is especially true when treating a diabetic patient requiring fingerstick blood testing while in the physical therapy department.)

Do you know how you initially came in contact with hepatitis?

(In this patient's case, the only possible cause he can postulate is a shot he received for influenza when he was travelling with a singing group in a rural area of the United States. This information is inconclusive in assisting the physician to establish a direct causative factor.) Other considerations requiring further questioning may include:

- Illicit drug use
- Poor sanitation in close quarters with travel companion
- Ingestion of contaminated food, water, milk, or seafood
- Recent blood transfusion or contact with blood/blood products
- For type B: modes of sexual transmission

What type of hepatitis did you have?

Give the patient a chance to respond, but you may have to prompt with "type A," "type B," or "non-A," "non-B." (Remember that hepatitis A is communicable before the appearance of any observable clinical symptoms [i.e., during the

CASE STUDY

initial and icteric stages that usually last from 1 to 6 weeks]. Hepatitis B can persist in body fluids indefinitely requiring necessary precautions by you.)

Medical Treatment

Did you receive any medical treatment? (In this case, the patient and the members of his travelling group received gamma globulin shots.)

How soon after you were diagnosed did you receive the gamma globulin shots?

(Gamma globulin shots are considered most effective in producing passive immunity for 3 to 4 months when administered as soon as possible after exposure to the hepatitis virus, but within 2 weeks after the onset of jaundice.)

Are you currently receiving follow-up care for your hepatitis through a local physician?

(This information will assist you in determining the appropriate medical source of further information if you need it and, in a case like this, assist you in choosing further follow-up questions that may help you to determine whether this person requires additional medical follow-up. If the patient is receiving no further medical follow-up [especially if no gamma globulin was administered initially*], consider these follow-up questions):

Associated Symptoms

What symptoms did you have with hepatitis?

Do you have any of those symptoms now?

Are you experiencing any unusual fatigue or muscle or joint aches and pains?

Have you noticed any unusual aversion to foods, alcohol, or cigarettes that you did not have before?

Have you had any problems with diarrhea, vomiting, or nausea?

Have you noticed any change in the color of your stools or urine?
(One to 4 days before the icteric stage, the urine darkens and the stool lightens.)

Have you noticed any unusual skin rash developing recently?

When did you notice the headaches developing?
(Try to correlate this with the onset of hepatitis because headaches can be persistent symptoms of hepatitis A.)

---

* Persons who have been treated with human immune serum globulin (ISG) may not develop jaundice, but those who have not received the gamma globulin usually develop jaundice.

References

Alyn, I.B.: Disturbances in hepatic function. *In* Jones, D.A., Dunbar, C.F., and Jirovec, M.M. (eds): Medical-Surgical Nursing, 2nd ed. New York, McGraw-Hill Book Company, 1982, pp. 717–743.

Andreoli, T., Carpenter, C., Plum, F., and Smith, L.C.: Essentials of Medicine. Philadelphia, W.B. Saunders Company, 1986.

Boyer, J.L., and Miller, D.J.: Chronic hepatitis. *In* Schiff, L., and Schiff, E.R. (eds): Diseases of the Liver, 5th ed. Philadelphia, J.B. Lippincott, 1982, pp. 771–811.

Buchan, P.C.: Pathogenesis of neonatal hyperbilirubinemia after induction of labour with oxytocin. Br. Med. J., *2*:1255, 1979.

Conn, H.O.: Cirrhosis. *In* Schiff, L., and Schiff, E.R. (eds): Diseases of the Liver, 5th ed. Philadelphia, J.B. Lippincott, 1982, pp. 847–977.

Edmondson, H.A., and Peters, R.L.: Neoplasms of the liver. *In* Schiff, L., and Schiff, E.R. (eds): Diseases of the Liver, 5th ed. Philadelphia, J.B. Lippincott, 1982, pp. 1101–1156.

Foster, J.H.: Cancer and the liver. *In* Gitnick, G.L. (ed): Current Hepatology, Vol. 2. New York, John Wiley & Sons, 1982, pp. 233–272.

Gitnick, G.L. (ed): Current Hepatology, Vol. 2. New York, John Wiley & Sons, 1982.

Given, B.A., and Simmons, S.J.: Gastroenterology in Clinical Nursing. Baltimore, C.V. Mosby, 1979.

Gocke, D.J.: Systemic manifestations of viral liver disease. *In* Gitnick, G.L. (ed): Current Hepatology, Vol. 2. New York, John Wiley & Sons, 1982, pp. 273–288.

Koff, R.S., and Galambos, J.: Viral hepatitis. *In* Schiff, L., and Schiff, E.R. (eds): Diseases of the Liver, 5th ed. Philadelphia, J.B. Lippincott, 1982, pp. 461–610.

Luckmann, J., and Sorensen, K.: Medical-Surgical Nursing: A Psychophysiologic Approach, 3rd ed. Philadelphia, W.B. Saunders Company, 1987.

Miller, B.F., and Keane, C.B.: Encyclopedia and Dictionary of Medicine, Nursing, and Allied Health, 4th ed. Philadelphia, W.B. Saunders Company, 1987.

Moertel, C.G.: Medical management of liver cancer. *In* Schiff, L., and Schiff, E.R. (eds): Diseases of the Liver, 5th ed. Philadelphia, J.B. Lippincott, 1982, pp. 1159–1164.

Nursing 81: Diseases. Horsham, PA, Intermed Communications, 1981.

Nursing 84: Gastrointestinal Disorders. Springhouse, PA, Springhouse Corporation, 1984.

Nursing 88: Clinical Pocket Manual: Signs and symptoms. Springhouse, PA, Springhouse Corporation, 1988.

Ockner, R.: Approaches to the diagnosis of jaundice. *In* Wyngaarden, J., and Smith, L.: Cecil Textbook of Medicine, 18th ed. Philadelphia, W.B. Saunders Company, 1988, pp. 817–818.

Overby, L.R.: Serology of liver diseases. *In* Gitnick, G.L. (ed): Current Hepatology, Vol. 2. New York, John Wiley & Sons, 1982, pp. 55–94.

Popper, H., and Schaffner, F.: Liver: Structure and Function. New York, McGraw-Hill Book Company, 1974.

Purtilo, D.T.: A Survey of Human Diseases, 2nd ed. Boston, Little, Brown, 1989.

Ross Laboratories: Hyperbilirubinemia in the newborn. Report of the Eighty-fifth Ross Conference on Pediatric Research. Columbus, OH, Ross Laboratories, 1983.

Schiff, L: Jaundice. *In* Blacklow, R.S. (ed): MacBryde's Signs and Symptoms, 6th ed. Philadelphia, J.B. Lippincott, 1983, pp. 423–440.

Sherlock, S: Diseases of the Liver and Biliary System, 7th ed. Chicago, Year Book Medical Publishing Inc., 1985.

Singhi, S., and Singh, M.: Pathogenesis of oxytocin-induced neonatal hyperbilirubinemia. Arch. Dis. Child., *54*:400, 1979.

Stewart, J.S., Farrow, J.L., Clifford, R.E., et al: A three-year survey of viral hepatitis in West London. Q. J. Medicine, *187*:365, 1978.

Tan, E.G.C., and Warren, K.W.: Diseases of the gallbladder and bile ducts. *In* Schiff, L., and Schiff, E.R. (eds): Diseases of the Liver, 5th ed. Philadelphia, J.B. Lippincott, 1982, pp. 1507–1559.

Van Dyke, R.W., Keefe, E.B., Gollan, J.L., and Scharschmidt, B.F.: Cholestasis, bile flow, and hyperbilirubinemia: Current clinical and pathophysiologic perspectives. *In* Gitnick, G.L. (ed): Current Hepatology, Vol. 2. New York, John Wiley & Sons, 1982, pp. 327–363.

Way, L.W.: Abdominal pain. *In* Sleisenger, M.H., and Fordtran, J.S. (eds): Gastrointestinal Disease, 2nd ed. Philadelphia, W.B. Saunders Company, 1983, pp. 207–221.

Zieve, L.: Hepatic encephalopathy. *In* Schiff, L., and Schiff, E.R. (eds): Diseases of the Liver, 5th ed. Philadelphia, J.B. Lippincott, 1982, pp. 433–459.

Zimmerman, H.J., and Maddrey, W.C.: Toxic and drug-induced hepatitis. *In* Schiff, L., and Schiff, E.R. (eds): Diseases of the Liver, 5th ed. Philadelphia, J.B. Lippincott, 1982, pp. 621–692.

Zimmerman, H.Y.: Hepatotoxicity: The Adverse Effects of Drugs and Other Chemicals on the Liver. New York, Appleton-Century-Crofts, 1978.

Bibliography

Jackson, G., and Whitfield, P.: Digestion: Fueling the System. New York, Torstar Books, 1984.

Jones, D.A., Dunbar, C.F., and Jirovec, M.M. (eds): Medical-Surgical Nursing, 2nd ed. New York, McGraw-Hill Book Company, 1982.

Leevy, C.M.: Evaluation of Liver Function in Clinical Practice. Indianapolis, IN, The Lilly Research Laboratories, 1974.

Wright, R., Millward-Sadler, K.G.M.M., and Karran, S.: Liver and Biliary Diseases, 2nd ed. Philadelphia, W.B. Saunders Company, 1986.

Zakim, D., and Boyer, T.D.: Hepatology: A Textbook of Liver Disease. Philadelphia, W.B. Saunders Company, 1982.

Chapter 9

Overview of Endocrinology and Metabolic Disorders: Signs and Symptoms

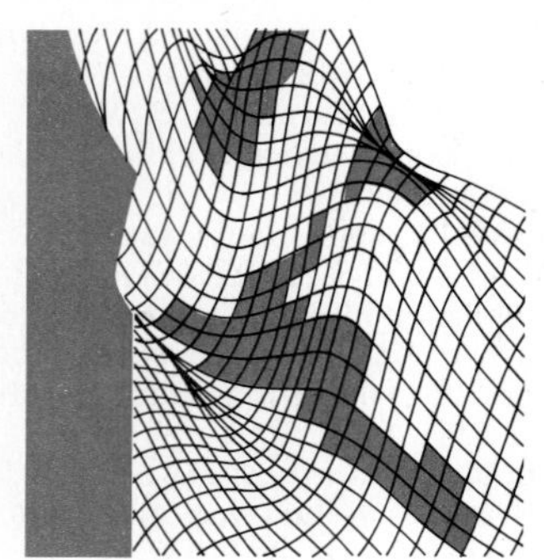

☐ ***Clinical Signs and Symptoms of:***

- Diabetes Insipidus
- Addison's Disease
- Cushing's Syndrome
- Goiter
- Thyroiditis
- Hyperthyroidism
- Hypothyroidism
- Thyroid Carcinoma
- Untreated or Uncontrolled Diabetes Mellitus
- Diabetic Ketoacidosis
- Hyperglycemia, Hyperosmolar, Nonketotic Coma (HHNC)
- Hypoglycemia
- Dehydration or Fluid Loss
- Water Intoxication
- Edema
- Metabolic Alkalosis
- Metabolic Acidosis
- Gout
- Paget's Disease

Endocrinology is the study of ductless (endocrine) glands that produce hormones that are released directly into the bloodstream permitting effects at distant sites called target glands (Table 9–1). A hormone acts as a chemical agent that is transported by the bloodstream to target tissues, where it regulates or modifies the activity of the target cell.

The pituitary (hypophysis), thyroid, parathyroids, adrenals, and the pineal are glands of the endocrine system whose functions are solely endocrine. Other glands in the body have dual functions. For example, the pancreas produces the hormone insulin from its islet cells, but it also produces digestive enzymes, which are carried by ducts and are thus exocrine.

The endocrine system cannot be understood fully without consideration of the nervous system's effects on the endocrine

Table 9–1. ENDOCRINE GLANDS: SECRETION, TARGET, AND ACTIONS

When reading a patient's chart, it is important to know basic hormone functions or effects that may have an impact on physical therapy treatment. At least 30 different hormones have been identified, but only those most common to physical therapy patients are included here.

Gland	Hormone	Target	Basic Action
Pituitary Gland			
ANTERIOR LOBE			
	Somatotropin (growth hormone [GH])	Bones, muscles, organs	Retention of nitrogen to promote protein anabolism
	Thyroid stimulating hormone (TSH)	Thyroid	Promotes secretory activity
	Follicle stimulating hormone (FSH)	Ovaries, seminiferous tubules	Promotes development of ovarian follicle, secretion of estrogen and maturation of sperm
	Luteinizing hormone	Follicle, interstitial cell	Promotes ovulation and formation of corpus luteum, secretion of progesterone, and secretion of testosterone
	Prolactin (Luteotrophic hormone)	Corpus luteum, breast	Maintains corpus luteum and progesterone secretion; stimulates milk secretion
	Adrenocorticotrophic hormone (ACTH)	Adrenal cortex	Stimulates secretory activity
POSTERIOR LOBE			
	Antidiuretic hormone (ADH)	Distal tubules of kidney	Reabsorption of water
	Oxytocin	Uterus	Stimulates contraction
Thyroid			
	Thyroxine (T4) Triiodothyronine (T3)	Widespread	Regulates oxidation rate of body cells and growth and metabolism; influences gluconeogenesis, mobilization of fats, and exchange of water, electrolytes, and protein
	Calcitonin	Skeleton	Calcium and phosphorus metabolism
Parathyroids			
	Parathyroid hormone (PTH)	Bone, kidney, intestinal tract	Essential for calcium and phosphorus metabolism and calcification of bone
Adrenal Gland			
CORTEX			
	Mineralocorticoid (aldosterone)	Widespread, primarily kidney	Maintains fluid/electrolyte balance; reabsorbs sodium chloride; excretes potassium
	Glucocorticoids (cortisol)	Widespread	Concerned with food metabolism and body response to stress; preserves carbohydrates and mobilizes amino acids; promotes gluconeogenesis; suppresses inflammation
	Sex hormones (testosterone, estrogen, progesterone)	Gonads	Ability to influence secondary sex

Table 9–1. ENDOCRINE GLANDS: SECRETION, TARGET, AND ACTIONS *Continued*

When reading a patient's chart, it is important to know basic hormone functions or effects that may have an impact on physical therapy treatment. At least 30 different hormones have been identified, but only those most common to physical therapy patients are included here.

Gland	Hormone	Target	Basic Action
MEDULLA			
	Epinephrine	Widespread	Vasoconstriction with increased blood pressure; increased blood sugar via glycolysis; stimulates ACTH production
	Norepinephrine	Widespread	Vasoconstriction
Pancreas			
	Insulin	Widespread	Increased utilization of carbohydrate, decreased lipolysis, and protein catabolism; decreased blood sugar
	Glucagon	Widespread	Hyperglycemic factor; increases blood sugar via glycogenolysis
Gonads			
OVARIES			
	Estrogen	Widespread	Secondary sex characteristics; maturation and sexual function
	Progesterone	Uterus, breast	Preparation for and maintenance of pregnancy; development of mammary gland secretory tissue
TESTIS			
	Testosterone	Widespread	Secondary sex characteristics; maturation and normal sex function

system. The hypothalamus in the brain can synthesize and release hormones from its axon terminals into the blood circulation. These *neurosecretory cells* are so-called because the neurons have a hormone-secreting function (Marshall, 1986). Hormones that can stimulate the neural mechanism resulting in the release of hormones and chemicals, such as acetylcholine (a neurotransmitter that is released at synapses to allow messages to pass along a nerve network) have been described as *neurohormones.* The interlocking of the endocrine and neural systems can be considered to constitute the neuroendocrine system (Marshall, 1986).

ENDOCRINE SYSTEM PHYSIOLOGY

The endocrine system works with the nervous system to regulate metabolism, water and salt balance, blood pressure, response to stress, sex, and reproduction. The endocrine system is slower in response and takes longer to act than the nervous system when transferring biochemical information. The glands in Figure 9–1 are part of the endocrine system that secrete essential hormones (see Table 9–1) into the bloodstream. The pituitary gland has been called the "master gland," because its anterior lobe has direct control over

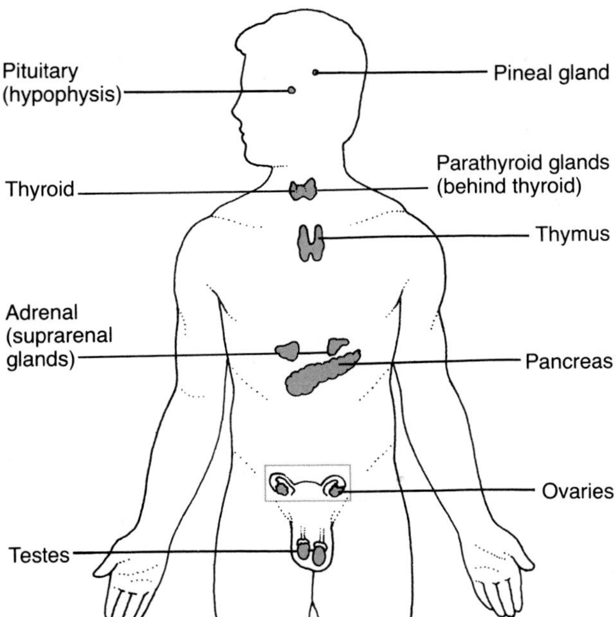

Figure 9–1. Location of the nine endocrine glands.

the thyroid gland (thyroid stimulating hormone [TSH]), adrenal cortex (adrenocorticotropic hormone [ACTH]), and the gonads (luteinizing hormone [LH] and follicle stimulating hormone [FSH]). The hypothalamus controls pituitary function and thus has an important, indirect influence on the other glands of the endocrine system (Muthe, 1981). Feedback mechanisms exist to keep hormones at normal levels.

Hypothalamus

The endocrine system meets the nervous system at the hypothalamic-pituitary interface. The hypothalamus regulates pituitary activity through two pathways: a neural and portal venous pathway. *Neural* pathways extend from the hypothalamus, where two hormones —antidiuretic hormone ([ADH] or vasopressin) and oxytocin—are synthesized, to the posterior pituitary lobe, where the hormones are stored and secreted. *Portal venous* pathways, which connect the hypothalamus to the anterior pituitary lobe, carry hypothalamic releasing and inhibiting hormones (Nursing 84, 1984).

Regulation of the secretion of hormones by the pituitary gland is maintained by the production and release of hypothalamic releasing or inhibiting hormones. These hormones act directly by inhibiting or by stimulating the release of specific hormones by the pituitary gland (Fig. 9–2) (Purtilo and Purtilo, 1989).

Pituitary Gland

The pituitary is an oval-shaped gland measuring approximately 1 cm in diameter. It is located at the base of the skull in an indentation of the sphenoid bone. The pituitary is joined to the hypothalamus by the pituitary stalk (neurohypophyseal tract). The pituitary gland consists of two parts: the anterior pituitary and the posterior pituitary. The anterior pituitary secretes six different hormones (see Table 9–1).

The posterior pituitary is a downward offshoot of the hypothalamus and contains many nerve fibers. The posterior pituitary produces

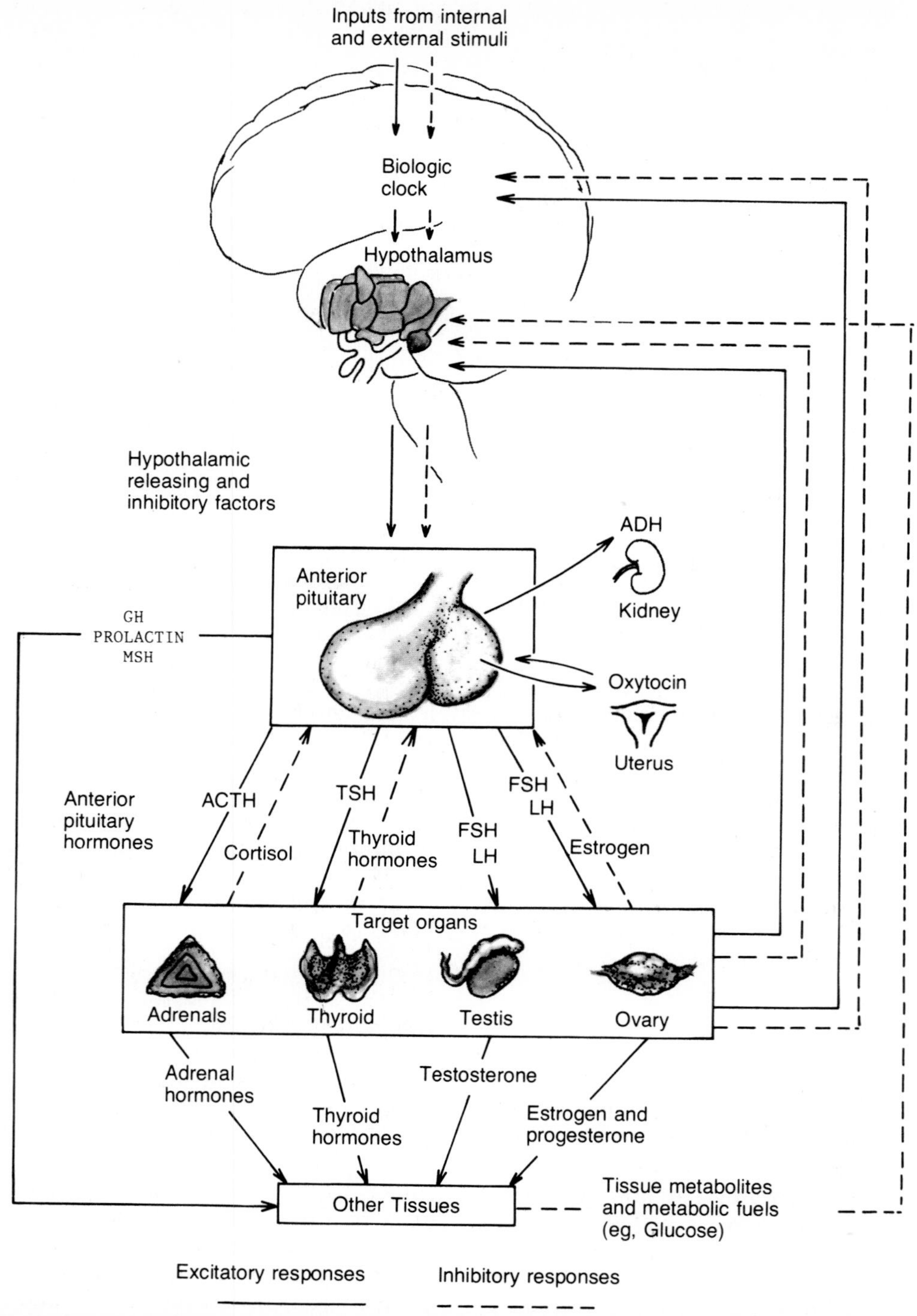

Figure 9–2. Control of the endocrine system by the nervous system. Note that the hypothalamus controls the pituitary gland through releasing and inhibiting factors. The anterior lobe of the pituitary gland then releases trophic hormones that act on target glands (thyroid, adrenals, and gonads). (From Purtilo, D.T. and Purtilo, R.B.: A Survey of Human Diseases, 2nd ed. Boston, Little, Brown, 1989.)

no hormones of its own. The hormones, which are produced in the hypothalamus and then stored and released by the posterior pituitary (ADH or vasopressin and oxytocin), pass down nerve fibers from the hypothalamus through the pituitary stalk to nerve endings in the posterior pituitary. These two hormones accumulate in the posterior pituitary during less active periods of the body. Transmitter substances, such as acetylcholine or norepinephrine, are thought to activate the release of these substances by the posterior pituitary gland when they are stimulated by nerve impulses from the hypothalamus (Muthe, 1981).

Adrenal Glands

The adrenals are two small glands located on the upper part of each kidney. Each adrenal gland consists of two relatively discrete parts: an outer cortex and an inner medulla. The outer cortex is responsible for the secretion of mineralocorticoids (steroid hormones that regulate fluid and mineral balance), glucocorticoids (steroid hormones responsible for controlling the metabolism of glucose), and androgens (sex hormones). The centrally located adrenal medulla is derived from neural tissue and secretes epinephrine and norepinephrine, which exert widespread effects on vascular tone, the heart, the nervous system, as well as affecting glucose metabolism. Together, the adrenal cortex and medulla are major factors in the body's response to stress (Marshall, 1986).

Thyroid Gland (Muthe, 1981)

The thyroid gland is located in the anterior portion of the lower neck below the larynx, on either side of and anterior to the trachea. The chief hormones produced by the thyroid are thyroxine (T4), and triiodothyronine (T3), and calcitonin. Both T3 and T4 regulate the metabolic rate of the body and increase protein synthesis (Marshall, 1986). Calcitonin affects calcium and phosphorus balance in the body. Thyroid function is regulated by the hypothalamus and pituitary feedback control, as well as by an intrinsic regulator mechanism within the gland itself.

Thyroid disorders affect women more often than men and develop from functional or structural changes of the thyroid gland, or both. Changes in the thyroid's ability to function normally result in excessive or deficient levels of thyroid hormone. Structural changes in the thyroid gland occur secondary to inflammatory, hyperplastic, or neoplastic disease (Nursing 84, 1984). With the exception of neoplasms, most of the common diseases of the thyroid gland arise from autoimmune disorders (Purtilo and Purtilo, 1989).

Basic thyroid disorders of significance to physical therapy practice include goiter, hyperthyroidism, hypothyroidism, and cancer. Alterations in thyroid function produce changes in hair, nails, skin, eyes, gastrointestinal (GI) tract, respiratory tract, heart and blood vessels, nervous tissue, bone, and muscle.

Parathyroid Glands

Two parathyroid glands are located on the posterior surface of each lobe of the thyroid gland. These glands secrete parathyroid hormone (PTH) which regulates calcium and phosphorus metabolism (Nursing 84, 1984). Parathyroid disorders include hyperparathyroidism and hypoparathyroidism.

Variations in location and color as well as the minute size of parathyroid glands makes identification very difficult and may result in their accidental removal during thyroid surgery. If two glands are removed, no functional change may result, but if three glands are removed, temporary hypoparathyroidism generally occurs. One gland, or even part of a gland, is capable of hypertrophying sufficiently to supply the necessary hormone (Muthe, 1981). The physical therapist will see patients with parathyroid disorders in acute-care and postoperative patients because these disorders can result from diseases and operations.

Pancreas

The pancreas is a fish-shaped organ that lies behind the stomach. Its head and neck are located in the curve of the duodenum, and its body extends horizontally across the posterior abdominal wall. The pancreas is usually 6 to 9 inches long and 1 to 1.5 inches wide. It varies in size, depending on the individual, and is larger in men.

The pancreas has dual functions. It acts as both an *endocrine gland,* secreting the hormones insulin and glucagon, and as an *exocrine gland,* producing digestive enzymes. The cells of the pancreas that function in the endocrine capacity are the islets of Langerhans. These cells consist of approximately 1 to 2% of the pancreatic mass.

Hormonal Action

The primary function of glucagon hormone is to increase the circulating blood glucose level. Glucagon is stimulated by a decreased blood glucose level and also by increased amino acid levels. When stimulated, glucagon converts stored glucose (primarily in the liver) to circulating glucose. When the need for glucose is greater than can be mobilized from the liver, glucagon promotes glucose formation utilizing both fat and protein. Glucagon is a counter-regulatory hormone to insulin as are the hormones epinephrine (adrenal medulla), growth hormones (anterior pituitary), and glucocorticoids (adrenal cortex). These hormones function together to restore low blood sugar to a normal level.

Insulin is a protein substance that affects the metabolism of glucose and fats by mobilizing circulating glucose to storage and use in the liver, fat cells, and muscle cells. Insulin, therefore, decreases the circulating blood glucose level. The effect of insulin on blood glucose level and the utilization of glucose in the cells of the body is thought to be the result of insulin's ability to change the permeability of cell membranes, thus allowing easier entry by glucose and promoting the use of glucose in those cells. The primary stimulus for insulin secretion is glucose, but intake of amino acids can also result in release of insulin. In the nondiabetic, insulin has an unstimulated continuous secretion that affects metabolism between meals (Cassmeyer, 1987).

ENDOCRINE PATHOPHYSIOLOGY

Disorders of the endocrine glands can be classified as primary or secondary diseases and are a result of either an excess (hyperfunction) or insufficiency (hypofunction) of hormonal secretions. *Primary dysfunction* of the endocrine system associated with excessive hormone production by a gland may be caused by a tumor or by another abnormal stimulus (e.g., antibodies mimicking hormonal stimulators). Endocrine hypofunction can result from congenital abnormalities, neoplasms, infarctions, infections, and autoimmune disorders affecting the gland itself.

Secondary dysfunction occurs when an abnormal stimulus causes excessive or insufficient hormone production by a target gland (i.e., a gland specifically affected by a pituitary hormone). For example, in chronic renal failure, abnormal levels of phosphate and calcium may cause secondary hyperparathyroidism, or chronic liver disease can affect both the pituitary gland and the testes, leading to decreased testosterone production and increased estrogen levels. Secondary dysfunction may also occur as a result of medical treatment (iatrogenic causes) by the effects of chemotherapy, surgical removal of glands, therapy for a nonendocrine disorder such as the use of large doses of corticosteroids resulting in Cushing's syndrome (see p. 222), or excessive therapy for an endocrine disorder (Nursing 84, 1984).

Pituitary Gland

Diabetes Insipidus

Vasopressin is the ADH secreted by the posterior pituitary gland. This hormone stimulates the distal tubules of the kidney to reabsorb water. Without ADH (vasopressin), water moving through the kidney is not reabsorbed, but is lost through the urine. Uncontrolled diuresis (increased urine excretion) and polyuria (excessive excretion of urine) occur. Deficiency of this hormone is called *diabetes insipidus* and can be a result of injury or loss of function of either the hypothalamus, the neurohyophyseal tract, or the posterior pituitary gland.

Primary diabetes insipidus is considered to be idiopathic and accounts for most cases, which have been related to subclinical encephalitis or to familial or congenital factors. Secondary diabetes insipidus can be caused by tumors, trauma, infections, or vascular lesions that affect the hypothalamus or pituitary system (Muthe, 1981).

CLINICAL SYMPTOMS OF DIABETES INSIPIDUS

- Polyuria (increased urination)
- Polydypsia (increased thirst, which occurs subsequent to polyuria in response to the loss of fluid)

Inadequate reabsorption of water by the kidney can result in a loss of as much as 20 L/day of urine and a specific gravity as low as 1.001 to 1.005 (normal: 1.01 to 1.03). If the patient is conscious and is able to respond appropriately to the thirst mechanism, hydration can be maintained. If, however, the patient is unconscious or confused and is unable to take in the necessary fluids to replace those fluids lost, rapid dehydration, shock, and death can occur. Because sleep is interrupted by the persistent need to void (nocturia), fatigue and irritability result. The onset of symptoms may be rapid and abrupt, and patients can often remember the exact time that the symptoms began. Another unusual feature of diabetes insipidus is the almost universal preference of the patient for ice water as a fluid replacement (Muthe, 1981).

Treatment is usually replacement of the ADH (vasopressin) by the use of exogenous (administered from an external source) vasopressin or a synthetic derivative (e.g., Desmopressin). Side effects of any type of ADH administration are very serious. ADH stimulates smooth muscle contraction of the vascular system (increased blood pressure), GI tract (diarrhea), and uterus (uterine cramps). Increases in blood pressure occur and can cause additional serious problems in some patients, particularly in patients with hypertension or coronary artery disease (CAD) and cerebrovascular disease (CVD).

Adrenal Glands

Addison's Disease (Muthe, 1981)

Chronic adrenocortical insufficiency (hyposecretion by the adrenal glands) is referred to as Addison's disease (hypofunction), named after the physician who first studied and described the associated symptoms. It can be treated by the administration of exogenous cortisol (one of the adrenocortical hormones). Addison's disease may be described as either *primary Addison's disease* or *secondary Addison's disease.* Primary Addison's disease occurs when the pathology of the gland itself results in decreased secretion of the ACTH.

In the past and in the Third World, the most common cause of Addison's disease is adrenal atrophy secondary to pulmonary or renal tuberculosis. The most frequent cause is now an autoimmune process that causes adrenocortical destruction (Marshall, 1986). Other conditions that may cause primary Addison's disease include:

- Infectious diseases
- Trauma
- Vascular occlusion
- Bilateral adrenalectomy
- Drugs, such as oral contraceptives or anticoagulants
- Abrupt withdrawal of high doses of corticosteroids (e.g., patients with rheumatoid arthritis)
- Metastatic cancer of the adrenal glands

- Hemorrhage and infarction secondary to septicemia (blood poisoning)
- Destruction by chemicals

Secondary Addison's disease refers to a dysfunction of the gland because of insufficient stimulation of the cortex from a lack of pituitary ACTH (Muthe, 1981).

Clinical manifestations of the disease do not occur until the adrenals are almost completely nonfunctioning. Diagnosis may not be made until a stress situation (when the need for the hormone becomes greater) causes more acute manifestations of the disease (Muthe, 1981). Most symptoms of Addison's disease arise from aldosterone and cortisol deficiency; very few symptoms are related to a deficiency of androgen.

CLINICAL SIGNS AND SYMPTOMS OF ADDISON'S DISEASE (Nelson, 1988b)

- Dark pigmentation of the skin, especially mouth and scars
- Hypotension (low blood pressure causing orthostatic symptoms)
- Progressive fatigue (improves with rest)
- Hyperkalemia: generalized weakness and paralysis
- GI disturbances
  - Anorexia and weight loss
  - Nausea and vomiting
- Arthralgias, myalgias (secondary Addison's disease)

The most striking physical finding in the patient with Addison's disease is the increased pigmentation of the skin and the mucous membranes. This may vary in the white population from a slight tan or a few black freckles to an intense generalized pigmentation, which has resulted in patients being mistakenly considered to be of a darker-skinned race. Melanin, the major product of the melanocyte, is largely responsible for the coloring of skin. In Addison's disease, the increase in pigmentation is initiated by the excessive secretion of melanocyte stimulating hormone (MSH) that occurs in association with increased ACTH (Wilson and Foster, 1985).

Most commonly, pigmentation is visible over extensor surfaces, such as the back of the hands, elbows, knees, creases of the hands, lips, and mouth. Increased pigmentation of scars formed after the onset of the disease is common. It is however possible for the patient with Addison's disease to demonstrate no significant increase in pigmentation (Nelson, 1988b). Members of darker-skinned races may develop a slate-gray color that is obvious only to the family members. Determining the presence of such changes in skin coloration requires that additional questions be asked of members of the family other than the patient.

Treatment of Addison's disease includes replacement of adrenocortical hormones and dietary measures to replace the lost sodium and fluid, and to replace potassium consumption. Too much adrenocortical hormone replacement can complicate Addison's disease with the development of Cushing's syndrome (Ford, 1987).

Cushing's Syndrome (Nelson, 1988a)

Cushing's syndrome (hyperfunction) is a general term for increased secretion of cortisol by the adrenal cortex. External administration of corticosteroids (e.g., hydrocortisone) reduces the body's secretion of cortisol and results in a cluster of signs and symptoms known as *Cushing's syndrome.* Cases caused by excess secretion of ACTH (e.g., from pituitary stimulation) are called *Cushing's disease.* Physical therapists often treat patients who have developed Cushing's syndrome after these patients have received large doses of cortisol (also known as hydrocortisone) for a number of inflammatory disorders. Gradual reduction of cortisol use returns the patient to normal (Purtilo and Purtilo, 1989).

Because cortisol suppresses the inflammatory response of the body, it can mask early signs of infection. *Any unexplained fever without other symptoms should be a warning to the physical therapist of the need for medical follow-up.*

CLINICAL SIGNS AND SYMPTOMS OF CUSHING'S SYNDROME (Fig. 9–3)

- "Moon" face (very round)
- Buffalo hump at the neck (fatty deposits)
- Protuberant abdomen with accumulation of fatty tissue and stretch marks
- Muscle wasting and weakness
- Decreased density of bones (especially spine)
- Kyphosis and back pain (secondary to bone loss)
- Easy bruising
- Psychiatric or emotional disturbances
- Impaired reproductive function (e.g., decreased libido and changes in menstrual cycle)
- Diabetes mellitus
- Slow wound healing
- For women: masculinizing effects (e.g., hair growth, breast atrophy, voice changes)

Cortisol Effects on Connective Tissue. Overproduction of cortisol or closely related glucocorticoids by abnormal adrenocortical tissue leads to a protein catabolic state. This overproduction causes liberation of amino acids from muscle tissue. The resultant weakened protein structures (muscle and elastic tissue) cause a protuberant abdomen; poor wound healing; generalized muscle weakness; and marked osteoporosis (demineralization of bone causing reduced bone mass), which is made worse by an excessive loss of calcium in the urine (Forsham, 1984).

Excessive glucose resulting from this protein catabolic state is transformed mainly into fat and appears in characteristic sites, such as the abdomen, supraclavicular fat pads, and facial cheeks (Forsham, 1984). The change in facial appearance may not be readily apparent to the patient or to the physical therapist, but pictures of the patient taken over a period of years may provide a visual record of those changes.

The effect of increased circulating levels of cortisol on the muscles of patients varies from slight to very marked. There may be so much muscle wasting that the condition simulates muscular dystrophy. Marked weakness of the quadriceps femoris often prevents affected patients from rising out of a chair unassisted. Patients with Cushing's syndrome of long duration almost always demonstrate demineralization of bone. In severe cases, this condition may lead to pathologic fractures, but results more commonly in wedging of the vertebrae, kyphosis, bone pain, and back pain.

Poor wound healing characteristic of this syndrome becomes a problem at the time that any surgical procedures are required. Inhibition of collagen formation with corticosteroid therapy is responsible for the frequency of wound breakdown in postsurgical patients.

Thyroid Gland

Goiter

Goiter, an enlargement of the thyroid gland, occurs in areas of the world where iodine (necessary for the production of thyroid hormone) is deficient in the diet. It is believed that when factors (e.g., a lack of iodine) inhibit normal thyroid hormone production, hypersecretion of TSH occurs because of a lack of a negative feedback loop. The TSH increase results in an increase in thyroid mass (Cassmeyer, 1987b). Pressure on the trachea and esophagus causes difficulty in breathing, dysphagia, and hoarseness. With the use of iodized salt, this problem has almost been eliminated in the United States. Although this is not present in the younger population in the United States, the elderly may have developed goiter during their childhood or adolescent years and may still have clinical manifestations of this disorder.

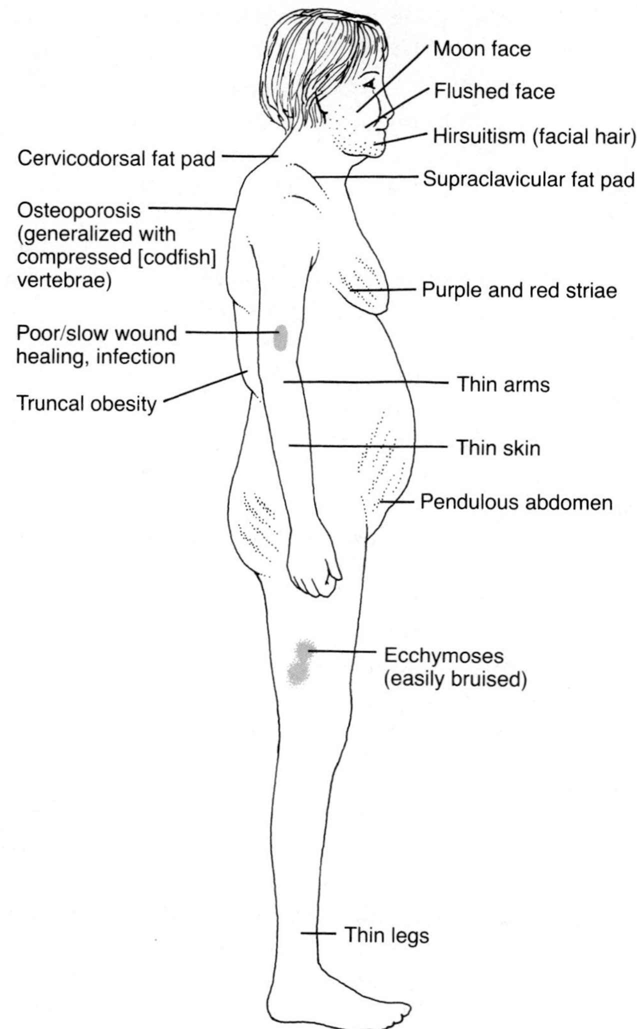

Figure 9–3. A composite of all the symptoms that occur as a result of hyperactivity of the adrenal cortex. (Based on Muthe, N.C.: Endocrinology: A Nursing Approach. Boston, Little, Brown, 1981, p. 147 and Meloni, R.C.: Obesity of Cushing's disease? Am. Fam. Physician, 5:93, 1972.)

CLINICAL SIGNS AND SYMPTOMS OF GOITER

- Increased neck size
- Pressure on adjacent tissue (e.g., trachea and esophagus)
- Difficulty in breathing
- Dysphagia
- Hoarseness

Thyroiditis (Cassmeyer, 1987b)

Thyroiditis is an inflammation of the thyroid gland. Causes can include infection and autoimmune processes. The most common form of this problem is a chronic thyroiditis called Hashimoto's thyroiditis. This condition affects women more frequently than men and is most often seen in the 30- to 50-year age group.

Hashimoto's thyroiditis causes destruction of the thyroid gland due to the infiltration of the gland by lymphocytes and antithyroid antibodies. This infiltration results in decreased serum levels of T3 and T4 and thus stimulates the pituitary gland to increase the production of TSH. The increased TSH causes hyperfunction of the tissue and goiter (enlargement of the gland) formation results.

Because some of the thyroid tissue has been destroyed, this increase in function helps to maintain a normal hormonal level for a period of time. Eventually, however, when enough of the gland is destroyed, hypothyroidism develops.

CLINICAL SIGNS AND SYMPTOMS OF THYROIDITIS

- Painless thyroid enlargement
- Dysphagia or choking

Both sides are usually enlarged, although one side may be larger than the other. Other symptoms are related to the state of function of the gland itself. Early involvement may cause mild symptoms of hyperthyroidism, whereas later symptoms are hypothyroid.

Treatment can include thyroid hormone or surgery depending on the severity of the problem. The goiter may become so large that it is disfiguring or pressing on adjacent structures, and surgery may be needed to correct this problem. No treatment is administered if the patient is asymptomatic and the disease is mild.

Hyperthyroidism

Hyperthyroidism (hyperfunction) or thyrotoxicosis refers to those disorders in which the thyroid gland secretes excessive amounts of thyroid hormone. Excessive thyroid hormone creates a generalized elevation in body metabolism. The effects of thyrotoxicosis occur gradually and are manifested in almost every system (Fig. 9–4; Table 9–2) (Nursing 84, 1984). Treatment for hyperthyroidism centers around drug therapy, radiation, and surgery.

Graves' disease is a type of excessive thyroid activity characterized by a generalized enlargement of the gland (or goiter leading to a swollen neck), and often, protruding eyes caused by retraction of the eyelids and inflammation of the ocular muscles (Marshall, 1986). Graves' disease accounts for more than 85% of cases of thyrotoxicosis. The cause of Graves' disease is unknown. Theoretically, the immune system may produce abnormal thyroid-stimulating antibodies, which, in turn, direct the thyroid gland to produce an excess of thyroid hormone.

SIGNS AND SYMPTOMS OF HYPERTHYROIDISM (Layzer, 1985)

- Lower extremity myopathy
- Upper extremity tremor
- Myokymia (persistent quivering of the muscles)
- Acute bulbar myopathy
  - Dsyphagia (difficulty in swallowing)
  - Hoarseness
  - Nasal voice
  - Weak cough
  - Weakness of muscle of the face, eye, and tongue
- Motor polyneuropathy
- Ocular myopathy (Graves' disease)

Proximal muscle weakness (most marked in the pelvic girdle and thigh muscles) accompanied by muscle atrophy known as myopathy has been shown to be a frequent complication of thyrotoxosis (Ramsay, 1965, 1966, 1974). The pathogenesis of the weakness is still a subject of controversy (Feibel and Campa, 1976; McComas et al, 1974). Studies by Ramsay (1966) showed that muscle power returned to normal in about 2 months after medical treatment, whereas muscle wasting resolved more slowly. In severe cases, normal strength may not be restored for months.

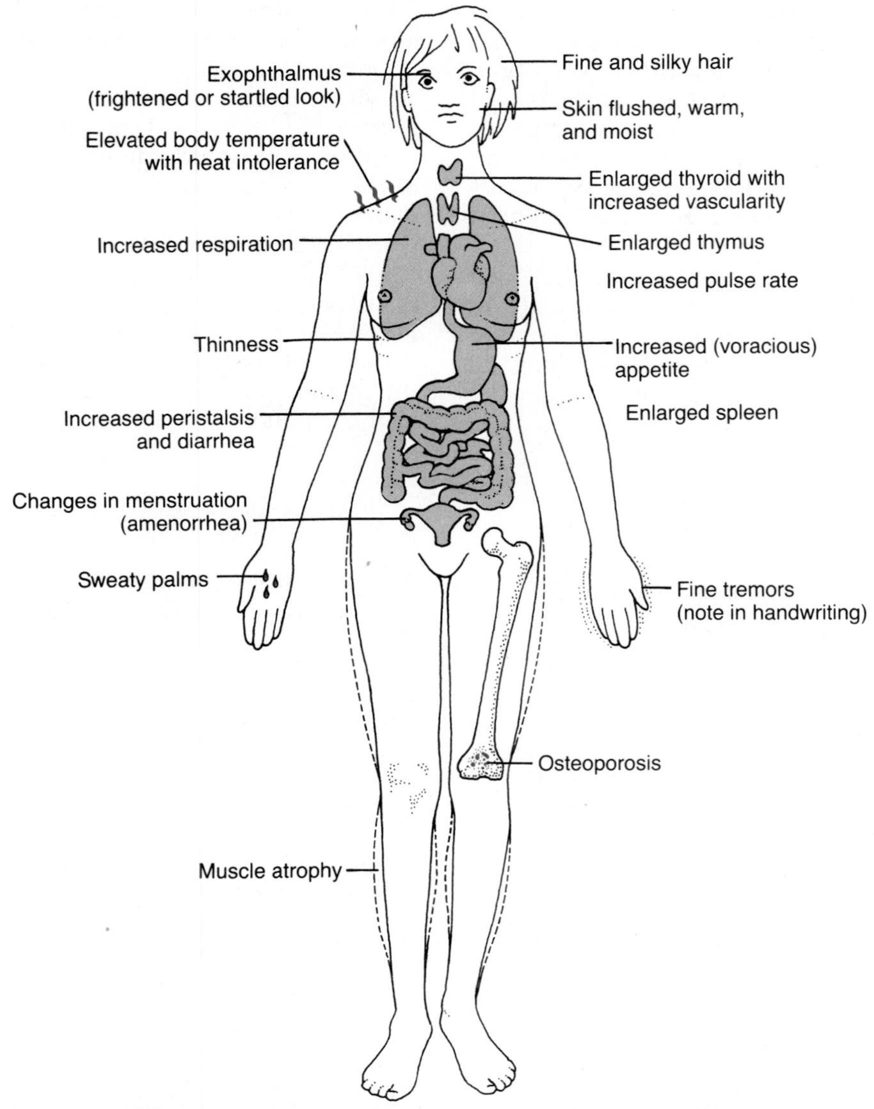

Figure 9–4. Various parts of the body are affected by the symptoms and pathophysiology of hyperthyroidism. (Adapted from Muthe, N.C.: Endocrinology: A Nursing Approach. Boston, Little, Brown, 1981, p. 93.)

ADDITIONAL SYMPTOMS OF HYPERTHYROIDISM

- Hyperactive, emotional, resulting in fatigue
- Eyelid lag
- Vitamin deficiency

Hypothyroidism

Hypothyroidism (hypofunction) results from insufficient thyroid hormone and creates a generalized depression of body metabolism. This condition may be classified as either being primary or secondary hypothyroidism.

Table 9–2. SYSTEMIC MANIFESTATIONS OF HYPERTHYROIDISM

CNS Effects	Cardiovascular and Pulmonary Effects	Integumentary Effects	Ocular Effects	GI Effects	GU Effects
Tremors Hyperkinesis (abnormally increased motor function or activity) Nervousness Emotional lability Weakness and muscle atrophy	Increased pulse rate/tachycardia/palpitations Dysrhythmias (palpitations) Weakness of respiratory muscles (breathlessness, hypoventilation)	Capillary dilatation (warm, flushed, moist skin) Heat intolerance Oncholysis (Separation of the fingernail from the nail bed) Easily broken hair and increased hair loss Hard, purple area over the anterior surface of the tibia with itching, erythema, and occasionally pain	Weakness of the extraocular muscles (poor convergence, poor upward gaze) Sensitivity to light Visual loss Spasm and retraction of the upper eyelids, lid tremor	Hypermetabolism (increased appetite with weight loss) Diarrhea, nausea, and vomiting	Polyuria (frequent urination) Amenorrhea (absence of menses) Female infertility

Primary hypothyroidism results from reduced functional thyroid tissue mass or impaired hormonal synthesis or release. Reduced thyroid mass may occur after treatment of thyrotoxicosis with radioactive iodine, from surgery, or from a metastasizing tumor. Impairment of hormone synthesis and release may result from iodine deficiency, prolonged lithium therapy (psychotropic drug), and impaired secretion of thyroid hormone (Nursing 84, 1984).

Secondary hypothyroidism (which accounts for a small percentage of all hypothyroidism) occurs as a result of inadequate stimulation of the gland because of pituitary disease (e.g., tumor, pituitary insufficiency, postpartum necrosis of the pituitary) (Nursing 84, 1984).

As with all disorders affecting the thyroid and parathyroid glands, clinical signs and symptoms affect many systems of the body that are outlined in Table 9–3 (Utiger, 1988). Of particular interest to the physical therapist is the concept that clinically, any compromise of the energy metabolism of muscle aggravates and perpetuates myofascial trigger points (TPs). Hypothyroid patients have only temporary pain relief with specific myofascial therapy until supplemented by thyroid hormone (Travell and Simons, 1983).

Neuromuscular symptoms are among the most frequent manifestations of hypothyroidism (Layzer, 1985). Characteristically, the muscular complaints of the patient with hypothyroidism are muscular aches and pains, cramps or stiffness of muscles, associated with muscle hypertrophy. The involved muscles are particularly likely to develop persistent TPs. Chronic fatigue, which may approach lethargy, is noticeable on arising in the morning and is usually worst during midafternoon. These patients are "weather conscious"; muscular pain increases with the onset of cold, rainy weather (Layzer, 1985; Travell and Simons, 1983).

Table 9–3. SYSTEMIC MANIFESTATIONS OF HYPOTHYROIDISM

CNS Effects	Musculoskeletal Effects	Cardiovascular Effects	Integumentary Effects	GI Effects
Slowed speech and hoarseness Slow mental function (loss of interest in daily activities, poor short-term memory) Fatigue and increased sleep Headache	Muscular weakness, cramps, myalgia, and stiffness Prolonged deep tendon reflexes (especially Achilles) Subjective report of paresthesias without supportive objective findings Muscular and joint edema Back pain	Bradycardia Congestive heart failure Poor peripheral circulation (pallor, cold skin, intolerance to cold, hypertension)	Thickened, cool, and dry skin Scaly skin (especially elbows and knees) Carotenosis (yellowing of the skin) Coarse, thinning hair Intolerance to cold Nonpitting edema of hands and feet Poor wound healing	Anorexia Constipation Weight gain disproportionate to caloric intake

CLINICAL SIGNS AND SYMPTOMS OF HYPOTHYROIDISM (Layzer, 1985)

- Mild, progressive, proximal muscle weakness
- Muscle aches
- Stiffness and slowness of movement
- Muscle cramps
- Acroparesthesias (abnormal sensation)
- Slow or prolonged reflexes
- Myoedema (knot of muscle)
- Muscular hypertrophy (enlargement; more common in children)
- Carpal tunnel syndrome
- Constipation

Acroparesthesias are usually due to median nerve compression at the wrist (carpal tunnel syndrome). The paresthesias are almost always located bilaterally in the hands. Most patients do not require surgical treatment because the symptoms respond to thyroid replacement; however, in long-standing cases, the presence of fat and fibrosis may require surgical treatment (Layzer, 1985).

Neoplasms* (Ingbar and Woeber, 1981)

Cancer of the thyroid is not uncommon and is often the incidental finding in patients being treated for other disorders (e.g., musculoskeletal disorders involving the head and neck). Thyroid tumors are generally slow-growing and are readily treated by surgery, administration of radioactive iodine, or suppression of tumor growth with thyroid hormone. Thyroid cancers seldom metastasize beyond regional lymph nodes of the neck; thus, the prognosis is good for all patients except those with the most aggressive types of cancer (Marshall, 1986). Benign neoplasms of the thyroid gland are called adenomas. Almost all malignant neoplasms of the thyroid are epithelial in origin and are therefore considered carcinomas.

* Primary cancers of other endocrine organs are rare and are unlikely to be encountered by the clinical therapist.

CLINICAL SIGNS AND SYMPTOMS OF THYROID CARCINOMA

- Presence of asymptomatic nodule or mass in thyroid tissue
- Nodule is firm, irregular, painless
- Hoarseness
- Dyspnea

Parathyroid Glands

Hyperparathyroidism

Hyperparathyroidism (hyperfunction) or the excessive secretion of PTH disrupts calcium, phosphate, and bone metabolism. The primary function of PTH is the maintenance of a normal serum calcium level. Elevated PTH causes release of calcium by the bone and accumulation of calcium in the bloodstream. Symptoms of hyperparathyroidism are related to this release of bone calcium into the bloodstream. This causes demineralization of bone and subsequent loss of bone strength and density. At the same time, the increase of calcium in the bloodstream can cause many other problems within the body.

Hyperparathyroidism may be classified as primary, secondary, tertiary, or ectopic. The major cause of primary hyperparathyroidism is adenoma of a parathyroid gland. Secondary hyperparathyroidism results from chronic renal disease: the excessive loss of calcium in the urine stimulates the parathyroid glands to undergo hyperplasia. The resultant metabolic effects are identical to those of primary hyperparathyroidism (Purtilo and Purtilo, 1989). Tertiary hyperparathyroidism may occur after chronic parathyroid stimulation in renal failure, and ectopic hyperparathyroidism occurs most commonly with lung or kidney carcinomas (Nursing 84, 1984).

Many systems of the body are affected by hyperparathyroidism, which is seen in the extensive list of signs and symptoms (Table 9–4) (Aurbach et al, 1985b). Proximal muscle weakness and fatigability are common findings.

A chief concern in hyperparathyroidism is damage to the kidneys from calcium deposits, which can result eventually in extensive renal damage. This condition may produce hypertension and eventual death from heart failure or uremia (renal failure). Hyperparathyroidism can also cause GI problems, pancreatitis, bone decalcification, and psychosis paranoia (Fig. 9–5). Treatment for primary hyperparathyroidism is surgical removal (parathyroidectomy). The prognosis for treatment is good if the condition is identified and treated early. Presence of kidney pathology is irreversible

Table 9–4. SYSTEMIC MANIFESTATIONS OF HYPERPARATHYROIDISM

Early CNS Symptoms	Musculoskeletal Effects	GI Effects	GU Effects
Lethargy, drowsiness, paresthesia Slow mentation, poor memory Easily fatigued Hyperactive deep tendon reflexes) Occasionally glove-and-stocking distribution sensory loss	Mild-to-severe proximal muscle weakness of the extremities Muscle atrophy Bone decalcification (bone pain, especially spine; pathologic fractures; bone cysts) Gout and pseudogout Arthralgias involving the hands Myalgia and sensation of heaviness in the lower extremities Joint hypermobility	Peptic ulcers Pancreatitis Nausea, vomiting, anorexia Constipation	Renal colic associated with kidney stones Hypercalcemia (polyuria, polydipsia, constipation) Kidney infections

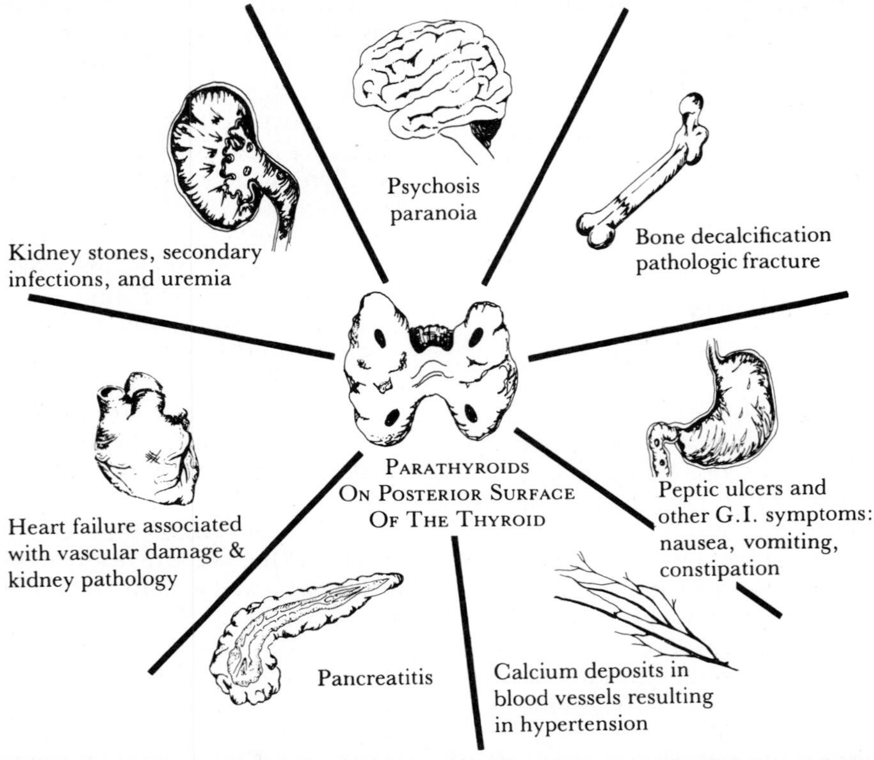

Figure 9–5. The pathologic processes of body structures as a result of excess parathyroid hormone. (From Muthe, N.C.: Endocrinology: A Nursing Approach. Boston, Little, Brown, 1981, p. 115.)

and tends to progress even with treatment for excess PTH.

Hypoparathyroidism

Hypoparathyroidism (hypofunction; insufficient secretion of PTH) results from the destruction of the absence of the parathyroid gland and disrupts mineral metabolism. It may be surgically induced (e.g., purposeful or inadvertent removal of functioning parathyroid tissue in anterior neck surgery) or result from chronic suppression of the gland after pathologic tissue is removed (Nursing 84, 1984). Any factor that limits the availability of vitamin D without compensatory treatment may cause hypoparathyroidism (e.g., GI surgery, pancreatitis, hepatic or renal disease, drugs such as phenobarbital and phenytoin). Hypocalcemia occurs when the parathyroids become inactive. The resultant deficiency of calcium in the blood alters the function of many tissues in the body, which is described by the systemic manifestations of *signs and symptoms* associated with hypoparathyroidism (Table 9–5).

Pancreas

Diabetes Mellitus

Diabetes mellitus (DM) is a chronic, multifaceted disorder caused by deficient insulin or defective insulin action. It is characterized by hyperglycemia (excess of glucose in the blood) and disruption of the metabolism of carbohydrates, fats, and proteins. Over time, it results in serious small and large vessel vascu-

Table 9-5. SYSTEMIC MANIFESTATIONS OF HYPOPARATHYROIDISM

CNS Effects	Musculoskeletal Effects	Cardiovascular Effects	Integumentary Effects	GI Effects
Personality changes (irritability, agitation, anxiety, depression)	Hypocalcemia (neuromuscular excitability and muscular tetany, especially involving flexion of upper extremity) Spasm of intercostal muscles and diaphragm compromising breathing Positive Chvostek's sign (twitching of facial muscles with tapping of the facial nerve in front of the ear)	Cardiac arrhythmias Eventual heart failure	Dry, scaly, coarse, pigmented skin Tendency to have skin infections Thinning of hair, including eyebrows and eyelashes Fingernails and toenails become brittle and form ridges	Nausea and vomiting Constipation or diarrhea Neuromuscular stimulation of the intestine (abdominal pain)

lar complications and neuropathies. This disease is ranked third as the cause of death from disease in the United States and is the leading cause of blindness (Muthe, 1981).

Since 1979, diabetes has been classified according to the various types of glucose abnormalities.* This classification system not only provides for the insulin-dependent diabetes mellitus (IDDM) and noninsulin-dependent diabetes mellitus (NIDDM), but also includes persons with impaired glucose tolerance, previous history of glucose abnormalities, and persons with potential for glucose abnormalities (Cassmeyer, 1987).

This text primarily focuses on the IDDM and NIDDM classifications, because these types of DM are more common and are more likely to be encountered by the physical therapist in the clinical setting.

Pathology. In DM, insulin is either insufficient in amount or ineffective in action. There is a difference in the pathology related to insulin response and secretion in IDDM and NIDDM. Some form of true deficiency in insulin secretion usually occurs with IDDM and results from a lack of, or destruction of, the pancreatic beta cells. In NIDDM, insulin levels may be depressed, normal, or increased, but the available insulin is ineffective in some way. Many factors contribute to the problem of ineffective insulin that include (Cassmeyer, 1987a):

- Islet cell defects, resulting in slowed or delayed insulin response
- Abnormalities or changes in insulin receptor sites
- Cellular resistance to insulin action

A defect in the alpha cell function of the pancreas is present in the individual with DM, so that glucagon function is also impaired. Glucagon does not respond normally to changes in blood glucose levels. This results in a chronically increased glucagon level, which, in turn, contributes to hyperglycemia (Cassmeyer, 1987a).

There are specific physiologic changes that occur when insulin is lacking or ineffective.

* This was categorized earlier as juvenile-onset and adult-onset DM. The guidelines for classifying DM are derived from the NIH National Diabetes Data Group: Classifications and diagnosis of diabetes mellitus and other categories of glucose intolerance. Diabetes, *28* (1042), 1979.

Normally, after a meal, the blood glucose level rises. A large amount of this glucose is taken up by the liver for storage or for use by other tissues, such as skeletal muscle and fat. When insulin function is impaired, the glucose in the general circulation is not taken up or removed by these tissues; thus, it continues to accumulate in the blood. Because new glucose has not been "deposited" into the liver, the liver synthesizes more glucose and releases it into the general circulation, which increases the already elevated blood glucose level (Cassmeyer, 1987a).

Protein synthesis is also impaired because amino acid transport into cells requires insulin. The metabolism of fats and fatty acids is altered and, instead of fat formation occurring, fat breakdown begins in an attempt to liberate more glucose (Cassmeyer, 1987a). The oxidation of these fats causes the formation of ketone bodies. Because the formation of these ketones can be rapid, they can build quickly and reach very high levels in the bloodstream. When the renal threshold for ketones is exceeded, the ketones appear in the urine as acetone (ketonuria).

The accumulation of high levels of glucose in the blood creates a hyperosmotic condition in the blood serum. This highly concentrated blood serum then "pulls" fluid from the interstitial areas, and fluid is lost through the kidneys (osmotic diuresis). Because large quantities of urine are excreted (polyuria), serious fluid losses occur and the conscious individual becomes extremely thirsty and drinks large amounts of water (polydypsia). In addition, the kidney is unable to reabsorb all the glucose so that glucose begins to be excreted in the urine (glycosuria).

CLINICAL SIGNS AND SYMPTOMS OF UNTREATED OR UNCONTROLLED DIABETES MELLITUS (Cassmeyer, 1987a; Muthe, 1981)

The classic clinical signs and symptoms of untreated or uncontrolled diabetes mellitus usually include one or more of the following:

- *Polyuria:* increased urination due to osmotic diuresis
- *Polydypsia:* increased thirst in response to polyuria
- *Polyphagia:* increased appetite and ingestion of food
- *Weight loss* in the presence of polyphagia; weight loss due to improper fat metabolism and breakdown of fat stores (usually only in IDDM)
- *Hyperglycemia:* increased blood glucose level (fasting= >140 mg/dl)
- *Glycosuria:* presence of glucose in the urine
- *Ketonuria:* presence of ketone bodies in urine (byproduct of fat catabolism)

It is important to note that certain medications can cause or contribute to hyperglycemia. Corticosteroids taken orally have the greatest glucogenic effect. Any diabetic patient taking corticosteroid medications needs to be monitored for changes in blood glucose levels. Oral contraceptives also have an effect on the stabilization of blood glucose levels. These drugs affect reproductive hormone production and can increase corticosteroid production. Antihypertensive diuretics, such as furosemide, thiazides, and ethacrynic acid, can affect blood glucose levels in already compromised patients (Lumley, 1988).

Physical Complications of Diabetes Mellitus. The patient with DM may present with a variety of serious physical problems. Infection and atherosclerosis are the two primary long-term complications of this disease and are the usual causes of severe illness and death in the diabetic patient.

Blood vessels and nerves sustain major pathologic changes in the diabetic patient. Atherosclerosis in both large vessels (macrovascular changes) and small vessels (microvascular changes) develop at a much earlier age and progress much faster in the diabetic patient. The precise mechanism underlying the development of these fatty plaques is unknown at this time, but may involve the interaction of several factors, such as abnormal lipid metabolism, hormonal imbalances, hyperglycemia, and abnormal platelet function (Foster, 1983). The blood vessel changes result in decreased blood vessel lumen size, compromised blood flow, and resultant tissue ischemia. The pathologic end-products are CVD, CAD, renal artery stenosis, and peripheral vascular disease (Cassmeyer, 1987a).

Microvascular changes, characterized by the thickening of capillaries and damage to the basement membrane, result in diabetic nephropathy (kidney disease) and retinopathy (disease of the retina). Again, the exact mechanism of pathology is unknown, but these changes are considered to be due to uncontrolled diabetes (Cassmeyer, 1987a).

Poorly controlled DM can lead to various tissue changes that result in impaired wound healing. Loss of fat deposits under the skin, loss of glycogen, and catabolism of body proteins can diminish the ability of tissue to repair itself. Catabolism of body proteins and resultant protein loss hamper the inflammatory process. Phagocytosis, migration of leukocytes, and bacterial killing are also impaired in the diabetic patient and result in increased susceptibility to tissue infections. In addition, decreased circulation to the skin can further delay or diminish healing (Cassmeyer, 1987).

Diabetic Neuropathy. Neuropathy is the most common chronic complication of long-term DM. Neuropathy in the diabetic patient is thought to be related to the accumulation in the nerve cells of sorbitol, a byproduct of improper glucose metabolism. This accumulation then results in abnormal fluid and electrolyte shifts and nerve cell dysfunction (Cassmeyer, 1987a). Diminished circulation to nervous system tissue due to blood vessel blockage is also believed by some people to contribute to this problem, but there is still much controversy regarding the precise etiology of diabetic neuropathy.

Neuropathy may affect the central nervous system (CNS), peripheral nervous system, or the autonomic nervous system. The most common form of diabetic neuropathy is polyneuropathy, which affects peripheral nerves in distal lower extremities, causes burning and numbness in feet, and can result in muscle weakness, atrophy, and foot drop.

The large and small vessel changes that occur with DM contribute to the changes in the feet of diabetics. Sensory neuropathy, which may lead to painless trauma and ulceration, can progress to infection. Neuropathy can result in drying and cracking of the skin, which creates more openings for bacteria to enter. The combination of all these factors can lead ultimately to gangrene and eventually to amputation. Prevention of these problems by meticulous care of the diabetic foot can reduce the need for amputation by 50 to 75% (Cassmeyer, 1987a).

Whether or not poorly controlled blood glucose is a causative factor in the development of the long-term physical complications of diabetes is still controversial (Cassmeyer, 1987a; Foster, 1983). It does seem clear, however, that these complications increase with the duration of the disease.

Diagnosis and Treatment. Diagnosis of DM occurs through a variety of laboratory tests that are used to measure blood glucose levels either at random or during a fasting state. Frequent self-glucose monitoring is also important in the long-term management of DM. This is most often accomplished by using a direct blood sampling by fingerstick technique.

Medical management of the diabetic patient is directed primarily toward maintenance of blood glucose values within the normal range (e.g., 80 to 120 mg/dl). The three primary treatment modalities used in the management of DM are diet, exercise, and medication (insulin and oral hypoglycemic agents) (Table 9-6). Although tight glucose control is still a controversial issue, more studies on patients are suggesting that long-term complications of the disease may be minimized if the blood glucose levels can be maintained consistently within this range (Hughes, 1987).

Severe Hyperglycemic States

There are two primary life-threatening metabolic conditions that can develop if un-

Table 9–6. INSULIN ACTION (average for classifications)

Type	Onset (Hrs)	Peak (Hrs)	Duration (Hrs)
RAPID ACTING (e.g., regular insulin, Semi lente)	½–1	2–6	5–12
INTERMEDIATE ACTING (e.g., NPH, Lente)	1–3	6–12	16–24
LONG-ACTING (e.g., Ultralente, protamine zinc)	4–8	16–18	36+

controlled or untreated DM progresses to a state of severe hyperglycemia (>400 mg/dl). These conditions are diabetic ketoacidosis (DKA) and hyperglycemic, hyperosmolar, nonketotic coma (HHNC) (Table 9–7).

DKA occurs with severe insulin deficiency either due to undiagnosed DM or to a situation in which the insulin needs of the patient become greater than usual (e.g., infection, trauma, emotional upsets). It is most often seen in the patient with IDDM, but can, in rare situations, occur with the patient with NIDDM (Cassmeyer, 1987a). Medical treatment is most often intravenous (IV) insulin, IV bicarbonate for buffering, and fluid and electrolyte replacement.

CLINICAL SIGNS AND SYMPTOMS RELATED TO DIABETIC KETOACIDOSIS

- Dry mouth
- Hot, dry skin
- Elevated body temperature from a fluid deficit
- Fruity (acetone) odor to the breath
- Overall weakness
- Confusion/lethargy/coma
- Deep, rapid respirations (Kussmaul respirations, a compensatory response of the lungs to neutralize acidosis)*
- Muscle and abdominal cramps (due to a loss of electrolytes)

* Dyspnea characterized by increased respiratory rate (above 20/min), increased depth of respiration, panting, and labored respiration typical of air hunger (Miller and Keane, 1987).

HHNC occurs most commonly in the elderly patient with NIDDM. This complication is extremely serious and, in many cases, is fatal. Factors that can precipitate this crisis are:

- Infections (e.g., pneumonia, pyelonephritis)
- Medications that elevate the blood glucose level (e.g., corticosteroids)
- Procedures, such as dialysis, surgery, or total parenteral nutrition (TPN)

There are specific clinical features that identify HHNC. Some of these features are similar to those of DKA, such as severe hyperglycemia (1,000 to 2,000 mg/dl) and dehydration. The major differentiating feature between DKA and HHNC, however, is the absence of ketosis in HHNC. Treatment of this problem includes insulin therapy and fluid and electrolyte replacement (Cassmeyer, 1987a).

CLINICAL SIGNS AND SYMPTOMS OF HYPERGLYCEMIC, HYPEROSMOLAR, NONKETOTIC COMA (HHNC)

- Severe polyuria (usually combined with poor fluid intake)
- Decreased temperature
- Signs of severe dehydration
- Lethargy/confusion/coma
- Seizures
- Gastric distention (paralysis of the intestine due to severe electrolyte losses)

Because it is likely that the physical therapist will work with diabetic patients in the

Table 9–7. CLINICAL SYMPTOMS OF LIFE-THREATENING GLYCEMIC STATES

Hyperglycemia		Hypoglycemia
Diabetic Ketoacidosis (DKA)	***Hyperglycemic, Hyperosmolar, Nonketotic Coma (HHNC)***	***Insulin Shock***
Gradual Onset	*Gradual Onset*	*Sudden Onset*
Headache Thirst Hyperventilation Fruity odor to breath Lethargy/confusion Coma Abdominal pain and distention Dehydration Polyuria Flushed face Elevated temperature	Thirst Polyuria leading quickly to decreased urine output Volume loss from polyuria leading quickly to renal insufficiency Severe dehydration Lethargy/confusion Seizures Coma Abdominal pain and distention	Pallor Perspiration Piloerection Increased heart rate Palpitation Irritability/nervousness Weakness Hunger Shakiness Headache Double/blurred vision Slurred speech Fatigue Numbness of lips/tongue Confusion Convulsion/coma

clinical setting, it is imperative that the clinical symptoms of DM and its potentially life-threatening metabolic states be understood. *If any diabetic patient arrives for a clinical appointment in a confused or lethargic state or exhibiting changes in mental function, fingerstick glucose should be performed. Immediate physician referral is necessary.*

Hypoglycemia Associated with Diabetes Mellitus

Hypoglycemia (blood glucose of <70 mg/dl) is a major complication of insulin or oral hypoglycemic agents. Hypoglycemia is usually the result of a decrease in food intake or an increase in physical activity in relation to insulin administration. It is a potentially lethal problem. The hypoglycemic state interrupts the oxygen consumption of nervous system tissue. Repeated or prolonged attacks can result in irreversible brain damage and death (Cassmeyer, 1987a).

Hypoglycemia during or after exercise can be a problem for any diabetic patient. When the circulating insulin level is high (which occurs during peak activity of the medication), the liver production of glucose induced by exercise is suppressed. Hypoglycemia results as glucose is utilized by the working muscles. The degree of hypoglycemia depends on such factors as:

- Pre-exercise blood glucose levels
- Duration and intensity of exercise
- Blood insulin concentration

CLINICAL SIGNS AND SYMPTOMS OF HYPOGLYCEMIA (Cassmeyer, 1987a)

The signs and symptoms of hypoglycemia are related to two body responses: increased sympathetic activity and deprivation of CNS glucose supply.

- Sympathetic activity
  - Pallor
  - Perspiration
  - Piloerection (erection of the hair)
  - Increased heart rate
  - Heart palpitation
  - Nervousness and irritability
  - Weakness

    - Shakiness/trembling
    - Hunger
- CNS activity
    - Headache
    - Blurred vision
    - Slurred speech
    - Numbness of the lips and tongue
    - Confusion
    - Euphoria
    - Convulsion
    - Coma

The severity and number of signs and symptoms depends on the individual patient and or the rapidity of the drop in blood glucose. The clinical manifestations of a rapid drop in blood glucose are primarily sympathetic in origin. A more gradual decrease in glucose can be a result of the use of longer-acting insulins and oral hypoglycemics. Symptoms in this situation are most often CNS-related. If a rapid drop is allowed to continue, both sympathetic and CNS manifestations may develop (Cassmeyer, 1987a).

It is important to note that patients can exhibit signs and symptoms of hypoglycemia when their blood glucose level drops rapidly from an elevated range to a range that is still elevated (e.g., 400 to 200 mg/dl). The *rapidity* of the drop is the stimulus for sympathetic activity, thus even though a blood glucose level appears elevated, patients may still have hypoglycemia (Cassmeyer, 1987a).

Patients receiving beta adrenergic blockers (e.g., propranolol) can be at special risk for hypoglycemia by the actions of this medication. These beta blockers inhibit the normal physiologic response of the body to the hypoglycemic state or block the appearance of the sympathetic manifestations of hypoglycemia (Lumley, 1988). Patients may also have hypoglycemia during nighttime sleep (most often related to the use of intermediate and long-acting insulins given more than once a day) with the only symptoms being (Cassmeyer, 1987a):

- Nightmares
- Sweating
- Headache

Hypoglycemia can be treated in the conscious patient by immediate administration of sugar. It is always safer to give the sugar, even when in doubt concerning the origin of symptoms (DKA and HHNC can also present with similar CNS symptoms). Most often 10 to 15 g of carbohydrate are sufficient to reverse the episode of hypoglycemia. Some examples of immediate-acting glucose sources that should be kept in every physical therapy department include (Cassmeyer, 1987a):

- 1/2 cup fruit juice
- 1/2 cup sugared cola
- 1/2 cup gelatin dessert
- 4 cubes or 2 packets of sugar
- 2 to 3 pieces of hard candy
- 2-oz tube of cake decorating gel

Most diabetic patients carry a rapid-acting source of carbohydrate so that it is readily available for use if a hypoglycemic episode occurs. Intramuscular glucagon is also used by some diabetic patients. If the patient loses consciousness, emergency personnel will need to be notified, and glucose will be administered intravenously. Any episode or suspected episode of hypoglycemia must be treated promptly and must be reported to the patient's physician. It is important to question each diabetic patient regarding his or her individual response to hypoglycemia. Information regarding individual symptoms, frequency of episodes, and precipitating factors may be invaluable to the physical therapist in preventing or minimizing a hypoglycemic attack.

Hypoglycemia

As discussed earlier in this text, hypoglycemia is the state in which blood glucose drops to below normal levels (<70 mg/dl). The clinical severity of the drop depends on several factors, including rapidity, duration, and individual tolerance. There are two classifications of hypoglycemia:

- Fasting hypoglycemia
- Reactive hypoglycemia

Fasting hypoglycemia is commonly manifested as a side effect of insulin or oral hypoglycemic medication. It can also be the result of pathologies that cause an underproduction of glucose (e.g., hormonal deficiencies of ACTH, cortisol, glucagon, and catecholamines), or it can be the result of an overproduction of insulin or insulinlike material (e.g, tumors such as insulinomas, autoimmune disease) (Cassmeyer, 1987a).

Reactive hypoglycemia (functional hypoglycemia) occurs after the intake of a meal and occurs usually as a result of stomach or duodenal surgery. After certain types of gastric surgery (e.g., gastectomy), food is emptied rapidly into the jejunem and does not undergo the usual dilutional changes that occur in the stomach. The blood glucose level rises rapidly as glucose is quickly absorbed into the bloodstream, but then falls rapidly to below normal levels as an exaggerated response of insulin output develops. This rapid drop in blood glucose results in symptoms of hypoglycemia. The cause of reactive hypoglycemia unrelated to gastric surgery is unknown, and this condition is called *idiopathic reactive hypoglycemia.* Diagnosis in this situation is usually difficult because the criteria for diagnosis is inconsistent among medical practitioners, and the condition is frequently overdiagnosed (Cassmeyer, 1987a).

Clinical signs and symptoms of both *fasting* and *reactive hypoglycemia* are the same as those described earlier for hypoglycemia related to DM. Treatment consists of glucose replacement for immediate symptom management and then treatment of the underlying cause, if applicable (e.g., surgery for tumors; correction of hormonal or hepatic problems; discontinuation of drugs that induce hypoglycemia, such as alcohol, salicylates). The patient is warned to avoid fasting and simple sugars. Some dietary modifications, such as low carbohydrate, high-protein diets have been suggested, but the effectiveness of these measures is largely unproven (Cassmeyer, 1987).

INTRODUCTION TO METABOLISM (Miller and Keane, 1987)

As noted earlier, the endocrine system works with the nervous system to regulate and integrate the body's metabolic activities (Nursing 84, 1984). Metabolism is the physical and chemical processes of the body broken down into two phases:

- Anabolic phase
- Catabolic phase

The anabolic, or constructive, phase is concerned with the conversion of simpler compounds derived from nutrients into living, organized substances that the body cells can use. In the catabolic, or destructive, phase these organized substances are reconverted into simpler compounds, with the release of energy necessary for the proper functioning of body cells.

The rate of metabolism can be increased by exercise, by elevated body temperature (e.g., high fever), by hormonal activity (e.g., thyroxine, insulin, epinephrine), and by specific dynamic action that occurs after the ingestion of a meal.

Although acid-base metabolism is not in itself a sign or a symptom, the consequences of disordered acid-base metabolism can result in many signs and symptoms. Physical therapists are unlikely to evaluate someone with a primary musculoskeletal lesion that reflects an underlying metabolic disorder. However, many inpatients in hospitals and some outpatients may be affected by disturbances in acid-base metabolism and other specific metabolic disorders. Only those conditions that are likely to be encountered by a physical therapist are included in this text.

Fluid Imbalances (Table 9–8)

The human body consists of approximately 45 to 60% water. The amount and distribution of body water varies with age, sex, and body fat content. The body of the newborn infant con-

Table 9–8. FLUID IMBALANCES

Imbalance	Symptoms
Fluid Deficit (Dehydration)	
INCREASED SOLUTES, DECREASED H_2O/ DECREASED SOLUTES, DECREASED H_2O	Thirst Weight loss Dryness of mouth, throat, face Poor skin turgor Decreased urine output Absence of sweat Postural changes from lying to standing Increased pulse (10 beats/min) Decreased blood pressure (10 mm Hg systolic when standing) Dizziness when standing Confusion
Fluid Excess	
INCREASED H_2O, DECREASED SOLUTES (water intoxication)	Decreased mental alertness Sleepiness Anorexia Poor motor coordination Confusion Convulsions Sudden weight gain Hyperventilation Warm, moist skin Increased intracerebral pressure Decreased pulse Increased systolic blood pressure Decreased diastolic blood pressure Mild peripheral edema
INCREASED H_2O, INCREASED SOLUTES (edema)	Weight gain Dependent edema Pitting edema Increased blood pressure Neck vein engorgement Effusions Pulmonary Pericardial Peritoneal Congestive heart failure

tains about 75% water, whereas the body water of the adult female is 50% and that of the adult male is 60%. Body water also decreases with increased body fat, because fat is free of water.

Body water contains the electrolytes that are essential to human life. This life-sustaining fluid is found within various body compartments including:

- Interstitial compartment
- Intravascular compartment
- Transcellular compartment

Fluid found inside cells (intracellular fluid [ICF]) comprises about 60% of the total amount of body fluid, whereas the fluid found outside cells (extracellular fluid [ECF]) comprises the remaining 40%. The ECF is contained in the interstitial compartment (space between cells) and in the intravascular compartment (vascular spaces). A third compartment called the transcellular compartment consists of fluid that is present in the body but is separated from body tissues by a layer of epithelial cells. This fluid includes digestive juices, water, and solutes in the renal tubules and bladder, intraocular fluid, and cerebrospinal fluid (Soltis and Cassmeyer, 1987).

Because there are many situations in the body that cause both normal and abnormal fluid shifts, it is important to have a clear understanding of fluid compartments. The recognition of pathologic conditions, such as edema, dehydration, ketoacidosis, and various types of shock can depend on the understanding of these concepts.

There are many functions of body fluids including digestion, gas and nutrient transport, elimination of wastes, temperature regulation, and chemical function within the cells. In the healthy body, fluid and electrolytes are constantly lost or exchanged between compartments. This balance must be maintained for the body to function properly. Fluids are lost daily from the GI tract, skin, respiratory tract, and renal system. The amount of fluid used in these functions depends on factors such as humidity, temperature, physical activity, and metabolic rate. Balance is achieved through fluid intake and dietary consumption.

Movement of fluid and solutes between body compartments occurs by one of three ways:

- Diffusion
- Osmosis
- Active transport

Diffusion

Diffusion is the movement of solutes or particles from an area of greater concentration to an area of lesser concentration (along the concentration gradient) through a semipermeable membrane. This action does not require any use of energy, but may, sometimes, require a carrier substance to transport the solute across the cell membrane (e.g., insulin is a "carrier" for glucose transport into the cell).

Osmosis

Osmosis is the movement of *water* from an area of low solute concentration (high water concentration) to an area of high solute concentration (low water concentration) across a semipermeable membrane. A solution with a high water concentration and a low solute concentration is a *hypotonic* solution. A solution that consists of a large amount of solute and a small amount of water is called *hypertonic.* If a solution contains both water and solutes in the same concentration as that of the fluid in the body, it is called an *isotonic* solution.

Active Transport

Active transport is a mechanism that moves *solutes* from an area of low concentration to high concentration (against the concentration gradient) and requires energy expenditure. This mechanism regulates the movement of sodium (Na^+) and potassium (K^+) into and out of the cell. It is the major factor in the maintenance of Na^+ and K^+ concentrations in the cells and is a primary factor in maintaining appropriate cellular electrical potential.

Fluid Deficit

Fluid deficit can occur as a result of two primary types of imbalance. There is either a loss of water without loss of solutes or a loss of both water and solutes.

The loss of body water without solutes results in the excess concentration of body solutes within the interstitial and intravascular compartments. To preserve equilibrium, water will then be forced to shift by osmosis from inside cells to these outside compartments. If the hypertonic state persists, large amounts of body water will be shifted and excreted (osmotic diuresis) and severe cellular dehydration will result. This type of imbalance can occur as a result of several conditions:

- Decreased water intake (e.g., unavailability, unconsciousness)
- Water loss without proportionate solute loss (e.g., prolonged hyperventilation, diabetes insipidus)
- Increased solute intake without proportionate water intake (tube feeding)

- Excess accumulation of solutes (e.g., high glucose levels such as in DM)

The second type of fluid imbalance results from a loss of *both* water and solutes. This is called an isotonic or volume-related fluid loss. This loss is restricted to the extracellular compartment and does not cause fluid shifting from the intracellular spaces.

Causes of the loss of both water and solutes include:

- Hemorrhage
- Profuse perspiration (marathon runners)
- Loss of GI tract secretions (vomiting, diarrhea, draining fistulas, ileostomy)

Severe losses of water and solutes can lead to hypovolemic shock. It is important for the physical therapist to be aware of possible fluid losses or water shifts in any patient who is already compromised by advanced age or by a situation such as an ileotomy or tracheostomy that results in a continuous loss of fluid. Because the response to fluid loss is highly individual, it is important to recognize the early clinical symptoms of fluid loss and to carefully monitor patients who are at risk.

CLINICAL SIGNS AND SYMPTOMS OF DEHYDRATION OR FLUID LOSS

Early clinical signs and symptoms

- Thirst
- Weight loss

As the condition worsens, other symptoms may include:

- Poor skin turgor
- Dryness of the mouth, throat, and face
- Absence of sweat
- Increased body temperature
- Low urine output
- Postural changes (increased heart rate by 10 beats/min and decreased systolic or diastolic blood pressure by 20 mm Hg when moving from a supine to a sitting position.
- Dizziness when standing
- Confusion

Athletes and normal adults may experience orthostatic hypotension when slightly dehydrated, especially when intense exercise increases the core body temperature. The normal vascular system can accommodate to this effectively.

Laboratory tests reveal increased hematocrit (blood becomes depleted of fluid, thus the percentage of red blood cells (RBCs) to fluid appears to be higher). Treatment consists of water or solute replacement and correction of the underlying problem. The patient under medical care is carefully assessed for hydration level, fluid intake, and urine output.

Fluid Excess Imbalances

Fluid excess can occur in two major forms:

- Water intoxication (excess of water without an excess of solutes)
- Edema (excess of both solutes and water)

Because the etiology, symptoms, and outcomes related to these problems are substantially different, these fluid imbalances are discussed separately.

Water Intoxication. Water intoxication is an excess of extracellular water in relationship to solutes. The ECF becomes diluted and water must then move into cells to equalize solute concentration on either side of the cell membrane. Water excess can be caused by an accumulation of solute-free fluid. An increase in solute-free fluid can occur for several possible reasons, which can include (Solis and Cassmeyer, 1987):

- Psychogenic polydypsia (psychologic problem that involves the intake of large amounts of tap water)
- Intake of only tap water after vomiting (many patients can tolerate water when experiencing vomiting and thus ingest water without solutes to replace lost fluid; this is an inadequate source of electrolytes)

- Excess secretion of ADH or vasopressin (e.g., stress, anesthesia, tumors, endocrine disorders)
- Poor renal function (water reabsorbed inappropriately)
- Solute loss without water loss (e.g., GI or biliary drainage, severe dietary sodium restriction)

CLINICAL SYMPTOMS OF WATER INTOXICATION

- Decreased mental alertness

Other accompanying symptoms

- Sleepiness
- Anorexia
- Poor motor coordination
- Confusion

In a severe imbalance, other symptoms may include:

- Convulsions
- Sudden weight gain
- Hyperventilation
- Warm, moist skin
- Signs of increased intracerebral pressure
  - Slow pulse
  - Increased systolic blood pressure (>10 mm Hg)
  - Decreased diastolic blood pressure (>10 mm Hg)
- Mild peripheral edema
- Low serum sodium

Laboratory results reveal low hematocrit (blood serum diluted so that the percentage of RBCs appears to be less). Treatment is usually careful restriction of water with possible sodium and solute replacement.

Edema. Excess of solutes and water is called an isotonic volume excess. The excess fluid is retained in the extracellular compartment and results in fluid accumulation in the interstitial spaces *(edema).* Edema can be produced by many different situations including (Soltis and Cassmeyer, 1987):

- Vein obstruction (e.g., thrombophlebitis, varicose veins)
- Increased aldosterone (e.g., Cushing's, steroid therapy, renal impairment)
- Loss of serum protein (e.g., decreased dietary intake, burns, renal impairment, decreased production in the liver, allergic reactions)
- Decreased cardiac output (e.g., congestive heart failure [CHF])

CLINICAL SIGNS AND SYMPTOMS OF EDEMA

- Weight gain (primary symptom)
- Excess fluid (several liters may accumulate before edema is evident)
- Dependent edema (collection of fluid in lower parts of the body)
- Pitting edema (indentation of finger pressed into edematous area leaves a persistent depression in tissues)

The treatment of volume excess depends on the condition that caused it to develop. For example, diuretics and cardiac medications may be used to treat congestive heart failure and to remove excess fluid. Some restriction of sodium may also be a part of the treatment for edema and prevention of further fluid gain. Malnutrition and protein losses are treated with increased protein intake (Soltis and Cassmeyer, 1987).

Diuretic medications are used frequently to treat isotonic volume excess. Various diuretic medications may be used depending on the underlying cause of the problem and the desired effect of the drug. The most commonly used are the thiazide diuretics (e.g., chlorothiazide, hydrochlorothiazide). These medications inhibit sodium and water reabsorption by the kidneys. Potassium is usually also lost with the sodium and water so that continuous replacement of potassium is a major concern for any patient receiving non–potassium-sparing diuretics (Soltis and Cassmeyer, 1987).

It is essential to monitor patients who take diuretics for signs and symptoms of potassium depletion:

- Muscle weakness
- Fatigue
- Cardiac arrhythmias
- Abdominal distention
- Nausea and vomiting

It is also very important to check laboratory data for the potassium level in any patient taking diuretics, particularly before exercise. Any value below the normal range (<3.5 meq/l) could be potentially dangerous and could result in a lethal cardiac arrhythmia even with moderate cardiovascular exercise. In addition, it is important to assess patients who take diuretic therapy for potential fluid loss and dehydration by observing for clinical symptoms of both. Questions concerning the correlation of potassium levels with exercise and possible appearance of symptoms consistent with dehydration should be discussed with a physician before physical therapy treatment.

METABOLIC DISORDERS

Metabolic Alkalosis

Metabolic alkalosis results from metabolic disturbances that either cause an increase in available bases or a loss of nonrespiratory body acids. Blood pH rises to a level greater than 7.45 (Table 9–9).

Common causes of metabolic alkalosis include (Stroot et al, 1980):

- Excessive vomiting (loss of stomach acids)
- Ingestion of large quantities of base (sodium bicarbonate preparations used as stomach antacids)
- Upper GI tract intubation and suctioning (loss of stomach acids)
- Use of diuretics (loss of hydrogen and chloride ions)
- Prolonged hypercalcemia (relationship unknown)
- Cushing's syndrome

PRIMARY CLINICAL SIGNS AND SYMPTOMS OF METABOLIC ALKALOSIS

- Nausea
- Prolonged vomiting
- Diarrhea
- Confusion
- Irritability
- Agitation, restlessness
- Muscle twitching and muscle cramping
- Muscle weakness
- Paresthesias
- Convulsions
- Eventual coma
- Slow, shallow breathing

Decreased respirations may occur as the respiratory system attempts to compensate by buffering the basic environment. The lungs attempt to retain carbon dioxide (CO_2) and thus hydrogen ions (H^+).

Treatment of alkalosis is correction of the underlying cause and neutralization of the increased pH. Losses of potassium and chloride that occur through the loss of the stomach acids and use of diuretics should be replaced. The medication acetazolamide (Diamox) can be used to increase renal excretion of bicarbonate. Acidic solutions (e.g., ammonium chloride) can be given to add hydrogen ions and to decrease pH.

It is important for the physical therapist to ask patients regarding the use of antacids, because symptoms of alkalosis can affect muscular function by causing muscle fasciculation and cramping. Prevention of problems related to alkalosis may be accomplished by education of the patient regarding antacid use.

Table 9–9. LABORATORY VALUES: UNCOMPENSATED AND COMPENSATED METABOLIC ACIDOSIS AND ALKALOSIS

Arterial Blood	*pH(7.35–7.45)*	*Pco_2(35–45 mm Hg)*	*HCO_3(22–26 meq/l)*	Signs/Symptoms
METABOLIC ACIDOSIS (uncompensated)	<7.35	Normal	<22	Headache Fatigue Nausea, vomiting
COMPENSATED	Normal	<35	<22	Diarrhea Muscular twitching Convulsions, coma Hyperventilation
METABOLIC ALKALOSIS (uncompensated)	>7.45	Normal	>26	Nausea Vomiting Diarrhea
COMPENSATED	Normal	>45	>26	Confusion Irritability Agitation Muscle twitch Muscle cramp Muscle weakness Paresthesias Convulsions Slow breathing

Metabolic Acidosis

Metabolic or nonrespiratory acidosis is an accumulation of fixed (nonvolatile) acids or a deficit of base. This condition is due primarily to an alteration in the utilization and metabolism of various nutrients and chemical compounds. Blood pH decreases to a level below 7.35 (see Table 9–9).

Common causes of metabolic acidosis include (Stroot et al, 1980):

- Diabetic ketoacidosis
- Renal failure
- Lactic acidosis
- Severe diarrhea
- Chemical intoxication (e.g, salicylate poisoning)

For example, ketoacidosis occurs because insufficiency of insulin for the proper use of glucose results in increased breakdown of fat. This accelerated fat breakdown produces ketones and other acids. These acids accumulate to high levels. While the body attempts to neutralize these increased acids, the plasma bicarbonate (HCO_3) is used up. Renal failure results in acidosis because the failing kidney is not only unable to rid the body of excess acids, but also cannot produce necessary bicarbonate. Lactic acidosis occurs as excess lactic acid is produced during strenuous exercise or when oxygen is insufficient for proper use of carbohydrate (CHO), glucose, and water (H_2O). Intestinal and pancreatic secretions are highly alkaline so that severe diarrhea depletes the body of these necessary bases. Metabolic acidosis can also result from ingestion of large quantities of acetylsalicylic acid (salicylates), and symptoms of possible metabolic acidosis should be carefully assessed in patients on high dose aspirin therapy (Stroot et al, 1980).

CLINICAL SIGNS AND SYMPTOMS OF METABOLIC ACIDOSIS

- Headache
- Fatigue

- Drowsiness, lethargy
- Nausea, vomiting
- Diarrhea
- Muscular twitching
- Convulsions
- Coma (severe)
- Rapid, deep breathing (hyperventilation)

Hyperventilation may also occur as the respiratory system attempts to rid the body of excess acid by increasing the rate and depth of respiration. The result is an increase in the amount of carbon dioxide and hydrogen excreted through the respiratory system.

Acidosis is usually treated by correction of the underlying cause of the condition. Sodium bicarbonate may also be used if the acidosis is severe and requires immediate treatment.

Gout

Primary gout is the manifestation of an inherited inborn error of purine metabolism characterized by an elevated serum uric acid (hyperuricemia). Uric acid is a waste product resulting from the breakdown of purines that are commonly found in foods. Uric acid is usually dissolved in the blood until it is passed into the urine through the kidneys. In patients with gout, the uric acid changes into crystals that deposit in joints (causing gouty arthritis) and other tissues such as the kidneys, causing renal disease.

Gout may occur as a result of another disorder or of its therapy. This is referred to as secondary gout. Secondary gout may be associated with other metabolic disorders, such as DM and hyperlipidemia (excess serum lipids). Gout affects men predominantly, and the usual form of primary gout is uncommon before the third decade with its peak incidence in the forties and fifties. Attacks may be precipitated by conditions that produce metabolic acidosis and a decrease in the excretion of uric acid in the urine. These conditions may include surgery, minor trauma, fatigue, emotional stress, infection, starvation (even the relative starvation resulting from crash diets), administration of drugs (e.g., penicillin, insulin, or thiazide diuretics), and dietary or alcoholic excesses (Hall, 1983). Additionally, secondary gout may occur as a side effect of chemotherapy for tumors, impairment of clearance due to the use of hypertensive drugs (e.g., hydrochlorthiazide), or due to the use of low-dose aspirin (Miller and Keane, 1987).

Gouty arthritis results in periarticular and subcutaneous deposits of sodium urate (or urate salts) referred to as tophus (tophi). The peripheral joints of the hands and feet are involved with 90% of gouty patients having attacks in the metatarsophalangeal joint of the great toe. Other typical sites of initial involvement (in order of frequency) are the instep, ankle, heel, knee, and wrist, although any joint in the body may be involved (Wyngaarden and Kelley, 1983). These deposits produce an acute inflammatory response that then leads to acute arthritis and later to chronic arthritis (Purtilo, 1978; Salter, 1983). Enlarged tophi on the joints of the hands and feet may erupt and discharge chalky masses of urate crystals (Berkow, 1987).

Onset of pain is sudden and severe and increases in intensity in one or more joints. The pain usually reaches its maximum intensity within 12 hours after its onset. There is exquisite tenderness accompanied by swelling of the inflamed joint, and any pressure (even the touch of clothes or bedsheets) on the joint is intolerable. The untreated attack lasts from 10 days to 2 weeks. Without treatment, the attacks tend to occur closer and closer together. In the early stages of the disease, the attacks are separated by asymptomatic periods that may last for months to years. In later stages, there is continual discomfort, attacks are often polyarticular, more severe, and may be accompanied by fever (Hall, 1983; Wyngaarden and Kelley, 1983).

CLINICAL SIGNS AND SYMPTOMS OF GOUT

- Tophi: lumps under the skin or actual eruptions through the skin of chalky urate crystals

- Joint pain and swelling
- Fever and chills
- Malaise

Metabolic Bone Disease

Connective tissue disorders represent a group of diseases with certain clinical and histologic features that are manifestations of connective tissue; that is, tissues that provide the supportive framework (musculoskeletal structures) and protective covering (skin and mucous membranes and vessel linings) for the body (Miller and Keane, 1987). Of the metabolic disorders involving connective tissue, muscle, and bone, only Paget's disease and osteogenesis imperfecta are included as the most commonly presented diseases in a physical therapy practice.

Paget's Disease (Salter, 1983)

Paget's disease (osteitis deformans) (named after Sir James Paget circa mid-1880s) is a relatively common disorder of bone remodeling that affects men more often than women (3:2 ratio). Although Paget's disease affects approximately 3% of the population over 40 years of age, it is most commonly seen in the elderly population (10% over 70 years of age), most of whom are asymptomatic.

This metabolic bone disorder is characterized by slowly progressive enlargement and deformity of multiple bones associated with unexplained acceleration of both deposition and resorption of bone. Although originally thought to be an inflammatory process, it is now considered to be caused by a "slow virus." During the early and more active phase, resorption exceeds deposition, and the bone, although enlarged, becomes sponge-like, weakened, and deformed. This osteolytic phase is followed by an osteosclerotic phase in which the deposition of bone results in enlarged, thick, and dense bones.

The bones most commonly involved include (in decreasing order): pelvis, lumbar spine, sacrum, femur, skull, shoulders, thoracic spine, cervical spine, and ribs (Guyer, 1981). Inadequate tensile strength of involved bone may lead to deformities, typically bowing of the femur or tibia, which may impair walking (Aurbach et al, 1985a).

Complications of this disease process include progressive deformities due to the enlargement and bending of bones in the osteolytic phase, pathologic fractures, and occasionally malignant change in the hyperactive osteoblasts resulting in osteogenic sarcoma (malignant and fatal). The femur and the humerus are the most common sites of malignant transformation, which may be signalled by increased pain and rapid soft tissue swelling. No specific medical treatment for Paget's disease exists, although therapeutic agents (e.g., calcitonin, diphosphonates, mithramycin) have been shown to reduce both bone resorption and bone formation and thus reduce the associated bone pain.

Although this disorder is often asymptomatic, when symptoms do develop, they occur insidiously (gradually). Bone pain is described as aching, deep, and occasionally severe. The patient may have pain at night, awaken with pain, and be unable to go back to sleep despite all efforts. This night pain occurs especially in the person who has developed an osteogenic sarcoma associated with Paget's disease.

CLINICAL SIGNS AND SYMPTOMS OF PAGET'S DISEASE

Clinical signs and symptoms of Paget's disease depend on the location and severity of the bone lesions, but may include:

- Pain and stiffness
- Fatigue
- Headaches and dizziness
- Deformity
  - Bowing of long bones
  - Increased size and abnormal contour of clavicles
  - Osteoarthritis of adjacent joints
- Periosteal tenderness

- Increased skin temperature over long bones*
- Decreased auditory acuity
- Compression neuropathy
  - Spinal stenosis
  - Paresis
  - Paraplegia
  - Muscle weakness

Osteogenesis Imperfecta (Pinnel and Murad, 1987; Salter, 1983)

Osteogenesis imperfecta (OI) is an inherited condition (occurring 1 in 20,000) characterized by abnormally brittle and fragile bones that are subject to gross pathologic fracture. This disorder is transmitted by an autosomal dominant gene. The underlying defect is an abnormality in collagen synthesis that leads to increased bone fragility and a variable incidence of extraskeletal manifestations (Aurbach et al, 1985a). Salter (1983) attributes the cause to a failure of periosteal and endosteal intramembranous ossification of unknown origin. As a result of an imbalance between bone deposition and bone resorption, the cortical bone and the trabeculae of cancellous bone are extremely thin.

There are six types of OI described by clinical and genetic features (Table 9–10). The severity of the defect, which varies considerably, is indicated by the age at which the fractures occur. The most common OI is the mild-to-moderate form (type I or infantile type). The afflicted infant has many gross fractures during early childhood (often at the time of standing and walking), which affect weight-

* Increased skin temperature over affected long bones is a typical finding and is explained by soft tissue vascularity surrounding the bones (Singer, 1987).

Table 9–10. OSTEOGENESIS IMPERFECTA*

Type	Inheritance	Fractures	Sclera	Dentinogenesis Imperfecta	Special Features
IA	Autosomal dominant	+	Blue	–	Birth/perinatal fractures are rare Joint hypermobility Easy bruising
IB	Autosomal dominant	+	Blue	+	Same as IA
II	Autosomal recessive	+++	Blue		Intrauterine or early infant death Intrauterine growth retardation Marked tissue fragility Beaded ribs Poor cranial calcification
III	Autosomal recessive	++	Blue at birth but less blue with age	+	Congenital fractures Postnatal growth retardation Kyphoscoliosis
IVA	Autosomal dominant	+	White	–	Kyphoscoliosis Postnatal growth retardation
IVB	Autosomal dominant	+	White	+	Same as IVA

* Adapted from Stanbury, J.B., Wyngaarden, J.B., Fredrickson, D.S., et al: The Metabolic Basis of Inherited Disease, 5th ed. New York, McGraw-Hill, 1983.

bearing bones. The infant develops severe limb deformities from bending of bones and may be stunted in growth.

In the most severe form (type II or fetal type), multiple fractures have already occurred in utero, and more fractures occur during the birth process. Type II is rare and is generally lethal, and associated mortality is high during early infancy. Although this disorder affects bones primarily, other connective tissue can be affected including tendons, ligaments, fascia, sclera, and dentin.

Extraskeletal manifestations of osteogenesis imperfecta may include:

- Blue sclerae (white of the eye)
- Deafness
- Thin skin
- Cardiac abnormalities (e.g., aortic or mitral valve insufficiency)

These extraskeletal features may be related to abnormal collagen synthesis. For example, the hearing loss may be due to abnormalities of bone conduction (as a result of ligamentous laxity) as well as abnormalities of nerve conduction. The extraskeletal anomalies listed occur more frequently in the milder type I form of OI. Abnormal, opalescent teeth due to abnormal dentin synthesis, dentinogenesis imperfecta, occur in subgroups within the various types of OI (see Table 9–7). Lax ligaments and joints are additional features. Short stature is probably secondary to repeated fracture and deformity (Aurbach et al, 1985a).

Frequency of fractures diminishes after puberty. This reduction is attributed to the hormonal influence on connective tissue metabolism. No medical treatment is currently effective, although surgery (internal fixation) to prevent deformity may be appropriate in selected cases. Physical therapists often treat those patients receiving protective long leg braces and for crutch and gait training after a fracture.

SUMMARY

This chapter on endocrine and metabolic signs and symptoms has included commonly encountered diseases of the endocrine organs, metabolic disorders, and connective tissue disorders. In the course of this discussion, we have attempted to provide an overview of:

- Endocrine system physiology and pathophysiology
  - Endocrine hormones
  - Diabetes insipidus
  - Addison's disease
  - Cushing's syndrome
  - Common thyroid and parathyroid disorders
  - DM and hypoglycemia
- Metabolic disorders
  - Fluid imbalances, including edema and dehydration
  - Metabolic alkalosis and acidosis
  - Gout
- Connective tissue disorders
  - OI
  - Paget's disease

Signs and Symptoms Requiring Physician Referral

- Abdominal cramps
- Abdominal distention
- Absence of sweat
- Acroparesthesias
- Arthralgias
- Buffalo hump
- Changes in appetite
- Changes in body or skin temperature
- Changes in skin pigmentation
- Coarse, dry skin
- Confusion/lethargy
- Constipation
- Deep, rapid respirations
- Dependent edema
- Diarrhea
- Dizziness
- Dry mouth, throat, face
- Dysphagia
- Dyspnea
- Ecchymosis
- Excessive sweating
- Fatigue
- Fever and chills
- Fruity breath odor
- Headaches
- Heart palpitations
- Hoarseness
- Low urine output
- Myalgias
- Myoedema
- Myokymia
- Nausea
- Night sweats
- Nightmares
- Nocturia
- Numbess (lips, tongue)
- Peripheral neuropathy

Pitting edema
Polydypsia
Polyphagia
Polyuria
Postural hypotension
Prolonged reflexes
Proximal muscle weakness
Shakiness/trembling
Striae
Tachycardia/palpitations
Weakness
Weight loss or gain

Diseases of the endocrine-metabolic system account for some of the most common disorders encountered in humans—diabetes, obesity, and thyroid abnormalities. In recent years, new laboratory techniques have greatly enhanced the physician's ability to diagnose these diseases. Nevertheless, in many cases, the disorder remains unrecognized until relatively late in its course; symptoms may be attributed to some other disease process or musculoskeletal disorder (e.g., weakness may be the major complaint in Addison's disease) (Frohman et al, 1987). Thus, any patient who has any of the preceding generalized symptoms without obvious or already known cause should be further evaluated by a physician.

SUBJECTIVE EXAMINATION

Special Questions to Ask

Endocrine and metabolic disorders may produce subtle symptoms that progress so gradually the patient may be unaware of the significance of such findings. This requires careful interviewing to screen for potential physical and psychologic changes associated with hormone imbalances or other endocrine or metabolic disorders.

As always, it is important to be aware of patient medications (whether over-the-counter or prescribed), the intended purpose of these drugs and any potential side effects.

- □ Have you noticed any decrease in your muscle strength recently? **(GH imbalance, FSH-LH deficiency, ACTH imbalance, Addison's disease, hyperthyroidism, hypothyroidism)**
- □ Do you frequently have unexplained fatigue? **(Hyperparathyroidism, hypothyroidism, GH deficiency, ACTH imbalance, Addison's disease)**
- □ What daily activities seem to be too difficult or tiring? **(Muscle weakness due to cortisol and aldosterone hypersecretion and adrenocortical insufficiency, hypothyroidism)**
- □ Do you notice general muscle and joint aches and pains that seem to persist despite rest? **(Hypothyroidism, Addison's disease)**
- □ Have you noticed tingling or spasms around the mouth, arms, or legs? **(Hypoparathyroidism, hypothyroidism)**
- □ Do you have frequent headaches? **(Tumor, primary aldosteronism)**

Subjective Exam

Special Questions to Ask

If yes, determine the location, frequency, intensity, duration, precipitating/relieving factors

- □ Have you ever undergone head/neck radiation or cranial surgery? **(Thyroid cancer, pituitary dysfunction)**
- □ Have you recently sustained a head injury? **(Pituitary dysfunction)**
- □ Have you noticed any disturbances in your vision such as blurred vision, double vision, loss of peripheral vision, sensitivity to light? **(Thyrotoxicosis, hypoglycemia, DM)**
- □ Have you had an increase in your thirst or the number of times you need to urinate? **(Aldosteronism, DM, diabetes insipidus)**
- □ Have you had an increase in your appetite? **(DM, hyperthyroidism)**
- □ Do you bruise easily? **(Cushing's syndrome, excessive secretion of cortisol causes capillary fragility; small bumps/injuries produce bruising)** (Nursing 84, 1984)
- □ When you injure yourself, do your wounds heal slowly? **(GH excess, ACTH excess, Cushing's syndrome)**
- □ Have you noticed any unusual intolerance to heat (sweat profusely) or cold? **(TSH imbalance)**
- □ Have you noticed any increase in your collar size (goiter growth), difficulty in breathing or swallowing? **(Goiter, Graves' disease, hyperthyroidism) To the physical therapist: observe also for hoarseness.**
- □ Have you noticed any changes in skin color? **(Addison's disease)** (e.g., overall skin color has become a darker shade of brown or bronze, occurrence of black freckles, darkening of palmar creases, tongue, mucous membranes)

For the Patient Known to be Taking Corticosteroids

- □ Have you ever been told that you have osteoporosis or brittle bones, fractures, or back problems? **(Wasting of bone matrix in Cushing's syndrome)**
- □ Have you ever been told that you have Cushing's syndrome?
- □ Do you have any difficulty in going up stairs or getting out of chairs? **(Muscle wasting secondary to large doses of cortisol)**

For the Patient with Diagnosed DM:

- □ What type of insulin do you take? (see Table 9–3)
- □ What is your schedule for taking your insulin? **To the physical therapist: coordinate exercise programs according to the time of peak insulin action. Do not schedule exercise during peak times.**

Subjective Exam

Special Questions to Ask

□ Do you ever have episodes of hypoglycemia or insulin reaction?

If yes, please describe the symptoms that you experience.

□ Do you carry a source of sugar with you in case of an emergency?

If yes, what is it and where do you keep it in case I need to retrieve it?

□ Have you ever had diabetic ketoacidosis ("diabetic coma")?

If yes, please describe any symptoms you may have had that I can recognize if this occurs during therapy.

□ Do you use the fingerstick method for testing your own blood glucose levels? **To the physical therapist: you may want to ask the patient to bring the test kit for use before or during exercise.**

□ Do you have difficulty in maintaining your blood glucose levels within acceptable ranges (80 to 120 mg/dl)?

If yes, **to the physical therapist: you may want to take a baseline of blood glucose levels before initiating an exercise program.**

□ Do you ever have burning, numbness, or a loss of sensation in your hands or feet? **(Diabetic neuropathy)**

PHYSICIAN REFERRAL

Disorders of the endocrine and metabolic systems may present with recognizable clinical signs and symptoms, but almost always require a combination of clinical and laboratory findings to identify them accurately. The physical therapist is encouraged to complete a thorough *Patient/Family History* form, augmented by the interview with the patient and careful clinical observations in order to provide the physician with as much information as possible when making a referral.

In most cases, the patient who has suffered from an endocrine disorder has already been diagnosed and may have been referred to physical therapy for some other musculoskeletal complaint. These patients may have musculoskeletal problems that can be affected by symptoms associated with hormone imbalances (see Table 9–2).

In the case of a known diabetic, any patient demonstrating signs of confusion, lethargy, or changes in mental alertness and function should undergo an immediate fingerstick glucose test with a subsequent follow-up visit on the same day to the physician. Likewise, any episode or suspected episode of hypoglycemia must be treated promptly and reported to the diabetic patient's physician.

It is important to monitor any patient taking diuretics to assess for signs or symptoms of potassium depletion or fluid dehydration before exercising the patient. Consultation with the physician is advised.

CASE STUDY

Referral

Mr. Paul Martin, a 45-year-old diabetic patient with IDDM, has been receiving whirlpool therapy for a foot ulcer during the last 2 weeks. Today, when he came to the clinic , he appeared slightly lethargic and confused. He indicated to you that he has had a "case of the flu" since early yesterday and that he had vomited once or twice the day before and once that morning before coming to the clinic. His wife, who had driven him to the clinic, said that he seemed to be "breathing fast" and urinating more frequently than usual. He has been thirsty, so he has been drinking "7-Up" and water, and those fluids "have stayed down okay."

What questions will you want to ask this patient?

When did you last take your insulin? (Patient may have forgotten due to his illness, forgetfulness, confusion, or just being afraid to take it while feeling sick with the "flu")

What type of insulin did you take?

Do you have a source of sugar with you? If yes, where do you keep it? (This question should be asked during the initial physical therapy interview.)

Have you contacted your physician about your condition?

Have you done a recent blood-glucose level (fingerstick)? If yes, when was the last time that this test was done?

What were the results?

To his wife. Your husband seems to be confused and is not himself; how long has he been like this? Have you observed any strong breath odor since this "flu" started? (Make your own observations regarding breath odor at this time.)

To the physical therapist. If possible, perform a fingerstick blood glucose test on this patient. This type of patient should be sent immediately to his physician without physical therapy treatment. If he is hypoglycemic (unlikely under these circumstances), this condition could be treated immediately. It is more likely that this patient is hyperglycemic and may have diabetic ketoacidosis. In either case, the patient should not be driving, and arrangements should be made for transport either to the physician's office or home.

References

Aurbach, G.D., Marx, S.J., and Spiegel, A.M.: Metabolic bone disease. *In* Wilson, J.B., and Foster, D.W. (eds): Williams' Textbook of Endocrinology, 7th ed. Philadelphia, W.B. Saunders Company, 1985a, pp. 1218–1255.

Aurbach, G.D., Marx, S.J., and Spiegel, A.M.: Parathyroid hormone, calcitonin and the calciferols. *In* Wilson, J.B., and Foster, D.W. (eds): Williams' Textbook of Endocrinology, 7th ed. Philadelphia, W.B. Saunders Company, 1985b, pp. 1137–1217.

Berkow, R. (ed.): The Merck Manual of Diagnosis and Therapy. Rahway, NJ, Merck Sharp & Dohme Research Laboratory, 1987.

Cassmeyer, V.: Interventions for persons with diabetes mellitus and hypoglycemia. *In* Phipps, W., Long, B., and Woods, N. (eds): Medical-Surgical Nursing: Concepts and Clinical Practice, 3rd ed. St. Louis, C.V. Mosby, 1987a, pp. 601–641.

Cassmeyer, V.: Interventions for persons with problems of the endocrine system: Pituitary, thyroid, parathyroid and adrenal glands. *In* Phipps, W., Long, B., and Woods, N. (eds): Medical-Surgical Nursing: Concepts and Clinical Practice, 3rd ed. St. Louis, C.V. Mosby, 1987b, pp. 549–600.

Feibel, J.H., and Campa, J.F.: Thyrotoxic neuropathy. J. Neurol. Neurosurg. Psychiatry, *39*:491, 1976.

Ford, R.D.: Patient Teaching Manual. Springhouse, PA, Springhouse Corporation, 1987.

Forsham, P.H.: Disorders of the adrenal glands. *In* Smith, D.R. (ed): General Urology, 11th ed. Los Altos, CA, Lange Medical Publications, 1984, pp. 444–463.

Foster, D.: Diabetes mellitus, *In* Stanbury, J., Wyngaarden, J., Fredrickson, D., et al: The Metabolic Basis of Inherited Disease, 5th ed. New York, McGraw-Hill, 1983, pp. 99–117.

Frohman, L.A., Felig, P., Broadus, A.E., and Baxter, J.D.: The clinical manifestations of endocrine disease. *In* Felig, P., Baxter, J.D., Broadus, A.E., and Frohman, L.A. (eds): Endocrinology and Metabolism, 2nd ed. New York, McGraw-Hill, 1987, pp. 23–34.

Guyer, P.B.: Paget's disease of bone: the anatomical distribution. Metabolic Bone Disease Rel. Res., *4*:239, 1981.

Hall, A.: Joint and periarticular pain. *In* Blacklow, R.S. (ed): MacBryde's Signs and Symptoms, 6th ed. Philadelphia, J.B. Lippincott, 1983, pp. 211–226.

Hughes, B.: Diabetes management: The time is right for tight glucose control. Nursing 87, *17*:63, 1987.

Ingbar, S.H.: The thyroid gland. *In* Wilson, J.B., and Foster, D.W. (eds): Williams' Textbook of Endocrinology, 7th ed. Philadelphia, W.B. Saunders Company, 1985, pp. 682–815.

Ingbar, S.H., and Woeber, K.A.: The thyroid gland. In Williams, R.H. (ed): Williams' Textbook of Endocrinology, 6th ed. Philadelphia, W.B. Saunders Company, 1981, pp. 117–248.

Layzer, R.B.: CNS (Contemporary Neurology Series) Neuromuscular Manifestations of Systemic Disease. Philadelphia, F.A. Davis, 1985.

Lumley, W.: Controlling hypoglycemia and hyperglycemia. Nursing 88, *18*:34, 1988.

Marshall, B.: The Endocrine System. New York, Torstar Books, 1986.

McComas, A.J., Sica, R.E.P., and McNabb, A.R. (eds): Evidence for reversible motor neuron dysfunction in thyrotoxicosis. J. Neurol. Neurosurg. Psychiatry, *37*:548, 1974.

Miller, B.F., and Keane, C.B.: Encyclopedia and Dictionary of Medicine, Nursing and Allied Health, 4th ed. Philadelphia, W.B. Saunders Company, 1987.

Muthe, N.C.: Endocrinology: A Nursing Approach. Boston, Little, Brown, 1981.

Nursing 84: Endocrine Disorders. Springhouse, PA, Springhouse Corporation, 1984.

Nelson, D.H.: Cushing's syndrome. *In* DeGroot, L.J. (ed): Endocrinology, Vol. 2, 2nd ed, New York, Grune & Stratton, 1988a, pp. 1179–1191.

Nelson, D.H.: Diagnosis and treatment of Addison's disease. *In* DeGroot, L.J. (ed): Endocrinology, Vol 2, 2nd ed. New York, Grune & Stratton, 1988b, pp. 1193–1201.

Nyhan, W.L.: Understanding inherited metabolic disease. Clinical Symposia, CIBA, *32*:1, 1980.

Pinnell, S.R., and Murad, S.: Disorders of collagen. *In* The Metabolic Basis of Inherited Disease, 5th ed. New York, McGraw-Hill, 1983, pp. 1425–1449.

Purtilo, D.T., and Purtilo, R.B.: A Survey of Human Diseases, 2nd ed. Boston, Little, Brown, 1989.

Ramsay, I.D.: Muscle dysfunction in hyperthyroidism. Lancet *11*:931, 1966.

Ramsay, I.D.: Thyroid Disease and Muscle Dysfunction. Chicago, Year Book Medical Publishers, 1974.

Ramsay, I.D.: Thyrotoxic myopathy—electromyography. Q. J. Med. *34*:255, 1965.

Salter, R.B.: Textbook of Disorders and Injuries of the Musculoskeletal System, 2nd ed. Baltimore, Williams & Wilkins, 1983.

Singer, F.R.: Metabolic bone disease. *In* Felig, P., Baxter, J.D., Broadus, A.E., and Frohman, L.A. (eds): Endocrinology and Metabolism, 2nd ed. New York, McGraw-Hill, 1987, pp. 1454–1499.

Soltis, B., and Cassmeyer, Y.: Fluid and electrolyte imbalance. *In* Phipps, W., Long, B., and Woods, N. (eds): Medical-Surgical Nursing: Concepts and Clinical Practice, 3rd ed, St. Louis, C.V. Mosby, 1987, pp. 215–253.

Stroot, V., Lee, B., and Schaper, H.: Fluids and Electolytes: A Practical Approach. Philadelphia, F.A. Davis, 1980.

Travell, J.G., and Simons, D.G.: Myofascial Pain and Dysfunction: The Trigger Point Manual. Baltimore, Williams & Wilkins, 1983.

Utiger, R.D.: Hypothyroidism. *In* DeGroot, L.J. (ed): Endocrinology, Vol. 2, 2nd ed, New York, Grune & Stratton, 1988, pp. 471–488.

Wilson, J.B., and Foster, D.W.: Williams' Textbook of Endocrinology, 7th ed. Philadelphia, W.B. Saunders Company, 1985.

Wyngaarden, J.B., and Kelley, W.N.: Gout. *In* Stanbury, J.B., Wyngaarden, J.B., Fredrickson, D.S., et al: The Metabolic Basis of Inherited Disease, 5th ed. New York, McGraw-Hill Book Company, 1983, pp. 1043–1114.

Bibliography

Bondy, P.K., and Rosenberg, L.E. (eds): Metabolic Control and Disease, 8th ed. Philadelphia, W.B. Saunders Company, 1980.

Blacklow, R.S. (ed): MacBryde's Signs and Symptoms, 6th ed. Philadelphia, J.B. Lippincott, 1983.

Christman, C., and Bennett, J.: Diabetes: New names, new test, new diet. Nursing 87, *17*:34, 1987.

DeGroot, L.J. (ed): Endocrinology, Vols. 1 and 2, 2nd ed. New York, Grune & Stratton, 1988.

Fischbach, F.A.: Manual of Laboratory Diagnostic Tests, 2nd ed. Philadelphia, J.B. Lippincott, 1988.

Greenspan, F.S., and Forsham, P.H.: Basic and Clinical Endocrinology, 2nd ed. Los Altos, CA, Lange Medical Publications, 1986.

Ingbar, S.H., and Braverman, L.E. (eds): Werner's: The Thyroid: A Fundamental and Clinical Text, 5th ed. Philadelphia, J.B. Lippincott, 1986.

Mitchel, T., Abraham, G., Schiffrin, A., et al: Hyperglycemia after intense exercise in IDDM subjects during continuous subcutaneous insulin infusion. Diabetes Care, *11*:311, 1988.

Richter, E., Ruderman, N., and Schneider, S.: Diabetes and exercise. Am. J. Med., *70*:201, 1981.

Schwartz, T.B., and Ryan, W.G. (eds): The Year Book of Endocrinology. Chicago, Year Book Medical Publishers, 1983.

Stanbury, J.B., Wyngaarden, J.B., Fredrickson, D.S., et al: The Metabolic Basis of Inherited Disease, 5th ed. New York, McGraw-Hill, 1983.

Tourian, A., and Sidbury, J.B.: Phenylketonuria and hyperphenylalaninemia. *In* Stanbury, J.B., Wyngaarden, J.B., Fredrickson, D.S., et al: The Metabolic Basis of Inherited Disease, 5th ed. New York, McGraw-Hill, 1983, pp. 270–286.

Chapter 10

Overview of Oncology: Signs and Symptoms

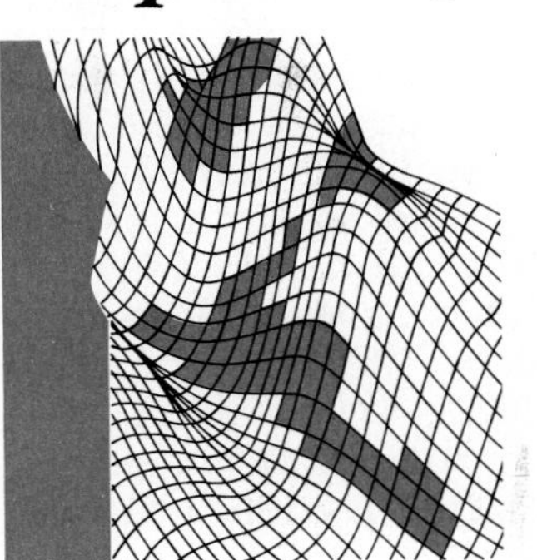

☐ ***Clinical Signs and Symptoms of:***

Acute Leukemia
Chronic Leukemia
Multiple Myeloma
Hodgkin's Disease
Non-Hodgkin's Lymphoma
Soft Tissue Neoplasm
Osteogenic Sarcoma
Ewing's Sarcoma
Paraneoplastic Syndromes
Brain Tumors

A 56-year-old man has come to you for an evaluation without a referral. He has not seen any type of physician for at least 3 years. He is seeking an evaluation on the insistence of his wife, who has noticed that his collar size has increased two sizes in the last year and that his neck looks "puffy." He has no complaints of any kind (including pain or discomfort), and he denies any known trauma; however, his wife insists that he has limited ability in turning his head when backing the car out of the driveway. What questions would be appropriate for your first physical therapy interview with this patient? What test procedures will you carry out during the first session? If you suggest to this man that he should see his physician, how would you make that recommendation? (See the Case Study at the end of the chapter.)

Cancer, in its early stages, is often asymptomatic, yet it is the second most common cause of death in the western world. About 700,000 Americans develop cancer each year; one in four Americans develop at least one cancer in his or her lifetime. Only heart disease claims more lives. In the past, cancer was invariably fatal. Today, however, treatment can cure many people. In fact, one in three people (more than 200,000 Americans each year) is cured with medical treatment (Glucksberg and Singer, 1982).

CANCER

Definition

Cancer is the uncontrolled growth and reproduction of cells. Cancer cells differ from normal cells in their structure, size, function, and rate of growth. In the cancerous, or malignant cell, normal restraints on growth are ineffective, and result in rapid cellular proliferation. The cause or causes of the genetic changes within a cell that result in malignancy are still poorly understood, but it is believed that the basic disturbance occurs in the regulatory functions of cellular deoxyribonucleic acid (DNA). This defect in growth regulation differentiates a malignant growth from one that is benign and from normal tissues. Benign tumors involve cellular proliferation of mature cells growing slowly in an encapsulated manner. A benign tumor does not usually invade the normal tissue around it and does not have the capacity to spread to other parts of the body.

The spread of cancer cells from their primary site to secondary sites is called metastasis. Cancer cells can spread throughout the body through the bloodstream, the lymphatic system, or by local invasion and infiltration into surrounding tissues. At secondary sites, the malignant cells continue to reproduce and new tumors or lesions develop.

Cancer describes a group of more than 100 disease processes characterized by uncontrolled growth and spread, eventually interfering with one or more vital functions of the host and possibly leading to death. Thus, cancer is not a singular, specific disease, but is instead a variable group of tissue responses.

Tissue Changes

Normal tissue contains cells of uniform size, shape, maturity, and nuclear structure. The nucleus of each normal cell contains the proper chromosomal number and composition for the species and when mitosis, or cell division, takes place, the splitting of the chromosomal material occurs in an orderly, sequenced process. Normal cells also have the characteristic of cell *differentiation.*

Differentiation refers to the specialized structure and function of any given cell and to the extent to which each cell resembles its normal parent cell. In malignant cells, differentiation is altered and may be lost completely so that the malignant cell may not be recognizable in relationship to its parent cell. In this case, it may become difficult or impossible to identify the malignant cell's tissue of origin.

Dysplasia

There are a variety of other tissue changes that can occur in the body. Some of these changes are benign and others denote a malignant or premalignant state. Dysplasia is a general category that indicates a disorganization of cells in which an adult cell varies from its normal size, shape, or organization. This is often due to chronic irritation and is seen with changes in cervical (uterine) epithelium owing to long-standing irritation of the cervix. Dysplasia may reverse itself or may progress to cancer.

Metaplasia

Metaplasia is the first level of dysplasia (early dysplasia), which is a reversible, benign, but abnormal change in which one adult cell changes from one type to another. For example, the most common type of epithelial metaplasia is the change of columnar epithelium of the respiratory tract to squamous epithelium (Hogan and Xistris, 1987). Although metaplasia usually gives rise to an orderly arrangement of cells, it may sometimes produce disorderly cellular patterns (i.e., cells varying in size, shape, and orientation to one another) (Upton, 1982).

Loss of cellular differentiation is called *anaplasia.* Anaplasia is the most advanced form of metaplasia and is a characteristic of malignant cells only.

Hyperplasia

Hyperplasia refers to an increase in the number of cells in a tissue or part of a tissue, resulting in increased tissue mass. This type of change can be a normal consequence of certain physiologic alterations *(physiologic hyperplasia),* such as increased breast mass during pregnancy, wound healing, or bone callus formation. *Neoplastic hyperplasia,* however, is the increase in cell mass due to tumor formation and is an abnormal process.

Tumors

Neoplasms (or tumors) are "new growths" and may be benign or malignant. The mass of tissue comprising the new growth is a neoplasm that enlarges at the expense of its host. It acts as a parasite by competing for nutrients and threatening the survival of the host. An example of a benign neoplasm is the common wart that does not invade or metastasize. A cancerous solid tumor is the classic example of a malignant neoplasm (Snyder, 1986). A *primary* neoplasm of a given structure arises from cells that are normally "local inhabitants" of that structure, whereas, a *secondary* neoplasm arises from cells that have metastasized from another part of the body. For example, a primary neoplasm *of* bone arises from within the bone structure itself, whereas, a secondary neoplasm occurs *in* bone as a result of metastasized cancer cells from another (primary) site.

Malignant tumors do not respond to the rules and regulations that govern normal tissue growth. However, there can be considerable differences in the rate of growth of malignant tumors. Some tumors are very slow-growing, even in a malignant state, and are easily removed. Other tumors may grow very rapidly initially and continue to grow rapidly; others may grow slowly at first, then undergo change and grow at a very fast rate later on. There are a variety of factors that affect the growth rate and pattern of tumors including host immunocompetence, the rate of individual cell replication, the proportion of total cell population that is actively dividing, and the rate of cell loss from the tumor (Hogan and Xistris, 1987).

Neoplasms are divided into three categories:

Benign tumors: Noninvasive and nonmetastatic
Characterized by a structure that is typical of the tissue of origin; well-differentiated and slow growing

Invasive tumors: Nonmetastatic (malignant)
Characterized by undifferentiated cells, consisting of a large percentage of dividing cells with many abnormal chromosomes

Metastatic tumors: Metastatic (malignant)
Able to invade and transfer disease from one organ to another organ not directly connected with the first organ

Within the categories of invasive and metastatic tumors, four large subcategories of malignancy have been identified. These subcategories are classified according to the cell type of origin.

Carcinomas: Arise from epithelial cells (e.g., breast, colon, and pancreas) and tend to be solid tumors

Sarcomas: Develop from connective tissues, such as muscle, bone, fat, cartilage, synovium, fibrous tissue

Lymphomas: Originate in lymphoid tissues

Leukemias: Cancers of the hematologic system

Tumors are also classified according to cellular maturity and cellular differentiation. When a tumor has completely lost identity with the parent tissue, it is considered to be undifferentiated. In general, the less differentiated a tumor becomes, the worse the patient's prognosis.

METASTASES

The biochemical basis for metastasis is unclear. One factor may be that malignant cells are less adherent to one another than are normal cells, possibly related to reduced calcium in the walls of the cancer cells. The reduced adherence may also be related to the high negative surface charge, thus resulting in a tendency for cancer cells to repel one another. Decreased adhesiveness enables the cells to break away from the primary tumor, invade nearby veins and lymphatics, and then travel to distant sites and develop into secondary tumors (Snyder, 1986).

Methods of Metastases

Routes of spread include local invasion, lymphatic spread, and distant spread by the bloodstream (Fig. 10–1). *Local invasion* refers to tumors that continue to grow at the original site of development. Tumors that remain localized are benign tumors and may not be troublesome unless they interfere mechanically with some body function. Some tumors invade nearby parts of the body that may include spread into major organs such as the bowel or bones. Tumors that grow rapidly and spread or destroy tissue are known as malig-

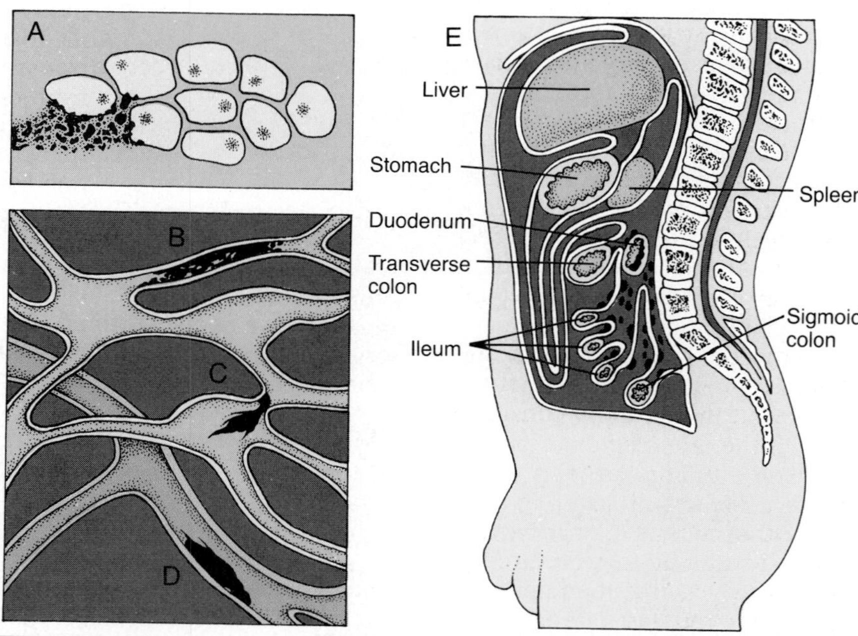

Figure 10–1. Modes of dissemination of cancer. Cancer spreads in many ways. *A,* Direct extension into neighboring tissue. *B,* Permeation along lymphatic vessels. *C,* Embolism via lymphatic vessels to the lymph nodes. *D,* Embolism via blood vessels. *E,* Invasion of a body cavity by diffusion. (Based on Phipps, J.S., et al (eds): Medical-Surgical Nursing: Concepts and Clinical Practice, 3rd ed. St. Louis, CV Mosby, 1987.)

nant tumors (American Medical Association, 1987).

The *lymph system* is a network of tiny vessels designed to remove excess fluid and unwanted substances, such as bacteria from the body's tissues. If a tumor invades locally into these abundant lymph vessels, it may spread along them to lymph nodes nearby. Lymph nodes (or glands) function to filter out foreign material by producing lymphocytes (a type of immune cell in the blood) that aid the lymph node in trapping cancer cells in the lymph node. Where lymph nodes drain into subclavian veins, cancer cells can enter the bloodstream (Williams and Williams, 1986).

Hematogenous spread (i.e., via the bloodstream) occurs as cells of malignant neoplasms penetrate thin-walled capillaries. If the tumor invades a blood vessel, then cancer cells may break off into the bloodstream and may be carried to other parts of the body. As blood vessels become progressively smaller, these cells become trapped and cancer may then develop at that point. The pattern of spread depends on the direction of the blood flow from the original tumor (Williams and Williams, 1986). Most cells released into the bloodstream are eliminated quickly, but the greater the number released by the primary tumor, the greater is the probability that some cells will survive to form metastases. Larger tumors release greater numbers of cells, which increases the chances of survival and metastasis (Fidler and Hart, 1985).

The usual mode of spread and eventual location of metastases vary with the type of cancer and the tissue from which the cancer arises. For example, prostatic carcinomas typically spread via the lymphatics to the bones of the pelvis and vertebrae. Primary cancers of the bone, such as osteogenic sarcoma, metastasize initially to the lungs. For some cancers, such as malignant melanoma, no typical pattern exists and metastases may occur anywhere (American Cancer Society, 1981).

Metastases usually reproduce the cellular structure of the primary growth well enough to enable a pathologist to determine the site of the primary tumor. For example, bone metastases from a carcinoma of the thyroid not only exhibit a microscopic structure similar to the original tumor, but may also produce thyroid hormone (American Cancer Society, 1981).

Central Nervous System Metastases

Many primary tumors may lead to CNS metastases. Lung carcinomas account for approximately half of all metastatic brain lesions. Breast carcinoma, the second leading type of primary tumor involved in brain metastases, accounts for approximately 15% of patients with metastases to the CNS (Gudas, 1987; Snyder, 1986). Metastatic disease in the brain is both life-threatening and emotionally debilitating. Metastatic brain tumors can increase intracranial pressure, obstruct the normal flow of cerebrospinal fluid, change mentation, and reduce sensory and motor function (Snyder, 1986).

Primary tumors of the CNS rarely develop metastases outside the CNS despite the highly invasive capacity of these tumors. When it does take place, spread occurs via the cerebrospinal fluid or by direct extension. Spinal cord and nerve root compression cause either insidious or rapid loss of neurologic function. This compression phenomenon occurs in approximately 5% of persons with systemic cancer caused by carcinomas of the lung, breast, prostate, and kidney. Lymphoma and multiple myeloma may also result in spinal cord and nerve root compression. The spinal cord is most often compressed anteriorly by direct growth of a tumor (Snyder, 1986).

Pulmonary System

Pulmonary metastases are the most common of all metastatic tumors because venous drainage of most areas of the body is through the superior and inferior vena cavae into the heart, making the lungs the first organ to filter malignant cells (Snyder, 1986). Parenchymal metastases are asymptomatic until tumor cells have expanded and reached the parietal pleura where pain fibers are stimulated.

Pleural pain and dyspnea may be the first two symptoms experienced by the patient. Tumor cells from the lung embolizing via the pulmonary veins and carotid artery can result in metastases to the CNS. Lung cancer is the most common primary tumor to metastasize to the brain. In any individual, any neurologic sign may be the presentation of a silent lung tumor (Gudas, 1987).

Hepatic System

Liver metastases are among the most ominous signs of advanced cancer. The liver filters blood coming in from the GI tract, making it a primary metastatic site for tumors of the stomach, colorectum, and pancreas. The patient has abdominal pain and tenderness with general malaise and fatigue.

Skeletal System

Bone metastases represent the initial site of metastatic disease in a large proportion of cancer cases and are generally ominous in terms of prognosis (Snyder, 1986). The primary symptom associated with bone metastases is pain. Although lung, breast, and prostate are the three primary sites responsible for most metastatic bone disease, tumors of the thyroid and kidney, lymphomas (cancer of the lymphatic system, including Hodgkin's disease), as well as melanoma (skin cancer), can also metastasize to the skeletal system. Metastatic involvement of the vertebrae may result in epidural spinal cord compression with resultant quadriplegia or paraplegia and possibly in death. The patient who presents with spinal cord symptomatology due to metastatic epidural disease and resultant compression may have only transient symptoms with proper medical treatment (Gudas, 1987).

CURRENT THEORIES OF ONCOGENESIS

Current cancer research has centered around the oncogene or "cancer gene," dysfunction of the immune system, and environmental features of oncogenesis.

Oncogene

The oncogene is a gene found in the chromosomes of tumor cells whose activation is associated with the initial and continuing conversion of normal cells into cancer cells (Miller and Keane, 1987). All cells contain oncogenes, which, when "turned on," produce a protein that causes the cell to begin growing in an abnormal fashion. Current research is centered on identifying factors that "switch on" the oncogenes (Holleb, 1986).

Because there may be thousands of factors that can activate oncogenes, many research scientists theorize that we have cancer cells forming in our bodies throughout life and that the change from normal to malignant cells may be a relatively common occurrence in the body. Because the malignant cells are different in character than normal cells, the body usually recognizes these cells as being different. Our immune system is on a constant alert to detect and eliminate these abnormal cells.

Dysfunction of the Immune System

Dysfunction of the immune system may predispose the body to the development of cancer. When the immune system response is altered, blocked, or overpowered by the number of malignant cells, recognition and subsequent "attack" may be ineffective or incomplete and cancer begins. People with genetic immune system defects are more likely to develop leukemia or lymphoma than are people who are immunocompetent. This theory is consistent with what happens when the immune system breaks down in patients with acquired immunodeficiency syndrome (AIDS). Likewise, people who have been immunosuppressed purposefully for organ transplants have an increased risk of cancer development. Several other commonly occurring factors alter normal immune function, such as stress, malnutrition, advancing age, and chronic disease (Snyder, 1986).

Cancer itself also appears to suppress the immune system both early and late in the progression of the disease. Although there is evidence to support involvement of the immune system in the etiology of cancer, at the present time, there are insufficient data to give strong support to this theory (Hogan and Xistris, 1987).

Environmental Causes of Oncogenesis

There may be many probable causes of tumor growth, and more than one precipitating factor may be needed to produce each individual tumor. *Environmental causes,* such as alcohol, cigarette smoking, water contamination, diet (food toxins or additives), occupation, background radiation, and genetic predisposition may contribute toward the development of specific cancers (Pitot, 1985). Viral carcinogens have been clearly demonstrated in animals, although no conclusive evidence has yet been documented in human cancers. Viruses are thought to contribute to the development of cancer by becoming incorporated into the host DNA or ribonucleic acid (RNA) and thus altering the host DNA or RNA with resultant cell proliferation (Pitot, 1985).

Genetic endowment, age, hormonal status, immunocompetence, and stress are thought to interact with and influence a person's vulnerability to potential oncogenic viruses (Snyder, 1986). The physical therapist must pay close attention to the patient's age in correlation with previous personal or family history of cancer (Table 10-1). For example, breast cancer shows a sharp increase after 45 years of age, testicular cancer peaks at 35 years of age, and acute lymphocytic leukemia has a bimodal distribution with peaks in infancy and in the elderly. The incidence of cancer doubles after 25 years of age with every 5-year increase in age. This correlation between age and incidence of cancer is thought to be due to an accumulation of premalignant changes over a long period.

EARLY WARNING SIGNS
(Holleb, 1986)

For many years, the American Cancer Society has publicized seven warning signs of cancer, the appearance of which could indicate the presence of cancer and the need for a medical evaluation. The following mnemonic is often used as a helpful reminder of these warning signs:

Changes in bowel or bladder habits
A sore that does not heal in 6 weeks
Unusual bleeding or discharge
Thickening or lump in breast or elsewhere
Indigestion or difficulty in swallowing
Obvious change in a wart or mole
Nagging cough or hoarseness

Table 10-1. DIFFERENTIATION OF COMMON MALIGNANT TUMORS BY AGE*

Age 0-8 Yrs	Age 8-40 Yrs	Age 40-55 Yrs	Age 55-75 Yrs
Neuroblastoma Ewing's sarcoma Lymphoma Osteogenic sarcoma	Osteogenic sarcoma Chondrosarcoma Ewing's sarcoma Lymphoma Secondary osteogenic or chondrosarcoma Metastatic carcinoma of the thyroid Metastatic carcinoma of the breast	Secondary osteogenic sarcoma Secondary chondrosarcoma Multiple myeloma Metastatic carcinoma of the breast Primary osteogenic sarcoma Neurogenic sarcoma	Metastatic carcinoma of the breast Metastatic carcinoma of the prostate Secondary osteogenic sarcoma Secondary chondrosarcoma Multiple myeloma Other metastatic tumors

* From D'Ambrosia, R.: Musculoskeletal Disorders: Regional Examination and Differential Diagnosis, 2nd ed. Philadelphia, J.B. Lippincott, 1986.

Awareness of these signals is useful, but it is generally agreed that these symptoms do not always reflect early curable cancer, nor does this list include all of the possible signs for the different types of cancer. For the physical therapist, idiopathic proximal muscle weakness may be an early sign of cancer. This syndrome of proximal muscle weakness is referred to as *carcinomatous neuromyopathy.* It is accompanied by a dimunition of two or more deep tendon reflexes (ankle jerk usually remains intact) (Croft and Wilkinson, 1965). Muscle weakness may occur secondary to hypercalcemia, which is typically found in patients with multiple myeloma, a form of plasma cell cancer that affects bone marrow.

Pain is rarely an early warning sign of cancer, even in the presence of unexplained bleeding. Bleeding is an important sign of cancer, but a cancer is generally well established by the time that bleeding occurs. Bleeding develops secondary to ulcerations in the central areas of the tumor or by pressure on or rupture of local blood vessels. As the cancer continues to grow, it may enlarge beyond its capacity to obtain necessary nutrients, resulting in devitalization of portions of the tumor. This process of invading and compressing local tissue, shutting off blood supply to normal cells, is called necrosis (American Cancer Society, 1981). Tissue necrosis leads ultimately to secondary infection, severe hemorrhage, and the development of pain when regional sensory nerves become involved. Other symptoms can include pathologic fractures, anemia, and thrombus formation.

SKIN AND BREAST CANCER

Skin cancer and breast cancer are two of the more common cancers about which patients will ask physical therapists for advice. During the observation/inspection portion of any examination, the physical therapist may observe skin lesions that may need further medical investigation. For these reasons, this special section on skin and breast cancer is included.*

* Other specific types of cancer affecting organ systems are discussed individually in each related chapter.

Likewise, the woman presenting with chest, breast, axillary, or shoulder pain of unknown etiology must be questioned regarding self-breast examinations. Any recently discovered lumps or nodules must be examined by a physician. The patient may need education regarding self-breast examination, and the physical therapist can provide this valuable information. Techniques of self-breast examination are commonly available in written form for the physical therapist or the patient who is unfamiliar with these methods (Williams and Williams, 1986).

Skin Cancer

Skin cancer is the most common cancer diagnosed in the United States and affects men and women equally, but seldom occurs in children before puberty. There is a higher incidence in whites than in blacks. Blondes and others with fair complexions are affected most frequently. Skin cancer tends to develop in sun-exposed areas of the body; women have a greater incidence on the arms, legs, and back; men on the head and trunk (American Cancer Society, 1981).

Although relatively rare, malignant melanoma is the most serious form of skin cancer that arises from pigmented cells in the skin called melanocytes. Melanomas spread early and rapidly via the lymphatics and the bloodstream. Although exposure to the sun has some relationship to this disease, melanomas may start in sites never exposed to the sun, such as inside the mouth, on the bottom of the feet, on the retina of the eye, or even inside the bowel (Glucksberg and Singer, 1982). In women, the most susceptible areas include the back, the face, and the lower legs. In men, the trunk is most often affected. The palms, soles, and under the nails are more common sites for black people. The lesions can vary a great deal in appearance. Some lesions are deeply pigmented (blue, black) with irregular borders and surfaces, and other lesions are irregularly pigmented (yellow, blue, black) with irregular borders and irregular surfaces (Long, 1987).

During observation and inspection, the

physical therapist should be alert to any potential signs of skin cancer. The major warning sign of melanoma is some change in a mole or "beauty mark." The Skin Cancer Foundation advocates the use of the ABCD method of early detection of melanoma and dysplastic (abnormal in size or shape) moles.

> **A: asymmetry:** (uneven edges, lopsided in shape, one half unlike the other half)
> **B: border:** irregularity, irregular edges, scalloped or poorly defined edges
> **C: color:** black, shades of brown, red, white, occasionally blue
> **D: diameter:** larger than a pencil eraser

Other *signs* that may be important include:

- Irritation and itching
- Tenderness, soreness or new moles developing around the mole in question

If any of these signs described are present in your patient and the patient's skin lesion(s) have not been examined by a physician, a medical referral is recommended. If the patient is planning a follow-up visit with the physician within the next 2 to 4 weeks, then the patient is advised to point out the mole or skin changes at that time. If no appointment is pending, then the patient is encouraged to make a specific visit either to the family/personal physician or to a dermatologist.

The more common squamous cell and basal cell carcinomas do not usually metastasize, but can affect layers of skin into bone and even the brain, causing disfigurement in advanced stages that could be prevented with early treatment. Squamous cell carcinoma arises from the top of the epidermis and appears usually as a pink opaque lump with an ulcerated or scabbed region in the center. This type of cancer develops in sun-exposed areas and may be related to arsenic (e.g, occupational, insecticides, drinking water) and radiation exposure, mainly in the form of therapeutic radiation used by physicians in the past to treat acne and other skin conditions. Squamous cell carcinoma can develop in scars from serious burns. If left untreated, these cancers can spread to lymph nodes nearby and from there to distant organs (Glucksberg and Singer, 1982).

Basal cell carcinoma involves the bottom layer of the epidermis (outermost layer of the skin) of the face, neck, arms, and other areas of the body exposed to the sun. This type of carcinoma may appear as a red spot with a bloody-like discharge, or a transluscent pink or white, pearly bump, or a smooth red spot with an indentation in the middle. A sore that keeps crusting and does not heal within 6 weeks is the most reliable sign.

Breast Cancer

Breast cancer is second to lung cancer as the most common site of cancer in American women today. Cancer of the breast appears to have a familial disposition in 15 to 20% of all new cases diagnosed, usually occurring at an earlier age than in the general population (Snyder, 1986).

Risk Factors

Heredity, race, hormonal influences, age, radiation, and diet are all being considered as scientific investigations continue to identify potential risk factors. The presence of any of these factors may become evident during the interview with the patient and alert the physical therapist to potential musculoskeletal complaints of a systemic origin that would require a medical referral.

First-degree relatives (daughters or sisters) of patients with breast cancer have two to three times the risk of developing breast cancer than the general female population; relatives of patients with bilateral breast cancer have five times the normal risk (Nursing 85, 1985). Women who have never been pregnant and women who have children after 30 years of age are at increased risk for the development of breast cancer. Women who have a full-term delivery before 18 years of age have only one third the risk of women who bear their first child after 30 years of age (Nursing 85, 1985). Other factors, such as women with a history of benign fibrocystic breast disease (who have four times the chances of developing breast cancer), can contribute to risk.

Breast cancer can occur in both premenopausal and postmenopausal women with the peak incidence occurring between 45 and 70 years of age. Age itself represents a risk factor, because breast cancer incidence is highest in women over 50 years of age. (When breast cancer appears in men, it is usually seen approximately 10 years later than in women at a mean age of 60).

Early menarche (onset of menstrual function) or late menopause increases the risk of breast cancer. However, an oophorectomy (removal of ovaries) before menopause decreases the risk by one third. There is still controversy with regard to whether certain noncontraceptive estrogen preparations increase the risk of developing breast cancer in postmenopausal women. There seems to be no increased risk observed in women using the estrogen-progesterone combinations prescribed for contraception (Molbo and Sun, 1987).

White people have a slightly higher incidence of breast cancer than blacks, and the obese, diabetic person seems to be at higher risk. The person exposed to ionizing radiation appears to have a higher risk of developing breast cancer. The risk increases with increasing doses of radiation (Fry, 1985). For example, survivors of the Japanese atomic bomb and women who received multiple fluoroscopies for tuberculosis or radiation treatment for mastitis during their adolescent or childbearing years are at increased risk.

Prevention

Regular self-examination and the use of mammography have become important tools in the early detection of breast cancer during its early stages (Scanlon and Strax, 1986). The patient may be questioned regarding the presence of the following warning signs (Williams and Williams, 1986):

INSPECTION	PALPATION
Unusual difference in size or shape of the breasts	Unusual discrete lump or nodule in any part of either breast
Alterations in the position of either nipple	
Retraction (turning in) of either nipple	
Puckering (dimple) of the skin surface	
Unusual rash on the breast or nipple	
Unusual prominence of the veins over either breast	

Any suspicious finding should be checked by a physician, especially in the case of the woman with identified risk factors (e.g., a previous personal or family history of breast cancer). For this reason, it is always important to ask the patient about risk factors identified in the text and previous history and to correlate this information with objective findings.

CANCERS OF THE BLOOD AND LYMPH SYSTEM

Cancers arising from the bone marrow include acute leukemias, chronic leukemias, multiple myeloma, and some lymphomas. These cancers are all characterized by the uncontrolled growth of blood cells. The major lymphoid organs of the body are the lymph nodes and the spleen (Fig. 10–2). Cancers arising from these organs are called malignant lymphomas and are categorized as either Hodgkin's disease or non-Hodgkin's lymphoma (Glucksberg and Singer, 1982).

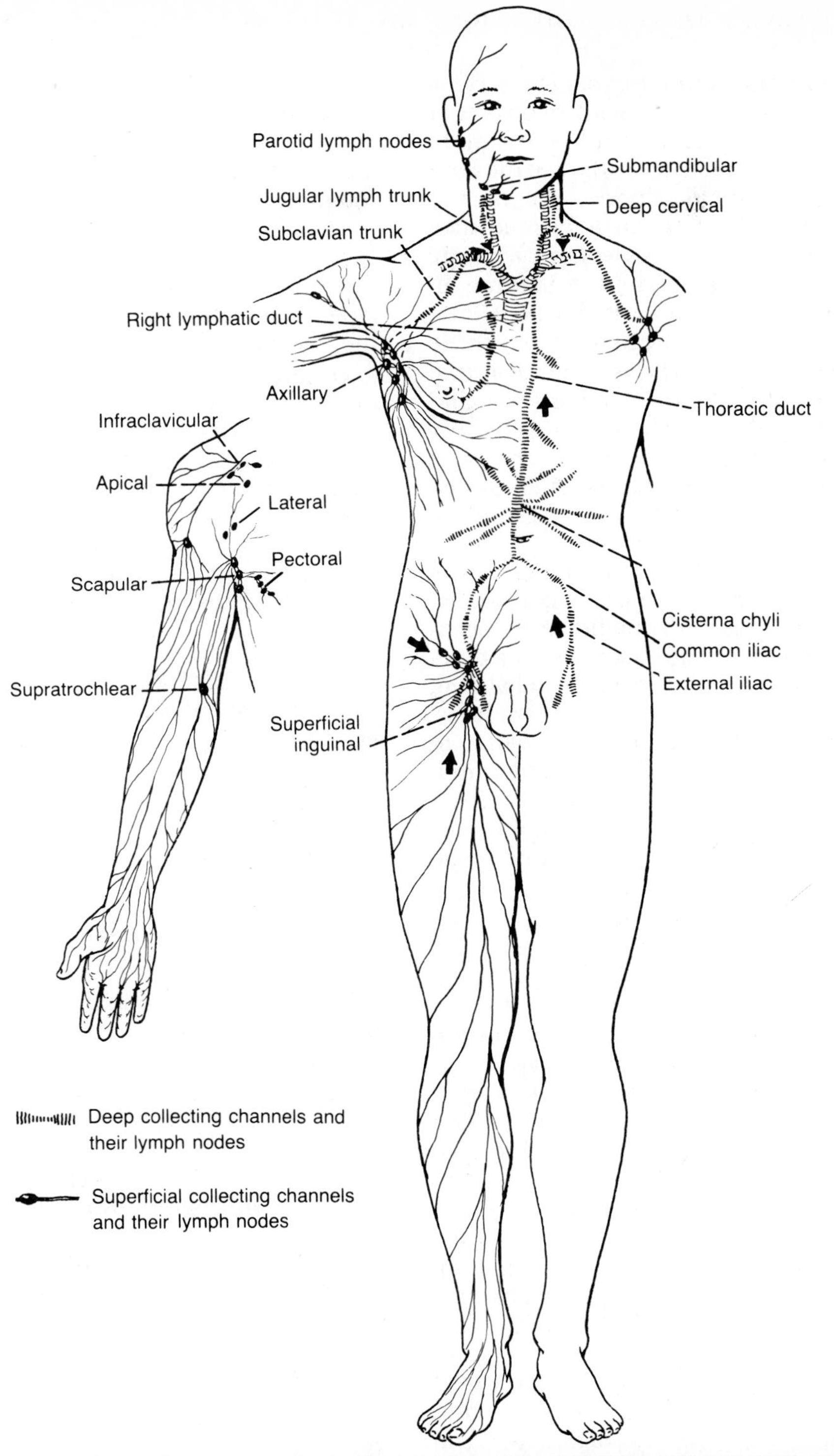

Figure 10–2. Major lymphoid organs of the body: lymph nodes and the spleen. (From Jacob, S.W., and Francore, C.A.: Elements of Anatomy and Physiology, 2nd ed. Philadelphia, W.B. Saunders Company, 1989.)

Like leukemia, lymphoma affects a body system that communicates with every other organ system. However, instead of arising in the blood system, this cancer arises in the lymphatic system, a network of nodes, vessels, and organs that provides a major defense against infection. The lymphatic vessels carry lymph, which is a clear, colorless fluid containing infection-fighting white blood cells (WBCs or leukocytes) throughout the body. Along these vessels, small oval glands (lymph nodes) trap and help to destroy foreign particles and agents that cause disease. Lymphoma usually originates in these nodes, but arises occasionally on other lymphoid tissues, such as the spleen or the intestinal lining (Nursing 85, 1985).

The cause of leukemia and lymphomas is not yet known. Among the predisposing factors of leukemia are ionizing radiation, occupational exposure to the chemical benzene, and exposure to drugs such as alkylating agents and nitrosoureas used in chemotherapy. Predisposing factors of lymphoma include ionizing radiation, infection, and immunologic defects resulting from illness or from medical treatment such as kidney transplants (Nursing 85, 1985). Diagnosis must be made by a biopsy.

Leukemia

Leukemia is a cancer that develops in the bone marrow and is characterized by abnormal multiplication and release of WBC precursors. The disease process originates during WBC development in the bone marrow or lymphoid tissue. With rapid proliferation of leukemic cells, the bone marrow becomes overcrowded with immature WBCs, which then spill over into the peripheral circulation. Crowding of the bone marrow by leukemic cells inhibits normal blood cell production. Decreased red blood cell (erythrocyte) production results in anemia and reduced tissue oxygenation. Decreased platelet production results in thrombocytopenia and risk of hemorrhage. Decreased production of normal WBCs results in increased vulnerability to infection, especially because leukemic cells are functionally unable to defend the body against pathogens. Leukemic cells may invade and infiltrate vital organs, such as the liver, kidneys, lung, heart, or brain (Snyder, 1986).

There are two general classes of leukemia (acute and chronic) that each have subclasses. The specific type of leukemia depends on the type of immature WBC that predominates in the peripheral blood (Nursing 83, 1983).

Prognosis for the acute leukemias depends on the patient's age, the level of total WBC counts, and the availability of treatment. With treatment, remission and cure are possible for some patients. The median survival for chronic leukemias is from 3 to 4 years after the onset of the disease. Bone marrow transplant has the potential to cure chronic myelogenous leukemia (Nursing 83, 1983).

CLINICAL SIGNS AND SYMPTOMS MOST COMMON TO ACUTE LEUKEMIA

- Abnormal bleeding
- Easy bruising of the skin
- Epistaxis (nosebleeds)
- Hematuria (blood in the urine)
- Rectal bleeding
- Infections

The abnormal bleeding is caused by a lack of blood platelets required for clotting. Infections are due to a depletion of WBCs needed to fight infection. For women, this abnormal bleeding may be prolonged menstruation leading to anemia. *Special Questions for Women* may elicit this kind of valuable information requiring medical referral. Other patients may experience easy bruising of the skin or abnormal bleeding from the nose, blood in the urine, or bleeding from the rectum.

CLINICAL SIGNS AND SYMPTOMS MOST COMMON TO CHRONIC LEUKEMIAS

- Fatigue
- Dyspnea

- Weight loss
- Loss of appetite
- Fevers and sweats
- Pain in the left abdomen (enlarged spleen)
- Occasionally epistaxis (nose bleeds) or bruising

Multiple Myeloma

Multiple myeloma, also known as plasma cell myeloma, is a primary malignant bony tumor associated with widespread osteolytic lesions (decreased areas of bone density), appearing radiographically as punched-out defects of bone (Miller and Keane, 1987). Excessive growth of plasma cells originating in the bone marrow destroy bone tissue. Plasma cells develop from lymphocytes and produce antibodies that fight infections. Because these patients cannot make normal antibodies, they are very susceptible to infections (Williams and Williams, 1986). This disease can develop at any age from young adulthood to advanced age, but peaks among people between the ages of 50 and 70 years.

CLINICAL SIGNS AND SYMPTOMS OF MULTIPLE MYELOMA

- Skeletal (bone) pain (especially back or thorax)
- Recurrent bacterial infections (especially pneumococcal pneumonias)
- Spontaneous fracture
- Anemia with weakness and fatigue
- Increased urination
- Loss of appetite
- Vomiting
- Carpal tunnel syndrome

The bone pain is caused by infiltration of the plasma cells into the marrow with subsequent destruction of bone. Initially, the skeletal pain may be mild and intermittent (comes and goes) or it may develop suddenly as a severe pain in the back, rib, leg or arm, often the result of an abrupt movement or effort that has caused a spontaneous (pathologic) bone fracture. As the disease progresses, more and more areas of bone destruction develop. If left untreated, this will result in skeletal deformities, particularly of the ribs, sternum, and spine. There may be a shortening of the spine (as much as 5 inches or more in stature) (Holleb, 1986).

Hypercalcemia, excessive calcium circulating in the blood, occurs secondary to the bone destruction. To rid the body of the excess calcium, the kidneys increase the output of urine, which can lead to serious dehydration if there is an inadequate intake of fluids. This dehydration may be compounded by vomiting. Patients who have symptoms of hypercalcemia (increased urination, loss of appetite, and vomiting) should seek immediate medical care, because this condition can be life-threatening. Patients with myeloma may also have excessive uric acid in the urine (hyperuricosuria) and increased uric acid in the blood (hyperuricemia). These can contribute to renal impairment due to the precipitation of urate and calcium crystals in the kidney (Osserman, 1986).

Approximately 10% of patients with myeloma have amyloidosis, deposits of insoluble fragments of a monoclonal protein resembling starch. These deposits cause tissues to become waxy and immobile and may affect nerves, muscles, and ligaments, especially the carpal tunnel area of the hand. Carpal tunnel syndrome with pain, numbness, or tingling in the hands and fingers may develop.

Hodgkin's Disease

Hodgkin's disease is a specific type of lymphoma that can occur at any age, but the most common age of incidence in the United States is in the young adult 15 to 35 years of age, with a second peak of frequency between 50 and 60 years of age. Hodgkin's disease arises in the lymph glands most commonly on one side of the neck or the groin and then metastasizes through the lymph system to other organs of the body, especially to the spleen, liver, lungs, bone, and bone marrow. Although many physical therapists are familiar with Hodgkin's disease as a type of cancer, it represents only about 1% of all cancers in the United States. This disease is one of the few cancers that can now be cured with treatment, whereas 25 years ago, the prognosis was poor and the disease was considered to be fatal.

CLINICAL SIGNS AND SYMPTOMS OF HODGKIN'S DISEASE

- Painless, progressive enlargement of unilateral lymph nodes, often in the neck

The physical therapist may palpate these nodes during a cervical spine examination. Enlarged lymph nodes refers to lymph nodes greater than 1.5 cm in diameter. Lymph nodes that are firm and rubbery in consistency and that persist for more than 4 weeks require a medical evaluation.

Other possible (although not always present) symptoms include:

- Fatigue
- Fever
- Night sweats
- Anorexia and weight loss
- Severe itching over entire body

The itching occurs more intensely at night and may result in severe scratches, because the patient is unaware of scratching during the sleep state. The fever typically peaks in the late afternoon, and night sweats occur when the fever drops during sleep.

Because lymph nodes enlarge in response to infections throughout the body, referral to a physician is not necessary upon finding enlarged lymph nodes unless these nodes persist and involve more than one area. However, the physician should be notified of your findings and the patient should be advised to have the lymph nodes checked at the next follow-up visit with the physician. If the nodes remain enlarged over a long period (4 weeks or more), then the patient should be encouraged to contact the physician to discuss the need for follow-up.

Non-Hodgkin's Lymphoma

This group of lymphomas affect lymphoid tissue and occur in people of all ages. Non-Hodgkin's lymphomas (NHLs) present a clinical picture broadly similar to that of Hodgkin's disease, except that the disease is usually initially more widespread. The most common manifestation is painless enlargement of one or more peripheral lymph nodes (Miller and Keane, 1987). As with all cancers of the lymph system, a biopsy is required to confirm the diagnosis with other follow-up tests, such as blood studies and bone marrow studies.

NHLs are classified on the basis of pattern (follicular or diffuse) and cytologic (cellular) composition into six different classifications. The most likely to be screened by the physical therapist include:

- Follicular (nodular) lymphomas
- Diffuse, aggressive lymphomas

The follicular lymphomas comprise the most common subgroup of patients with NHL. These lymphomas are often widespread at the time of diagnosis, and more than one half of the cases involve the bone marrow. Prognosis is good with treatment, although the disease is rarely eradicated. Aggressive lymphomas are usually less widespread on diagnosis, but grow rapidly and are fatal without treatment.

Diffuse, aggressive lymphomas share a common clinical presentation and natural history. These tumors tend to disseminate rapidly and involve the central nervous system (CNS). The prognosis is unfavorable unless intensive chemotherapeutic regimens can bring about a complete remission that can be maintained for more than 2 years (DeVita et al, 1985).

CLINICAL SIGNS AND SYMPTOMS OF NON-HODGKIN'S LYMPHOMA

- Enlarged lymph nodes
- Fever
- Night sweats
- Weight loss
- Bleeding
- Infection
- Red skin and generalized itching of unknown etiology

SOFT TISSUE TUMORS

Sarcoma

By definition, sarcoma is a fleshy growth and refers to a large variety of tumors arising in the soft tissues that are grouped together because of similarities in pathologic appearance and clinical presentation (Rosenberg et al, 1985). Soft tissues affected include

- Connective tissue such as bone and cartilage
- Muscle
- Fibrous tissue
- Fat
- Synovium

The different types of sarcomas are named for the specific tissues affected (e.g., fibrosarcomas are tumors of the fibrous connective tissue; osteosarcomas are tumors of the bone; and chondrosarcomas are tumors arising in cartilage [Table 10–2]).

As a general category, sarcoma differs from carcinoma in the origin of cells comprising the tumor. As mentioned, sarcomas arise in connective tissue, whereas carcinomas arise in epithelial tissue (i.e., cellular structures covering or lining surfaces of body cavities, small vessels, or visceral organs) (Rosenberg et al, 1985). Carcinomas affect structures such as the skin, large intestine, stomach, breast, and lungs. Generally, carcinomas tend to metastasize via the lymphatics, whereas sarcomas are more likely to metastasize hematogenously (Gudas, 1987).

Malignant neoplasms or new growths that develop as *primary* lesions in the musculoskeletal tissues are relatively rare, representing less than 1% of malignant disease of all age groups and 6.5% of all cancers in children under the age of 15. *Secondary* neoplasms that develop in bone as metastases from a primary neoplasm elsewhere (especially metastatic carcinoma) are common (Rosenberg et al, 1985).

CLINICAL SIGNS AND SYMPTOMS OF A SOFT TISSUE NEOPLASM

- Persistent swelling or lump in a muscle (most common finding)
- Pain
- Pathologic fracture
- Local swelling

Often, the neoplasm goes unnoticed until the patient has some trauma or injury that requires medical attention (e.g., x-ray to rule out fracture). The poor prognosis of most patients with soft tissue sarcomas is due to the tendency of these lesions to invade aggressively into surrounding tissues and to early hematogenous dissemination, generally to the lungs. Soft tissue sarcomas have a significant tendency to invade locally along nerve fibers, muscle bundles, fascial planes, and blood vessels (Rosenberg et al, 1985). Pain is the most significant symptom of rapidly growing neoplasms. Initially mild and intermittent, the pain from a neoplasm becomes progressively more severe and more constant.

A history of sudden onset of severe pain usually indicates the complication of a pathologic fracture (a break in an already weakened bone). Local swelling can be detected when the lesion protrudes beyond the normal confines of the bone. The swelling of a benign lesion is usually firm and nontender. In the presence of a rapidly growing malignant neoplasm, however, the swelling is more diffuse and is frequently tender (Fig. 10–3). The overlying skin may be warm due to the highly

Table 10–2. CLASSIFICATION OF SOFT TISSUE AND BONE TUMOR*

Tissue of Origin	Benign Tumor	Malignant Tumor
Connective Tissue		
Fibrous	Fibroma	Fibrosarcoma
Cartilage	Chondroma	Chondrosarcoma
Bone	Osteoma	Osteosarcoma
Bone marrow		Leukemia Multiple myeloma Ewing's sarcoma
Adipose (fat)	Lipoma	Liposarcoma
Synovial	Ganglion, giant cell of tendon sheath	Synovial sarcoma
Muscle		
Smooth muscle	Leiomyoma	Leiomyosarcoma
Striated muscle	Rhabdomyoma	Rhabdomyosarcoma
Endothelium (Vascular/Lymphatic)		
Lymph vessels	Lymphangioma	Lymphangiosarcoma Kaposi's sarcoma
Lymphoid tissue		Lymphosarcoma (lymphoma) Lymphatic leukemia
Blood vessels	Hemangioma	Hemangiosarcoma
Neural Tissue		
Nerve fibers and sheaths	Neurofibroma Neuroma Neurinoma (neurilemmoma)	Neurofibrosarcoma Neurogenic sarcoma
Glial tissue	Gliosis	Glioma
Epithelium		
Skin and mucous membrane	Papilloma Polyp	Squamous cell carcinoma Basal cell carcinoma
Glandular epithelium	Adenoma	Adenocarcinoma

* Data from Purtilo, D.T.: A Survey of Human Diseases. Menlo Park, CA, Addison-Wesley Publishing Company, 1978; Phipps, W., et al: Medical-Surgical Nursing: Concepts and Clinical Practice. St. Louis, C.V. Mosby, 1987.

vascularized nature of neoplasms. If the lesion is close to a joint, function in that joint may be disturbed with painful and restricted range of motion (Salter, 1983).

BONE TUMORS

Primary bone tumors are relatively rare, accounting for less than 1% of total deaths from cancer. Excluding multiple myeloma, the ratio of benign to malignant bone tumors is approximately 7 : 1. Primary bone cancer affects children and young adults most commonly, whereas, secondary bone tumors occur in adults with primary cancer (e.g., cancer of the prostate, breast, lungs, kidneys, thyroid). The two most common childhood sarcomas of the bone are osteogenic sarcoma and Ewing's sarcoma; both have a poor prognosis. This text is limited to the most common forms of bone tumors. The reader is referred to a more comprehensive text for a detailed discussion of all the soft tissue and bone tumors (DeVita et al, 1985).

Bone pain (especially pain on weight bearing) that persists for more than 1 week and grows worse at night, often awakening the patient, is usually the most common symptom of bone cancer. The pain is often associated with

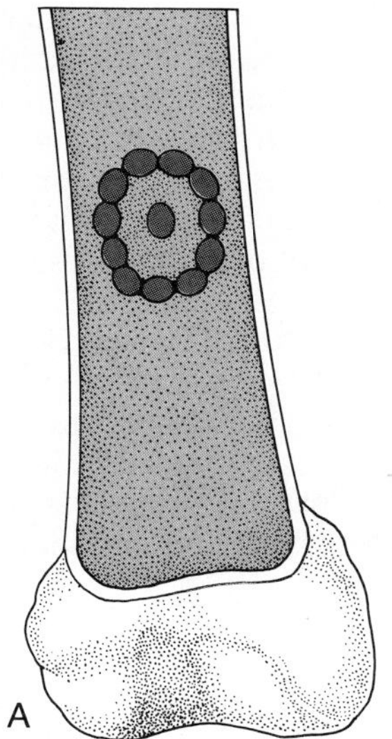

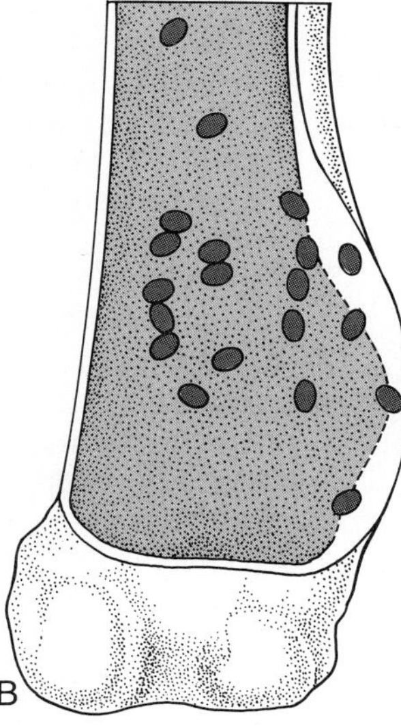

Figure 10–3. *A,* Benign bone tumors have a characteristic sclerotic rim around the periphery of the lesion. The lesion is usually well defined, and there is no evidence of the erosion of the cortex or soft-tissue mass. *B,* Malignant bone tumors can have lytic or sclerotic components. It is frequently difficult to know the extent of the lesion within the bone, because there is no well-defined sclerotic rim around the tumor. The destructive process is diffuse within the medullary cavity of the bone, and the tumor may break through the cortex of the bone, thus producing a Codman triangle. Frequently, there is an associated soft-tisse mass. Differential diagnosis of this lesion is between an osteogenic sarcoma and chondrosarcoma. (Adapted from DeVita, V.T., Jr., and Hellman, S. (eds): Cancer: Principles and Practice of Oncology. Philadelphia, J.B. Lippincott, 1982.)

trauma during a game or exercise and may be dismissed as "growing pains."

Occasionally, a growing bone mass is the first sign of disease (American Cancer Society, 1981). Diagnosis is made by x-ray and surgical biopsy, requiring immediate attention to suspicious symptoms by referral to the patient's physician.

Osteogenic Sarcoma

Osteogenic sarcoma (also known as osteosarcoma) is the most common type of bone cancer, occurring between the ages of 10 and 25 and is more common in boys. Although it can involve any bones in the body, because it arises from osteoblasts, the usual site is the epiphyses of the long bones, where active growth takes place (e.g., lower end of the femur, upper end of the tibia or fibula, and upper end of the humerus). The growth spurt of adolescence is a peak time for the development of osteosarcoma. Half of all osteosarcomas are located in the upper leg above the knee, where the most active epiphyseal growth occurs.

CLINICAL SIGNS AND SYMPTOMS OF OSTEOGENIC SARCOMA

- Pain and swelling of the involved body part
- Loss of motion and functional movement of adjacent joints
- Tender lump
- Pathologic fracture
- Occasional weight loss
- Malaise
- Fatigue

The pain is mild initially and intermittent, but becomes more severe and constant over time. A tender lump may be present, and a bone weakened by erosion of the metaphyseal cortex may break with little or no stress. This pathologic fracture often brings the patient into the medical system, at which time a diagnosis is established by x-ray and surgical biopsy. This neoplasm is highly vascularized so that the overlying skin is usually warm. Metastases to lungs, pleura, lymph nodes, kidney, brain, and other bones are common and occur early in the disease process (Snyder, 1986; Williams and Williams, 1986).

Ewing's Sarcoma

Ewing's sarcoma is a relatively rare, but malignant tumor of bones that is most common between the ages of 5 and 16 with slightly greater incidence in boys than girls. Almost any bone can be involved, but typically the pelvis, femur, tibia, ulna, and metatarsals are the most frequent sites for Ewing's sarcoma.

CLINICAL SIGNS AND SYMPTOMS OF EWING'S SARCOMA

- Increasing and persistent pain
- Increasing and persistent swelling over a bone (localized over the area of tumor)
- Decrease in movement if a limb bone is involved
- Fever

Ewing's sarcoma is a rapidly growing tumor that often outgrows its blood supply and quickly erodes the bone cortex, producing a soft, tender, palpable mass. Fever may occur when products of bone degeneration enter the bloodstream. In addition, the blood supply to local areas of bone may be compromised with resultant avascular necrosis of bone (Salter, 1983). Neurologic symptoms may occur secondary to nerve entrapment by the tumor. Prognosis depends greatly on whether metastatic disease is present at the time of diagnosis. Metastasis to the lungs, lymph nodes, and other bone usually occurs late in the disease process with poor survival statistics (Snyder, 1986; Williams and Williams, 1986).

Chondrosarcoma

Chondrosarcoma, unlike osteosarcoma and Ewing's sarcoma, occurs most often in middle-aged adults. It arises from cartilage and occurs most commonly in some part of the pelvic or shoulder girdles or long bones, such as the femur. Chondrosarcoma is usually a relatively slow-growing malignant neoplasm that arises either spontaneously in previously normal bone or as a result of malignant change in a pre-existing benign bone tumor (osteochondromas and enchondromas or chondromas) (American Cancer Society, 1981; Salter, 1983; Williams and Williams, 1986). Because chondrosarcoma grows relatively slowly, pain is not a prominent clinical feature, but rather, a large cartilaginous mass develops undetected. Metastases develop late so that the prognosis of chondrosarcoma is considerably better than that of osteosarcoma (Salter, 1983).

NEUROLOGIC MANIFESTATIONS OF MALIGNANCY (Minna and Bunn, 1985)

Neurologic problems occur frequently in patients with cancer. The most frequent neurologic complications are caused directly by tumor metastases to the brain; by endocrine, fluid, and electrolyte abnormalities; or by paraneoplastic syndromes or "remote effects" of tumors on the CNS.

When tumors produce signs and symptoms at a distance from the tumor or its metastasized sites, these "remote effects" of malignancy are collectively referred to as *paraneoplastic syndromes.* For example, when tumors secrete hormones, such as adrenocorticotropin (ACTH), which are distributed by the circulation and act on target organs at a site other than the location of the tumor, a paraneoplastic syndrome may occur. These syndromes are not rare, but less than 10% of all cancer patients have been reported to have neurologic paraneoplastic syndromes (Croft and Wilkinson, 1965). Paraneoplastic syndromes may be the first sign of a malignancy that allows its early detection in a curable state.

CLINICAL SIGNS AND SYMPTOMS OF PARANEOPLASTIC SYNDROMES

- Skin rash
- Clubbing of the fingers

- Pigmentation disorders
- Arthralgias
- Paresthesias
- Thrombophlebitis

Gradual, progressive muscle weakness during a period of weeks to months (especially of the pelvic girdle muscles) may occur. Proximal muscles are most likely to be involved. The weakness does stabilize. Reflexes of the involved extremities are present, but are diminished.

Primary Central Nervous System Tumors (Nursing 85, 1985)

Primary tumors of the CNS refer to tumors that arise within the CNS and include tumors that lie within the spinal cord (intramedullary), within the dura mater (extramedullary), or extradurally (outside the dura mater). About 80% of CNS tumors occur intracranially and 20% occur within the spinal canal. Of the intracranial lesions, about 60% are primary and the remaining 40% are metastatic lesions, often multiple and most commonly from lung, breast, kidney, and gastrointestinal (GI) tract.

CNS tumors are associated with a high mortality, despite advances in treatment with surgery and radiation. Brain tumors occur in people of all ages with peak incidence at 5 to 10 years of age and 50 to 55 years of age. They are second only to leukemia as a cause of death in children.

Virtually every cell type within the CNS can give rise to a neoplasm. However, tumors commonly develop from the neurons themselves. Glial (support) cells give rise to gliomas, and meningeal cells give rise to meningiomas. Gliomas comprise 40 to 50% of primary brain tumors. Less frequently, they occur within the spinal canal where the condition is predominantly benign.

Any CNS tumor, even if well-differentiated and histologically benign, is potentially dangerous due to the lethal effects of increased intracranial pressure and tumor location near critical structures. For example, a small, well-differentiated lesion in the pons or medulla may be more rapidly fatal than a massive liver cancer.

Primary CNS tumors rarely metastasize outside the CNS, because there is no lymphatic drainage available; hematogenous spread is also unlikely. In most cases, CNS spread is contained in the cerebrospinal axis, involving local invasion or CNS seeding through the subarachnoid space and the ventricles.

Brain Tumors

Headaches occur in 30 to 50% of persons with brain tumors and are usually bioccipital or bifrontal. The headache is characteristically worse on awakening due to differences in CNS drainage in the supine and prone positions and usually disappears soon after the person arises. It may be intensified or precipitated by any activity that increases intracranial pressure, such as straining during a bowel movement, stooping, lifting heavy objects, or coughing. Often, the pain can be relieved by aspirin, acetaminophen, or other moderate painkillers. Vomiting with or without nausea (unrelated to food) occurs in about 25 to 30% of patients with brain tumors and often accompanies headaches. If the tumor invades the meninges, the headaches will be more severe (Shapiro, 1986).

Focal manifestations of a space-occupying brain lesion are caused by the local compression or destruction of the brain tissue as well as by compression secondary to edema (Snyder, 1986). Specific symptoms depend on where the tumor is located. For example, if a tumor is growing in the motor cortex, the patient may develop isolated extremity weakness. If the tumor is developing in the cerebellum, coordination may be affected. Seizures occur in approximately one third of persons with metastatic brain tumors (Glucksberg and Singer, 1982).

Brain Tumors

CLINICAL SIGNS AND SYMPTOMS ASSOCIATED WITH BRAIN TUMORS

- Altered mentation
- Increased sleeping

- Difficulty in concentration
- Memory loss
- Increased irritability
- Poor judgment in decision making
- Headaches

OTHER CLINICAL SIGNS AND SYMPTOMS OF BRAIN TUMORS (Snyder, 1986):

- Seizures (without previous history)
- Sensory changes
- Muscle weakness
- Bladder dysfunction
- Positive Babinski reflex
- Increased lower extremity (LE) reflexes compared with upper extremity reflexes
- Decreased coordination
- Ataxia
- Paralysis
- Clonus (ankle or wrist)

LATE SIGNS OF INCREASED INTRACRANIAL PRESSURE MAY INCLUDE (Snyder, 1986):

- Pupillary change
- Changes in vital signs
- Elevated systolic blood pressure
- Bradycardia
- Slow, irregular respirations

If left untreated, the median survival for patients with brain lesions is 1 month after the appearance of neurologic signs and symptoms (Gudas, 1987). Medical intervention results in extension of the survival time to three to six months. Melanoma frequently metastasizes to the neuraxis (central nervous system) causing transient paralysis or paresis of motor and sensory function. In brain tumors as well as metastasized melanoma, a wide variety of neurological symptoms and syndromes may present, mimicking CVA victims with early return of function (Gudas, 1987).

Spinal Cord

Primary spinal cord tumors usually produce a slow onset of symptoms, whereas metastatic tumors are characterized by rapid development of symptoms. Spinal cord tumors compress the cord and produce symptoms in the body below the level of the tumor. Tumors most often occur in the thoracic spine because of its length, the proximity to the mediastinum, and proximity to direct metastatic extension from lymph nodes involved with lymphoma, breast, or lung cancer.

INITIAL SYMPTOM OF BOTH PRIMARY AND SECONDARY SPINAL CORD TUMORS

- Pain

Discomfort may be thoracolumbar back pain in a beltlike distribution, and the pain may extend to the groin or to the legs (Snyder, 1986). The pain may be constant or intermittent, a dull ache or a sharp, knifelike sensation. Pain location can be primarily at the site of the lesion or may refer down the ipsilateral extremity with radicular involvement (nerve root compression or irritation). For example, an extramedullary intradural tumor, such as a neurofibroma, may be restricted to one nerve route, producing radicular pain confined to that particular nerve root distribution. The pain occurs most often at rest and pain occurring at night can awaken an individual from sleep, with the patient reporting that it is impossible to go back to sleep.

ONCOLOGIC PAIN (Snyder, 1986)

Some patients fear the pain of cancer as much as or more than death. But generally, pain occurs only in the advanced stages and varies according to the type of cancer. For example, pancreatic cancer causes symptoms in up to 70% of affected patients. The more common cancers of the lung and breast cause pain in about 50% of cases, mainly because of the metastasis to bone. Primary bone cancer is associated with pain in as many as 85% of cases. Blood cancers and cancers of the lymph system give rise to pain in only 5% of cases. Overall, about 30% of cancer patients undergoing cancer treatment have pain, and the discomfort is readily managed by most patients (Holleb, 1986).

Signs and Symptoms Associated With Levels of Pain

The severity of pain varies from one patient to another, but certain signs and symptoms are characteristic of particular levels of pain. For example, in *mild-to-moderate superficial pain,* a sympathetic nervous system response is usually elicited with hypertension, tachycardia, and tachypnea. In *severe or visceral pain,* a parasympathetic nervous system response is more characteristic with hypotension, bradycardia, nausea, vomiting, tachypnea (rapid, shallow breathing), weakness, or fainting (Nursing 83, 1983; Snyder, 1986). Depression and anxiety may increase the patient's perception of pain requiring additional psychologic and emotional support.

Biologic Mechanisms of Cancer Pain (Glucksberg and Singer, 1982; Holleb, 1986; Snyder, 1986)

Five biologic mechanisms have been implicated in the development of chronic cancer pain. The characteristics of the pain depend on tissue morphology as well as on the involved mechanisms.

Bone Destruction

Bone destruction secondary to infiltration by malignant cells or resulting from metastatic lesions is the *first* and most common of the biologic mechanisms causing chronic cancer pain. Bone metastases cause increased release of prostaglandins and subsequent bone breakdown and resorption. The patient's pain threshold is reduced through sensitization of free nerve endings. Bone pain may be felt by the patient as mild to intense. Maladaptive outcomes of bone destruction may include sharp continuous pain that increases on movement or ambulation. The rich supply of nerves and tension or pressure on the sensitive periosteum or endosteum may cause bone pain. Other factors contributing to the intense discomfort reported by patients include limited space for relief of pressure, altered local metabolism, weakening of the bone structure, and pathologic fractures ranging in size from microscopic to large (Salter, 1983).

Obstruction

Obstruction of a hollow, viscus organ and ducts such as the bowel, stomach, or ureters is a *second* physiologic factor in the development of chronic cancer pain. Viscus obstruction is most often due to the obstruction of an organ lumen by tumor growth. In the GI or genitourinary tracts, obstruction results in either a severe, colicky, crampy pain or true visceral pain that is dull, diffuse, boring, and poorly localized. If a vein, artery, or lymphatic channel is obstructed, venous engorgement, arterial ischemia, or edema will result, respectively. In these cases, pain is described as being dull, diffuse, burning, and aching. Obstruction of the ducts leading from the gallbladder and pancreas is common in cancer of these organs, although jaundice is more frequently an earlier symptom than pain. Cancer of the throat or esophagus can obstruct these organs, leading to difficulties in eating or speaking.

Infiltration or Compression

Infiltration or compression of peripheral nerves is the *third* physiologic factor that produces chronic cancer pain and discomfort. Pressure on nerves from adjacent tumor masses and microscopic infiltration of nerves by tumor cells result in continuous, sharp, stabbing pain generally following the pattern of nerve distribution. The invading cells affect the conduction of impulses by the nervous system and sometimes result in constant, dull, poorly localized pain and altered sensation.

Blockage of the blood in arteries and veins, again both by pressure from tumor masses nearby and by infiltration, can decrease oxygen and nutrient supply to tissues. This deficiency can be perceived as pain similar in origin and character to cardiac pain, or angina pectoris, which is chest pain from insufficient supply of oxygen to the heart (Foley, 1986). Hyperesthesia or paresthesia may result.

Infiltration or Distention

Infiltration or distention of integument (skin or tissue) is the *fourth* physiologic phenomenon resulting in chronic, severe cancer pain. This type of pain is secondary to the skin or tissue being painfully stretched because of underlying tumor growth. This stretching produces severe, dull, aching, and localized pain with the severity of the pain increasing concurrently with increase of tumor size. Pain associated with headaches secondary to brain tumors is thought to be due to traction on pain-sensitive intracranial structures (Snyder, 1986).

Inflammation, Infection, and Necrosis of Tissue

Inflammation, infection, and necrosis of tissue may be the *fifth* and final cause of cancer pain. Inflammation with its accompanying symptoms of redness, edema, pain, heat, and loss of function may progress to infection, necrosis, and sloughing of tissue. If the inflammatory process alone is present, the pain is characterized by a sensitive tenderness. If, however, necrosis and tissue sloughing have occurred, pain may be excruciating.

OVERVIEW OF CANCER PRESENCE AND PAIN PATTERNS

Skin (Melanoma only)

Location:	Women: arms, legs, back, face
	Men: head, trunk
	Blacks: palms, soles, under the nails
Referral:	None
Description:	Usually painless
	Irritation and itching
	Tenderness and soreness around a mole
Intensity:	Mild
Duration:	Constant
Associated Signs and Symptoms:	None

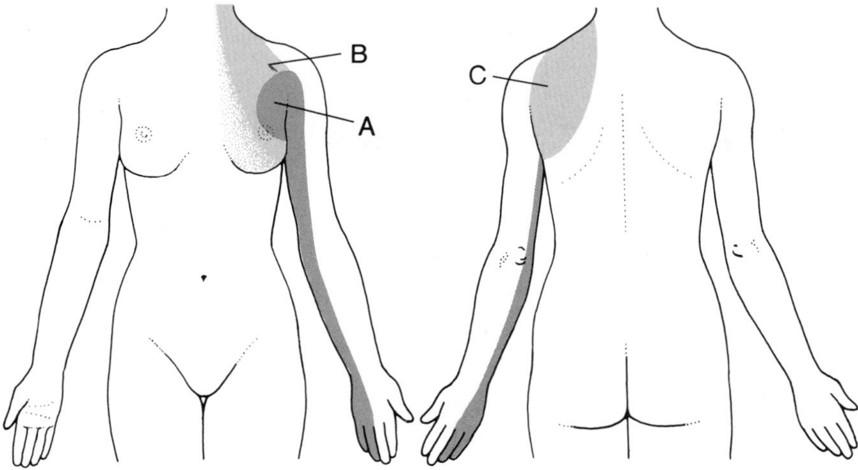

Figure 10–4. Pain arising from the breast showing *(A)* mammary pain referred into the axilla along the medial aspect of the arm; *(B)* referral pain to the supraclavicular level and into the neck; *(C)* breast pain may diffuse around the thorax through the intercostal nerves. Pain may be referred to the back and to the posterior shoulder.

Breast

Location (Fig. 10–4):	Changes or pain occur anywhere on the breast or nipple
Referral:	May be painless
	Around the chest into the axilla, to the back at the level of the breast, occasionally into the neck and posterior aspect of the shoulder girdle
	Along the medial aspect of the ipsilateral arm to the 4th and 5th digits
Description:	Usually painless
	Involvement of breast tissue may result in sharp cutting or sharp aching
Intensity:	Mild to severe
Duration:	Intermittent to constant
Associated Signs and Symptoms:	May have no other symptoms
	May report discharge or bleeding from the breasts or nipples
	Distorted shape of the breast or nipple
	Enlarged tender lymph nodes
	Dimpling of the skin surface over the breast
	Unusual rash on the breast or nipple
	Unusual prominence of the veins over the breast

Leukemia

Location:	Usually painless, may have pain in the left abdomen
Referral:	None
Description:	Dull pain in the abdomen and may occur only on palpation
Intensity:	Mild to moderate
Duration:	Intermittent (with applied pressure)
Associated Signs and Symptoms:	Unusual bleeding from the nose, rectum, or in urine Prolonged menstruation Easy bruising of the skin Fatigue Dyspnea Weight loss, loss of appetite Fevers and sweats

Multiple Myeloma

Location:	Skeletal pain, especially in the spine, sternum, rib, leg, or arm
Referral:	According to the location of the tumor
Description:	Sharp, knifelike
Intensity:	Moderate to severe
Duration:	Intermittent, progressing to constant
Associated Signs and Symptoms:	Hypercalcemia: dehydration (vomiting), polyuria Spontaneous bone fracture Carpal tunnel syndrome

Hodgkin's Disease

Location:	Lymph glands, usually unilateral neck or groin
Referral:	According to the location of the metastases
Description:	Usually painless, progressive enlargement of lymph nodes
Intensity:	Not applicable
Duration:	Not applicable

Associated Signs and Symptoms:	Fever peaks in the late afternoon, night sweats Anorexia and weight loss Severe itching over the entire body

Non-Hodgkin's Lymphoma

Location:	Peripheral lymph nodes
Referral:	Not applicable
Description:	Usually painless
Intensity:	Not applicable
Duration:	Not applicable
Associated Signs and Symptoms:	Fever Weight loss Bleeding Generalized itching and reddened skin

Soft Tissue Tumors

Location:	Any connective tissue (e.g., muscle, cartilage, fat, synovium, fibrous tissue)
Referral:	According to the tissue involved
Description:	Persistent swelling or lump, especially in the muscle
Intensity:	Mild, increases progressively to severe
Duration:	Intermittent, increases progressively to constant
Associated Signs and Symptoms:	Local swelling with tenderness and skin warmth

Bone Tumors

Location:	Can affect any bone in the body, depending on the specific type of bone cancer
Referral:	According to pattern and location of metastases
Description:	Sharp, knifelike, aching bone pain Occurs on movement, weight-bearing, and with pathologic fractures Pain at night preventing sleep
Intensity:	Initially mild, progressing to severe

Duration:	Usually intermittent, progressing to constant
Associated Signs and Symptoms:	Fatigue and malaise Weight loss Swelling over localized areas of tumor Soft, tender palpable mass over bone Loss of range or motion and joint function if limb bone is involved Fever

Primary Central Nervous System Tumors

Location:	Intramedullary (within the spinal cord) Extramedullary (within the dura mater) Extradurally (outside the dura mater) Thoracolumbar back pain in a beltlike distribution
Referral:	Pain may extend to the ipsilateral groin or to the legs with a radicular involvement
Description:	Dull ache or sharp, knifelike sensation Occurs at rest, pain at night prevents sleep
Intensity:	Mild to severe, progressive
Duration:	Intermittent progressing to constant
Associated Signs and Symptoms:	Altered mentation Increased sleeping Difficulty in concentrating Memory loss Increased irritability Poor judgment Headaches on awakening, which increase during any activity that increases intracranial pressure (e.g., straining during bowel movement, stooping, lifting heavy objects, coughing) Pain can be relieved by painkillers (e.g., aspirin, acetaminophen) Vomiting unrelated to food, accompanies headaches Seizures Neurologic findings Positive Babinski reflex Sensory changes Decreased coordination Ataxia Muscle weakness Increased LE reflexes Transient paralysis

SUMMARY

Cancer and its presenting clinical signs and symptoms of individual organs (e.g., lungs, liver, prostate) are covered in the related chapters concerning each system. In this chapter, we have attempted to provide an overview of:

- Definition of cancer and a description of cancer
- Definition and description of metastases
- Discussion of current theories regarding the biochemical and immunologic basis for the development of cancer
- Early warning signs of cancer
- Discussion of cancers that are not covered in chapters related to organ systems (e.g., skin and breast cancer, cancers of the blood and lymph system, soft tissue and bone cancer)
- Neurologic manifestations of malignancy
- Discussion of oncologic pain

Signs and Symptoms Requiring Physician Referral

The physical therapist is advised to ask the patient further questions whenever any of the following signs and symptoms are reported or observed, because they may indicate cancer or some other systemic disease. The patient should therefore be referred to a physician for further evaluation.

Arthralgias
Bleeding mole
Bone pain
Change in bowel habits
Change in urinary habits
Change in voice
Chronic cough
Clubbing of the fingers
Drowsiness/confusion
Dysphagia
Dyspnea
Epistaxis
Fatigue, general malaise
Fevers and sweats
Headache
Hemoptysis (blood in the urine)
Hoarseness
Itching/scratching
Loss of appetite
Lump or thickening
Pain at night disturbing sleep
Pain on weight bearing
Persistent nausea; vomiting and neurologic findings
Prolonged menstruation
(Proximal) muscle weakness
Restlessness
Sore that does not heal
Unusual bleeding
Unusual discharge
Unusual skin lesions or rash
Wheezing

SUBJECTIVE EXAMINATION

Special Questions to Ask

Special questions to ask will vary with each patient and the clinical signs and symptoms presented at the time of the evaluation. The physical therapist should refer to the specific chapter representing the patient's current complaints. The case study provided here is one example of how to follow-up with necessary questions to rule out systemic origin of musculoskeletal findings.

Previous history of drug therapy and current drug use may be important

Subjective Exam

Special Questions to Ask

information to obtain because prolonged use of drugs such as phenytoin (Dilantin) or immunosuppressive drugs, such as azathioprine (Imuran), may lead to cancer. Postmenopausal use of estrogens has been linked with endometrial cancer (Nursing 85, 1985).

Previous personal/family history of cancer may be significant, especially any history of breast, colorectal, or lung cancers that demonstrates genetic susceptibility.

Using the seven early warning signs of cancer as a basis for follow-up, one or all of these questions may be appropriate:

□ Have you noticed any changes in your bowel movement or in the flow of urination?

  If yes, ask pertinent follow-up questions as suggested in Chapter 7.

  If the patient answers "No," it may be necessary to provide prompts or examples of what changes you are referring to (e.g., difficulty in starting or stopping the flow of urine, numbness, or tingling in the groin or pelvis).

□ Have you noticed any sores that have not healed properly?

  If yes, where are they located? How long has the sore been present? Has your physician examined this area?

□ Have you noticed any unusual bleeding (for women: prolonged menstruation) or prolonged discharge from any part of your body?

  If yes, where? How long has this been present? Has your physician examined this area?

□ Have you noticed any thickening or lump of any muscle, tendon, bone, breast, or anywhere else?

  If yes, where? How long has this been present? Has your physician examined this area?*

  If no, (for women): do you examine your own breasts? How often do you examine them, and when was the last time that you did a self-breast examination?

□ Have you noticed any difficulty in eating or swallowing? Have you had a chronic cough, recurrent laryngitis, hoarseness, or any difficulty with speaking?

  If yes, how long has this been happening? Have you discussed this with your physician?

□ Have you had any change in digestive patterns? Have you had increasing indigestion or unusual constipation?

  If yes, how long has this been happening? Have you discussed this with your physician?

---

* An asymptomatic mass that has been present for years and causes only cosmetic concern is usually benign, whereas, a painful mass of short duration that has caused a decrease in function may be malignant (Wilkins and Sim, 1986).

Subjective Exam

Special Questions to Ask

- □ Have you had a recent, sudden weight loss, such as 10 to 15 lb in 2 weeks without really trying?
- □ Have you noticed any obvious change in color, shape, or size of a wart or mole?

    If yes, what have you noticed? How long has this wart or mole been present? Have you discussed this problem with your physician?

- □ Have you had any unusual headaches or changes in your vision?

    If yes, please describe. **(Brain tumors: bioccipital or bifrontal)**

    Can you attribute these to anything in particular?

    Do you vomit (unrelated to food) when your headaches occur? **(Brain tumor)**

- □ Have you been more tired than usual or experienced persistent fatigue during the last month?
- □ Can you think of any time during the past week when you may have bumped yourself, fallen, or injured yourself in any way? (Ask when in the presence of local swelling and tenderness, **bone tumors**)
- □ Have you ever been exposed to chemical agents or irritants, such as asbestos, asphalt, aniline dyes, benzene, herbicides, fertilizers, wood dust, or others? **(Environmental causes of cancer)**

PHYSICIAN REFERRAL

Early detection of cancer can save a patient's life when it is found and treated appropriately. Any suspicious sign or symptom discussed in this chapter should be investigated immediately by a physician. This is true especially in the presence of a positive family history of cancer, previous personal history of cancer, presence of environmental risk factors and/or in the absence of medical or dental (oral) evaluation during the previous year.

Any recently discovered lumps or nodules must be examined by a physician. Any suspicious finding by report, on observation, or by palpation should be checked by a physician. Finding enlarged, tender lymph nodes does not require a referral to a physician unless these lymph nodes persist and involve more than one area because lymph nodes enlarge in response to infections throughout the body.

However, the physician should be notified of your findings, and the patient should be advised to have the lymph nodes checked at the next follow-up visit with the physician. If the nodes remain enlarged over a long period (4 weeks or more), then the patient should be encouraged to contact the physician to discuss the need for follow-up. The exception is with patients who have enlarged, *painless* lymph nodes. These people should notify their physician of these findings and make an appointment for follow-up at the physician's discretion.

If any signs of skin lesions are described by the patient or if they are observed by the physical therapist, and the patient has not been examined by a physician, a medical referral is recommended. If the patient is planning a follow-up visit with the physician within the next 2 to 4 weeks, then that patient is advised to indicate the mole or skin changes at that time. If no appointment is pending, then the patient is encouraged to make a specific visit either to the family/personal physician or to a dermatologist.

CASE STUDY

Referral

A 56-year-old man has come to you for an evaluation without referral. He has not been examined by a physician of any kind for at least 3 years. He is seeking an evaluation on the insistence of his wife, who has noticed that his collar size has increased two sizes in the last year and that his neck looks "puffy." He has no complaints of any kind (including pain or discomfort), and he denies any known trauma, but his wife insists that he has limited ability in turning his head when backing the car out of the driveway.

A. What questions would be appropriate for your physical therapy interview with this patient?

First read the patient's *Personal/Family History* form with particular interest in his personal or family history of cancer, the presence of allergies or asthma, the use of medications or over-the-counter drugs, previous surgeries, available x-rays of the neck or spine, and/or history of cigarette smoking (tobacco use). An appropriate lead-in to the following series of questions may be, "Since you have not seen a physician before your appointment with me, I will ask you a series of questions to determine whether your symptoms may be more indicative of a medical problem that requires an examination by a physician than a true muscular or neck problem appropriate for treatment in this office."

Current Symptoms

What have you noticed different about your neck that brings you here today?

When did you first notice that your neck was changing (in size or shape)?

Can you remember having any accidents, falls, twists, or any other kind of potential trauma at that time?

Do you ever notice any pain, stiffness, soreness, or discomfort in your neck or shoulders?

If yes, please describe (as per outline in *the physical therapy interview*).

Does this or any other pain ever awaken you at night or keep you awake? **(Night pain associated with cancer)**

If yes, follow-up with appropriate questions. (See the physical therapy interview.)

Associated Symptoms

Have you noticed any numbness or tingling in your arms or hands?

Have you noticed any swollen glands, lumps, or thickened areas of skin or muscle in your neck, armpits, or groin? **(Cancer screen)**

Do you have any difficulty in swallowing? Do you have recurrent hoarseness, influenzalike symptoms, or a persistent cough or cold that never seems to go away? **(Cancer screen)**

Have you noticed any low-grade fevers or night sweats? **(Systemic disease)**

Have you had any recent unexplained weight gain or loss? Have you had a loss of appetite? (You may need to explain that you mean a gain or loss of 10 to 15 lb in as many days without dieting.) **(Cancer screen or other systemic disease)**

CASE STUDY

Do you ever have any difficulty with breathing or find yourself short of breath at rest or after minimal exercise? **(Dyspnea)**

Do you have frequent headaches or do you experience any dizziness, nausea, or vomiting? **(Systemic disease, carotid artery affected)**

Functional Capacity

What kind of work do you do?

Do you have any limitations caused by this condition that limit you in any way at work or at home? **(Occupational disease, limitations of activities of daily living (ADL) skills)**

Do you have difficulty when driving or turning your head?

Final Questions

How would you describe your general health?

Have you ever been diagnosed with cancer of any kind?

Is there anything that you would like to tell me that you think is important about your neck or your health in general?

B. What test procedures will you carry out during the first session to assess the musculoskeletal system?

Observation/Inspection. Observe for presence of swelling anywhere, tender or swollen lymph nodes (cervical and axillary), changes in skin temperature, unusual moles or warts. Perform a brief posture screen (general postural observations may be made while you are interviewing the patient). Palpate for carotid and upper extremity pulses. Check vital signs and **TAKE THE PATIENT'S ORAL TEMPERATURE!**

Cervical AROM/PROM. Assess for muscle tightness, loss of joint motion (including accessory movements if indicated by a loss of passive motion). Assess for compromise of the vertebral artery and, if negative, clear the cervical spine by using a quadrant test with overpressure (e.g., Spurling's test) and assess accessory movements of the cervical spine. Perform tests for thoracic outlet syndrome. Palpate anterior cervical spine for pathologic protrusion while the patient swallows.

Temporomandibular Joint (TMJ) Screen. Clear the joint above (i.e., TMJ) using AROM, observation, and palpation specific to TMJ.

Shoulder Screen. Clear the joint below (i.e., shoulder) by using a screening examination (e.g., AROM/PROM and quadrant testing).

Neurologic Screen. Deep tendon reflexes, sensory screen (e.g., gross sensory testing for light touch), manual muscle test (MMT) screening using break testing of the upper quadrant, grip strength. If test(s) are abnormal, consider further neurologic testing (e.g., balance, coordination, stereognosia, in-depth sensory examination, dysmetria).

It is always recommended that the physical therapist give the patient ongoing verbal feedback during the examination regarding evaluation results, such as "I notice that you can't turn your head to the right as fully as you can turn it to the left, but when I checked your muscles and the joints, it looks like this is just from muscle tightness and not from a true loss of joint movement." . . . or . . . "I

CASE STUDY

notice that your reflexes are not the same on both sides (the right arm moves faster and harder when I hit the tendon with my reflex hammer compared with the left arm). I'll check a few more things to see what this might be."

C. If you suggest to this man that he should see his physician, how would you make that recommendation?

I noticed on your intake form that you haven't listed the name of a personal or family physician. Do you have a physician?

If yes, when was the last time you saw your physician? Have you seen your physician for this current problem?

Give the patient a brief summary of your findings while making your recommendations; for example, Mr. X., I notice today that although you don't have any ongoing neck pain, the lymph nodes in the neck and armpit are enlarged but are not particularly tender. Otherwise, all of my findings are negative. Your loss of motion on turning your head is not unusual for a person your age and certainly would not cause your neck to increase in size or shape. It is more likely to be the other way around: Whatever is going on in your neck has caused a change in motion.

Given the fact that you have not seen a physician for almost 3 years, I strongly recommend that you see either a physician of your own choice or I can give you the names of several physicians to choose from. In either case, I think some medical tests are necessary to rule out any underlying medical problem. For example, a neck x-ray would be recommended before I would feel comfortable treating you.

If the patient has indicated a positive family history of cancer, it might be appropriate to suggest, "Given your positive family history of previous medical illnesses, the 3 years since you have seen a physician and the lack of musculoskeletal findings, I strongly recommend . . . etc." It is important to provide the patient with all the information available to you, but without causing undue alarm and emotional stress that could actually prevent the patient from seeking further testing.

If the patient does give the name of a physician, you may ask for written permission (disclosure release) to send a copy of your results to the physician. If the patient does not have a physician and requests recommendations from you, then you may offer to send a copy of your results to the physician with whom the patient makes an appointment. If you think that a problem may be potentially serious and you want this patient to receive adequate follow-up without causing alarm, you may offer to let the patient make the appointment from your office, suggest that your secretary or receptionist make the appointment for him, or even offer to make the initial telephone contact yourself.

Result

This patient did comply with the physical therapist's suggestion to see a physician and was diagnosed as having Hodgkin's disease (a cancer of the lymph system) without constitutional symptoms (i.e., without evidence of weight loss, fever, or night sweats). Medical treatment was initiated and physical therapy treatment was not warranted.

References

American Cancer Society: A Cancer Source Book for Nurses (Revised ed). New York, American Cancer Society Professional Education Publication, 1981.

American Medical Association: Cancer: Facts You Should Know. American Medical Association, Patient Information Service, 1987.

Croft, P.B., and Wilkinson, M.W.: The incidence of carcinomatous neuromyopathy with special reference to carcinoma of the lung and breast. *In* Brain, W.R., and Norris, F.H., Jr. (eds): The Remote Effects of Cancer on the Nervous System. New York, Grune & Stratton, 1965, pp. 44–54.

Croft, P.B., and Wilkinson, M.W.: The incidence of carcinomatous neuropathy in patients with various types of carcinoma. Brain, *88*:427, 1965.

DeVita, V.T., Jaffe, E.S., and Hellman, S.: Hodgkin's disease and non-Hodgkin's lymphomas. *In* DeVita, V.T., Hellman, S., and Rosenberg, S.A. (eds): Cancer: Principles & Practice of Oncology, Vols. 1 and 2, 2nd ed. Philadelphia, J.B. Lippincott, 1985, pp. 1623–1709.

Fidler, I.J., and Hart, I.R.: Principles of cancer biology: Cancer metastasis. *In* DeVita, V.T., Hellman, S., and Rosenberg, S.A. (eds): Cancer: Principles & Practice of Oncology, Vols. 1 and 2, 2nd ed. Philadelphia, J.B. Lippincott, 1985, pp. 113–124.

Foley, K.M.: Cancer and pain. *In* Holleb, A.I. (ed): The American Cancer Society Cancer Book. New York, Doubleday & Co, 1986, pp. 225–237.

Fry, R.J.M.: Principles of cancer biology: Physical carcinogenesis. *In* DeVita, V.T., Hellman, S., and Rosenberg, S.A. (eds): Cancer: Principles & Practice of Oncology, Vols. 1 and 2, 2nd ed. Philadelphia, J.B. Lippincott, 1985, pp. 101–112.

Glucksberg, H. and Singer, J.W.: Cancer Care. New York, Chas. Scribner's Sons, 1982.

Gudas, S.: The physical therapy challenge in disseminated cancer. Oncology Section Newsletter of the APTA, *5*:3, 1987.

Hogan, R., and Xistris, D.: Cancer. *In* Phipps, W., Long, B., and Woods, N. (eds): Medical-Surgical Nursing: Concepts and Clinical Practice, 3rd ed. St. Louis, C.V. Mosby, 1987, pp. 329–396.

Holleb, A.I. (ed): The American Cancer Society Cancer Book. New York, Doubleday & Co, 1986.

Long, B.: Interventions for persons with skin problems. *In* Phipps, W., Long, B., and Woods, N. (eds): Medical-Surgical Nursing: Concepts & Clinical Practice, 3rd ed. St. Louis, C.V. Mosby, 1987, pp. 1957–1982.

Miller, B.F., and Keane, C.B.: Encyclopedia and Dictionary of Medicine, Nursing, and Allied Health, 4th ed. Philadelphia, W.B. Saunders Company, 1987.

Minna, J.D., and Bunn, P.A.: Paraneoplastic syndromes. *In* DeVita, V.T., Hellman, S., and Rosenberg, S.A. (eds): Cancer: Principles & Practice of Oncology, Vols. 1 and 2, 2nd ed. Philadelphia: J.B. Lippincott, 1985, pp. 1797–1842.

Molbo, D., and Sun, C.: Problems of the breast. *In* Phipps, W., Long, B., and Woods, N. (eds): Medical-Surgical Nursing: Concepts and Clinical Practice, 3rd ed. St. Louis, C.V. Mosby, 1987, pp. 1855–1878.

Nursing 83: Helping Cancer Patients—Effectively. Springhouse, PA, Intermed Communications, 1983.

Nursing 85: Neoplastic Disorders. Springhouse, PA, Springhouse Publishing Co., 1985.

Osserman, E.F.: Multiple myeloma. *In* Holleb, A.I. (ed): The American Cancer Society Cancer Book. New York, Doubleday & Co, 1986, pp. 460–467.

Pitot, H.C.: Principles of cancer biology: Chemical carcinogenesis. *In* DeVita, V.T., Hellman, S., and Rosenberg, S.A. (eds): Cancer: Principles & Practice of Oncology, Vols. 1 and 2, 2nd ed. Philadelphia, J.B. Lippincott, 1985, pp. 79–100.

Rosenberg, S.A., Suit, H.D., and Baker, L.H.: Sarcomas of soft tissues. *In* DeVita, V.T., Hellman, S., and Rosenberg, S.A. (eds): Cancer: Principles & Practice of Oncology, Vols. 1 and 2, 2nd ed. Philadelphia, J.B. Lippincott, 1985, pp. 1243–1292.

Salter, R.B.: Textbook of Disorders and Injuries of the Musculoskeletal System, 2nd ed. Baltimore, Williams & Wilkins, 1983.

Scanlon, E.F., and Strax, P.: Breast cancer. *In* Holleb, A.I. (ed): The American Cancer Society Cancer Book. New York, Doubleday & Co, 1986, pp. 297–340.

Shapiro, W.R.: Tumors of the brain. *In* Holleb, A.I. (ed): The American Cancer Society Cancer Book. New York, Doubleday & Co, 1986, pp. 277–296.

Snyder, C.C.: Oncology Nursing. Boston, Little, Brown, 1986.

Upton, A.C.: Principles of cancer biology: Etiology and prevention of cancer. *In* DeVita, V.T., Hellman, S., and Rosenberg, S.A. (eds): Cancer: Principles & Practice of Oncology. Philadelphia, J.B. Lippincott, 1982, pp. 33–58.

Wilkins, R.M., and Sim, F.H.: Evaluation of bone and soft tissue tumors. *In* D'Ambrosia, R.D. (ed): Musculoskeletal Disorders: Regional Examination and Differential Diagnosis, 2nd ed. Philadelphia, J.B. Lippincott, 1986.

Williams, C., and Williams, S.: Cancer: A guide for patients and their families. New York, John Wiley & Sons, 1986.

Bibliography

Caldwell, D.S.: Musculoskeletal syndromes associated with malignancy. *In* Kelley, W.N., et al (eds): Textbook of Rheumatology, 2nd ed. Philadelphia, W.B. Saunders Company, pp. 1603–1619.

Edelhart, M.: Interferon: The new hope for cancer. Reading, MA, Addison-Wesley, 1981.

Hall, T.C.: The paraneoplastic syndromes. *In* Rubin, P. (ed): Clinical Oncology for Medical Students and Physicians, 4th ed. Rochester, NY, University of Rochester, 1974.

Layzer, R.B.: Neuromuscular Manifestations of Systemic Disease. Philadelphia, F.A. Davis, 1985.

Levenson, F.B.: The Causes and Prevention of Cancer. New York, Stein and Day, 1984.

Panem, S.: The interferon crusade. Washington, DC, The Brookings Institution, 1984.

Chapter 11

Overview of Immunology: Signs and Symptoms

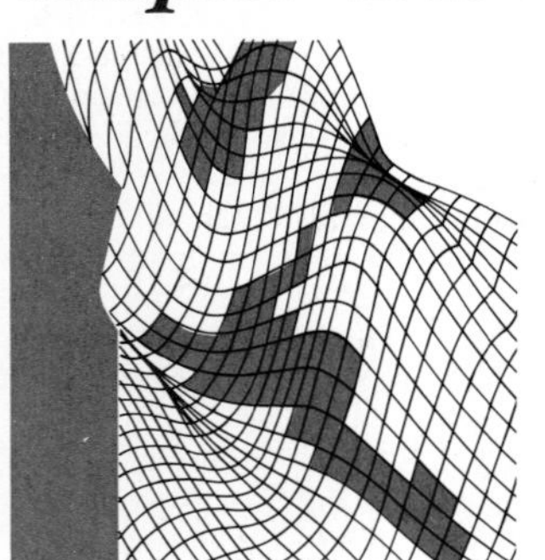

☐ ***Clinical Signs and Symptoms of:***

- AIDS Related Complex (ARC)
- Acquired Immunodeficiency Syndrome and the "Opportunistic Infections"
- Myasthenia Gravis
- Guillain-Barré Syndrome (or Acute Idiopathic Polyneuritis)
- Multiple Sclerosis
- Rheumatoid Arthritis
- Early Stages of Systemic Lupus Erythematosus
- Scleroderma
- Esophageal Involvement
- Gastrointestinal Involvement
- Lung Involvement
- Polymyositis/Dermatomyositis
- Mixed Connective Tissue Disease
- Ankylosing Spondylitis
- Reiter's Syndrome
- Psoriatic Arthritis

Immunology, one of the few disciplines with a full range of involvement in all aspects of health and disease, is one of the most rapidly expanding fields in medicine today. Keeping current is difficult at best with the volume of new immunologic information generated by clinical researchers each year (Nursing 85, 1985). The information presented here is a simplistic representation of the immune system and should be supplemented by the reader with any of the texts referenced.

Immunity denotes protection against infectious organisms (Nursing 85, 1985). The immune system is a complex network of specialized organs and cells that has evolved to defend the body against attacks by "foreign" invaders (National Institutes of Health, 1985). Immunity is provided by lymphoid cells residing in the immune system. This system consists of central and peripheral lymphoid organs (Fig. 11–1).

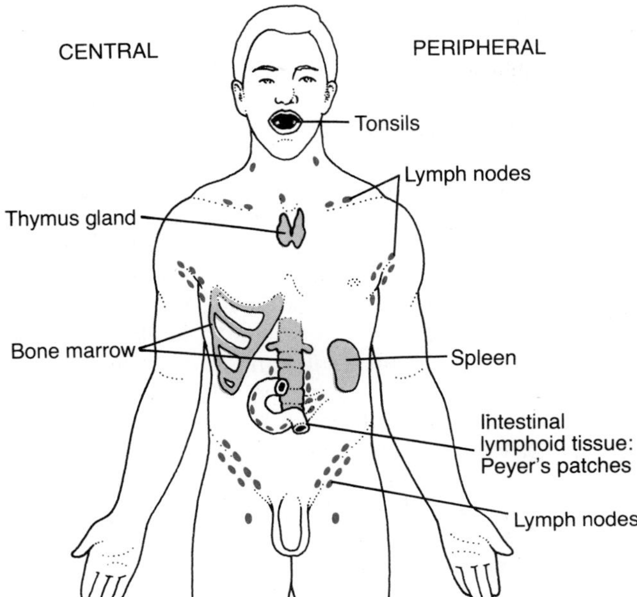

Figure 11–1. Organs of the immune system.

By circulating its component cells and substances, the immune system maintains an early warning system against both exogenous microorganisms (infections produced by bacteria, viruses, parasites, and fungi) and endogenous cells that have become neoplastic. Understanding the interactions of antigens and antibodies is basic to understanding how the immune system functions. These interactions are discussed later in this chapter.

Immunologic responses in humans can be divided into two broad categories: humoral immunity, which takes place in the body fluids (humors) and is concerned with antibody and complement activities; and cell-mediated or cellular immunity, which involves a variety of activities designed to destroy or at least contain cells that are recognized by the body as being alien and harmful. Both types of responses are initiated by lymphocytes and are discussed in the context of lymphocytic function (Miller and Keane, 1987).

PHYSIOLOGY OF THE IMMUNE SYSTEM

Organs of the Immune System

The lymphoid system includes organs and tissues in which lymphocytes predominate, as well as cells that circulate in peripheral blood. As mentioned earlier, central and primary organs include (Nursing 85, 1985):

- Bone marrow
- Thymus (see Fig. 11–1)

Peripheral or secondary organs include:

- Lymph nodes and lymph vessels of the lymphatic system (see Fig. 10–3)
- Spleen
- Tonsils
- Intestinal lymphoid tissue: Peyer's patches and appendix

Central Lymphoid Organs

The *bone marrow* and the *thymus gland* play a role in developing the principal cells of the immune system. The cells involved in the immune response are all derived from undifferentiated stem cells of the bone marrow. The stem cell has the potential for developing into any of the body's blood cells (Fig. 11–2). Various signals and influences within the body's replicative mechanism control this process.

The primary cells of the immune system develop from the lymphocytic cell population. One population of lymphocytic cells undergoes change and differentiation in the thymus gland (thymus-dependent). These cells are called *T-cells* and become responsible for mediating the cell-mediated immune responses. Another population of lymphocytes undergoes maturation in sites other than the thymus gland (thymus-independent) and are called *B-cells.* The B-cells are responsible for the production of the immunoglobulins (antibodies) and mediate the body's humoral response (Wright, 1987) (Fig. 11–3).

Peripheral Lymphoid Organs

Both B-cells and T-cells are distributed throughout the tissue of the peripheral lymphoid organs. *Lymph nodes,* small oval-shaped organs, are located throughout the body, most abundantly in the head and neck, axillae, abdomen, and groin (see Fig. 10–3). They contain lymphocytes (B-cells, T-cells) and macrophages and comprise webbed areas that filter and enmesh antigens (foreign substances). The nodes are linked by a network of lymphatic vessels similar in physical properties to blood vessels (National Institutes of Health, 1985). The lymph vessels carry lymph, a clear fluid derived from interstitial fluid that contains lymphocytes and flows from connective tissue spaces throughout the body via lymphatic capillaries (Hess, 1987). As the lymph passes through lymph nodes, antigens are filtered out and more lymphocytes are picked up. These lymphocytes are then carried to the bloodstream, which delivers them to tissues throughout the body and returns eventually to the lymphatic system where they are used again (National Institutes of Health, 1985).

The *spleen* is the chief site of the immune system's filtering response to antigens. It is rich in lymphocytes and cells of the monocyte-macrophage lineage and represents the single largest collection of lymphoid tissue in the body (Hess, 1987). In addition to its role of erythrocyte production in the fetus, the spleen acts as a reservoir for cellular elements of the peripheral blood (platelets, lymphocytes, and monocytes) and also acts to keep the blood free of unwanted substances, including wastes and infecting organisms. The blood is delivered to the spleen by the splenic artery and passes through smaller branch arteries into a network of channels lined with leukocytes known as phagocytes. These phagocytes clear the blood of old erythrocytes, damaged cells, parasites, and other toxic or foreign substances (Miller and Keane, 1987). Because of the remarkable phagocytic capacity of the spleen and its active participation in the host immune response to foreign antigen, the spleen is often responsible for many of the clinical and laboratory manifestations of a variety of infectious, malignant, autoimmune, and hereditary disorders (Hess, 1987).

The remaining peripheral lymphoid organs (tonsils, Peyer's patches, appendix) are masses of lymphoid tissue containing lymphocytes and thymus-dependent areas (Nursing 85, 1985). *Tonsils* are small, round masses of lymphoid tissue located on each side of the back of the throat. These tissues filter the circulating lymph of any bacteria or foreign material that may enter the body, especially through the mouth and nose (Miller and Keane, 1987). *Peyer's patches* consist of aggregates of lymphoid nodules located in the submucosa of the intestinal wall. A Peyer's patch contains a varying number of B-cells and T-cells as well as a collection of lymphocytes that do not demonstrate either B-cell or T-cell markers (Hess, 1987). The (vermiform) appendix, an appendage near the juncture of the small intestine and the large intestine, is lined with large lymphatic nodules that atrophy in adult life and apparently become nonfunctional.

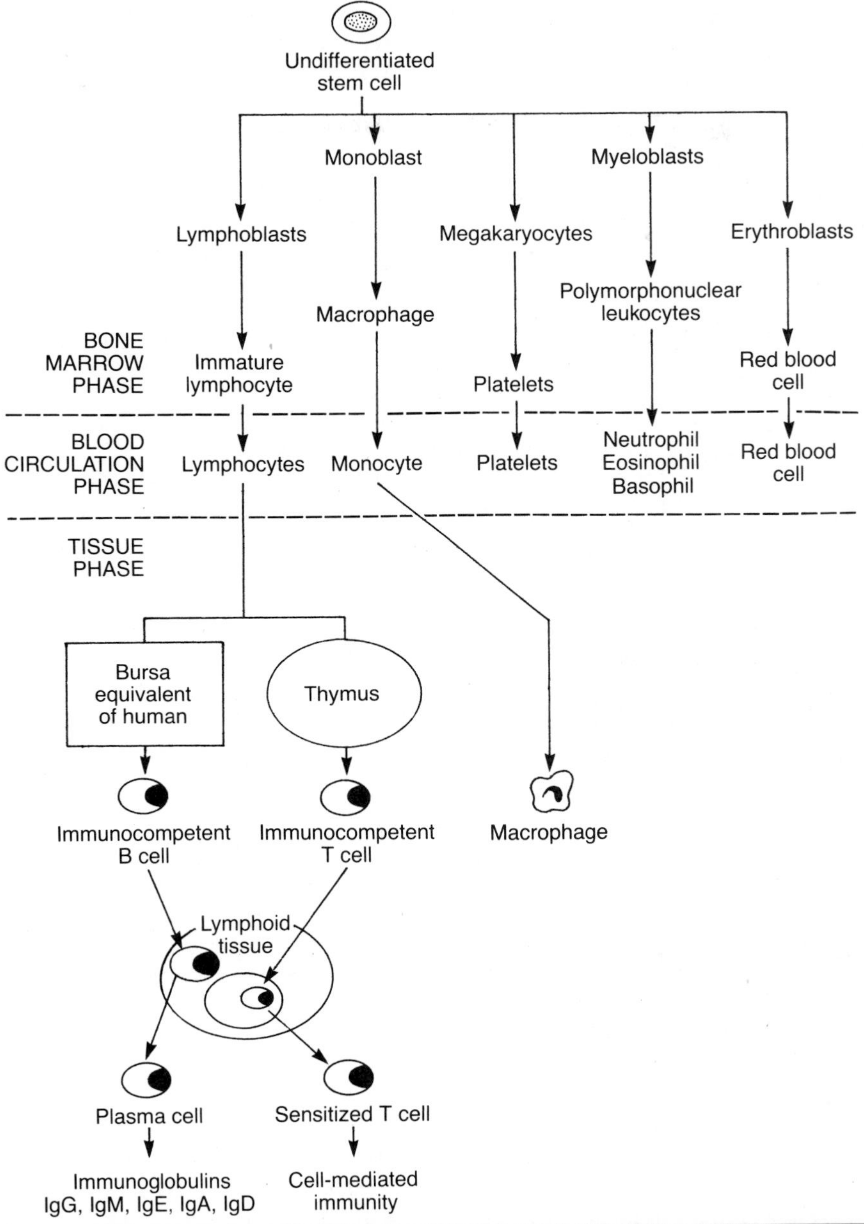

Figure 11–2. Development of cells of the immune system. (From Phipps, W., Long, B. and Woods, N.: Medical-Surgical Nursing: Concepts and Clinical Practice. St. Louis, C.V. Mosby, 1987, p. 1899.)

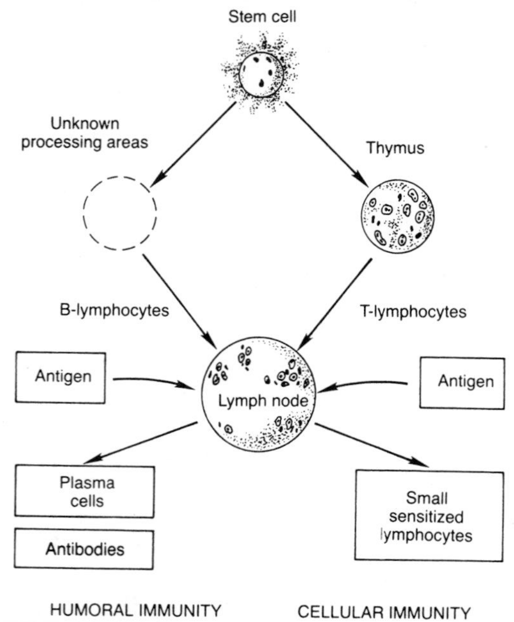

Figure 11–3. Origin of B-lymphocytes and T-lymphocytes responsible for cellular and humoral immunity. In response to antigens, B-lymphocytes and T-lymphocytes are sensitized by lymphoid tissue. (From Miller, B.F., and Keane, C.B.: Encyclopedia and Dictionary of Medicine, Nursing, and Allied Health, 4th ed. Philadelphia, W.B. Saunders Company, 1987, p. 727.)

Function of the Lymphoid System

The lymphoid system has four main functions (Nursing 85, 1985):

- To bring B-cells and T-cells to maturity
- To concentrate antigens from throughout the body into a few lymphoid organs
- To circulate lymphocytes through these organs so that any antigen is quickly exposed to antigen-specific lymphocytes
- To carry antigen-specific lymphocytes and antibodies to the blood and tissues

An *antigen* is any substance (exogenous or endogenous) capable of eliciting an immune response because the body recognizes it as being "foreign." Antigens are sometimes referred to as "nonself" molecules. The body recognizes molecules as being "self" or "nonself" by identifying epitopes (markers) that protrude from the molecule surface. An antigen is usually a protein, polysaccharide, or lipid that can be contained within microorganisms, such as fungi, parasites, bacteria, and viruses.

When an antigen enters the body, lymphoid cells function together to eliminate it. Within the lymph nodes, macrophages prepare or process antigens so that lymphocytes can mount a response to invasion. Synthesis of antibody by B-lymphocytes is one type of response to antigenic stimulation.

Antibodies are serum proteins produced by plasma cells (cells derived from B-lymphocytes). Antibodies bind to specific antigens and begin processes that induce lysis (destruction) or phagocytosis (engulfing) of an offending antigen. Another possible response to antigenic invasion is the growth of new T-lymphocytes that have receptors on their surfaces for the antigen. T-lymphocytes that have received an antigenic stimulus are called sensitized T-cell lymphocytes. In this situation, no circulating antibody is produced, but sensitized T-cells are released into the circulation. These cells then migrate to the site of the antigen's entrance and begin a direct attack on the invading antigen. Most antigens, however, do not cause purely one or the other of these reactions, but usually induce a combination of both. The type of antigen introduced will determine which of these immune responses will occur.

Cells of the Immune System: White Blood Cells (Table 11–1)

The immune system stockpiles a tremendous arsenal of immunocompetent cells. By storing just a few cells specific for each potential invader, it has room for the entire array. When an antigen appears, the few specifically matched cells of the immune system are stimulated to multiply (Purtilo and Purtilo, 1989).

Table 11–1. CATEGORIES OF WHITE BLOOD CELLS AND THEIR FUNCTIONS

Leukocyte Type	% in Normal Leukocytes	Function
Lymphocytes	34	
B-lymphocytes		Humoral immunity; production of specific antibodies against viruses, bacteria, and other proteins
T-lymphocytes		Cell-mediated immunity, including delayed hypersensitivity and graft rejection; regulation of immune response
Monocytes	4	Phagocytosis of microorganisms and cell debris; cooperation in immune response
Granulocytes		
Neutrophils	59	Phagocytosis and killing of bacteria; release of pyrogen that produces fever
Eosinophils	2.7	Phagocytosis of antigen-antibody complexes; killing of parasites
Basophils	0.3	Release of chemical mediators of immediate hypersensitivity

Lymphocytes

Lymphocytes are the white blood cells that bear the major responsibility for carrying out both cell-mediated and humoral immunity. The two major classes of lymphocytes are the *T-cells* (which are processed in the **t**hymus) and the *B-cells* (which grow to maturity in the **b**one marrow independent of the thymus). Both B-cells and T-cells include a number of different subsets, which all have different functions (Table 11–2).

B-cells are the precursors of antibody-producing plasma cells; and T-cell subclasses either promote or suppress the immune response, kill antigens directly, or participate in other immune responses, such as delayed hypersensitivity (Nursing 85, 1985). These reactions, which are often referred to as cell-mediated immune responses, are mediated by antigen-specific T-cells and are slow to develop, beginning 18 to 24 hours after antigen exposure. They reach maximum response by

Table 11–2. COMPARATIVE FUNCTIONS OF THE T-LYMPHOCYTES AND B-LYMPHOCYTES*

B-Lymphocytes *Short-Lived*	T-Lymphocytes *Long-Lived*
Humoral immunity	Cell-mediated immunity
Specific antigen recognition	Specific antigen recognition
Synthesis of antibody; most effective in pyrogenic infections and toxic reactions	Macrophage stimulation, complement activation, destruction of intracellular pathogens; graft rejection; immunologic surveillance; stimulation of B-cell antibody production by helper cells
Immediate hypersensitivity reaction (allergy)	Delayed hypersensitivity reactions (skin test to antigens)
Transferable by plasma	Transfer uncommon, occurs only via cells
Mostly in blood	Mostly in lymph tissue

* From Gurevich, I.: The competent internal immune system. Nurs. Clin. North Am., *20*:156, 1985.

48 hours and subside by 3 to 7 days (Hess, 1987).

Approximately two thirds of the lymphocytes circulating in the peripheral blood are T-lymphocytes, 15% are B-lymphocytes, and the remaining lymphocytes are made up of uncommitted lymphocytes (lymphocytes without surface antigens) called *null cells.* Such cells are seen in active systemic lupus erythematosus and other disease states discussed later in this chapter. All lymphocytes recirculate from the blood to the lymph nodes via the lymphatic vessels (Miller and Keane, 1987).

B-Cells. B-cells are responsible for humoral-mediated immunity and derive from hematopoietic stem cells that mature in the **b**one marrow (or in lymphoid organs other than the thymus). B-cells secrete soluble substances called antibodies. Every B-cell is programmed to make only one specific antibody that coats foreign cells or agents, making them susceptible to lymphocytotoxicity or neutrophil and macrophage ingestion. A given antibody exactly matches a specific invading antigen. Stimulation of B-cells to produce antibody is a complex process that usually requires interactions between macrophages, T-cells, and B-cells (Reich, 1984). The exact mechanism of this process is not clearly understood.

When the B-cell encounters its triggering antigen, the B-cell gives rise to many cells called plasma cells. Every plasma cell is essentially a factory for producing millions of identical antibodies. Scientists have identified five classes of antibodies or antigen-specific immunoglobulins: IgG, IgM, IgA, IgE, and IgD (National Institutes of Health, 1985). Special functions are served by each class of immunoglobulin.*

T-Cells. T-cells are responsible for cell-mediated immunity and are derived from hematopoietic stem cells at T-cell precursors that mature into T-cells within the thymus. T-cell subgroups include the regulatory helper and suppressor T-cells, which respectively enhance or suppress the development of immune responses, particularly antibody production. Helper T-cells stimulate B-cell proliferation and differentiation into antibody-secreting plasma cells. These helper cells also aid in B-cell activation by producing soluble, nonspecific mediators called lymphokines. Suppressor T-cells reduce the immune response by limiting the amount of T-cell help available to activate B-cells, thus protecting the body from the excesses of its own defense (Nursing 85, 1985). T-lymphocytes are capable of (Purtilo and Purtilo, 1989):

- Killing intracellular viruses, bacteria, and fungi
- Rejecting transplanted organs*
- Defending against neoplastic cells by providing immunologic surveillance that eliminates these cancer cells

Lymphokines. Lymphokines are soluble mediators that are produced by activated lymphocytes (through complex interactions among macrophages and subsets of T-cells). They facilitate intracellular communication between macrophages, B-cells, T-cells, and lymphoid cells (Nursing 85, 1985). The reader may appreciate the complexity of the immune system by noting the following identified lymphokines:

- Chemotactic factor (CF)
- Macrophage-activating factor (MAF)
- Migrating-inhibiting factor (MIF)
- Transfer factor (TF)
- Blastogenic factor (BF)
- Lymphotoxin, B-cell growth factor (BCGF)
- T-cell replacement factor (TRF)
- Interleukin-1 (IL-1): also known as lymphocyte-activating factor

* The reader is referred to an immunologic text for specific details concerning the known actions of these immunoglobulins.

* Tissues or cells from another individual, unless it is an identical twin, can also act as antigens; because a transplanted organ is seen as "foreign" or "nonself," the body's natural response is to reject it (National Institutes of Health, 1985).

- Interleukin-2 (IL-2): also known as T-cell growth factor
- Interferon

The nomenclature of these lymphokines generally describes their predominant biologic activity. For example, chemotactic and migratory inhibitory factors affect cell motility; activation factors enhance such cellular processes as phagocytosis and induce further mediator release. Mitogenic factors stimulate cell proliferation, whereas cytotoxic factors target cell lysis and death. Interferons are a heterogeneous group of glycoproteins secreted by a variety of human cell types in response to viral infection and a variety of other stimuli. Although described initially as antiviral factors, these glycoproteins have other biologic effects, particularly in immunoregulation. Once released, interferons interact with surrounding cells to induce the synthesis and secretion of other soluble factors that are actually responsible for the various activities ascribed to the interferons (Hess, 1987).

Monocytes and Macrophages
(Nursing 85, 1985)

Monocytes and macrophages are large cells that act as scavengers (or phagocytes), engulfing and digesting microorganisms, and other antigenic particles, such as bacteria, fungi, dead tissue, antigen-antibody complexes, and tumor cells. Originating in the stem cell, monocytes circulate in the blood for 24 hours before migrating to the tissues where they develop into macrophages. Macrophages line the lungs and intestines and are often referred to by different names depending on their location. For example, dendritic macrophages are found in lymph nodes; Kupffer's cells are found in the liver; and tissue histiocytes are found in connective tissue surrounding skin and muscle.

Macrophages are the chief cells of the mononuclear phagocyte system. Macrophages not only phagocytize foreign matter, but also play a crucial role in initiating the immune response by "presenting" antigens to T-cells in a special way that allows the T-cell to recognize them. In addition, macrophages and monocytes secrete powerful chemical substances called *monokines* that help to direct and regulate the immune response.

Granulocytes and Mast Cells

Granulocytes, like macrophages and monocytes, are phagocytes and are thus capable of enveloping and destroying invaders. They contain granules filled with potent chemicals that enable them to digest microorganisms. These chemicals also contribute to inflammatory reactions and are responsible for the symptoms of allergy. Neutrophils, eosinophils, basophils, and mast cells are examples of granulocytes (National Institutes of Health, 1985).

Along with the major immune cells (B-cells and T-cells and macrophages), granulocytes and mast cells participate in immunologic reactions. As discussed in Chapter 5, *granulocytes* (neutrophils, eosinophils, and basophils) are participants in phagocytosis, allergic reactions, and specific antibody (IgE) response important in anaphylactic reactions, respectively. *Mast cells* are thought to be derived from circulating basophils and are most abundant in organs or tissues that are exposed to the environment (e.g., skin and mucosa of the gastrointestinal and respiratory tracts). These cells serve an important role in the immediate hypersensitivity reaction to foreign antigen by releasing chemicals (e.g., histamine, heparin, hyaluronic acid) that produce the redness, warmth, and swelling of the inflammatory, allergic response (Hess, 1987).

Immune Response

When an antigen enters the body, a wide spectrum of response mechanisms can be activated. The specific response pattern depends on (Wright, 1987):

- Amount of antigen introduced
- Site of introduction
- Type of antigen introduced

Each immune response is a unique sequence of events determined by the nature of the antigen. Chemical toxins and a large number of inert environmental substances, such as asbestos and smoke particles, are normally attacked only by phagocytes and are handled efficiently at a local site. Organic antigens such as viruses, single-cell bacteria, protozoa, and fungi elicit the full range of immunologic responses. An excessively large, sustained antigen dose can overwhelm defenses at the local site and can exhaust the entire defense system (Jaret, 1986; Wright, 1987).

Microorganisms entering the body must find a route past the body's first line of defense: the outer protection of skin and mucous membranes; ciliated epithelium of the respiratory tract; and antimicrobial factors in tears, saliva, and breast milk. The second line of the body's defense includes the macrophages and neutrophils that do not react to specific antigens, but can recognize antigenic material and attempt to destroy it (Abernathy, 1987).

Once an antigen has overcome the first-line and second-line barriers, the immune response begins to function to destroy the antigen. There are two types of immunity that can be summoned for use: immunity occurring in the blood and tissue fluid outside the cells, provided by B-lymphocyte cells that produce antibodies (humoral immunity), and immunity taking place inside or on the surface of cells, provided by T-lymphocyte cells (cell-mediated immunity). These two distinct mechanisms usually work together to provide a defense against immunologic threats.

When an antigenic substance is introduced into the body, it is taken directly to a regional lymphoid tissue where it is processed and then presented to reactive B-cells or T-cells in the regional lymph node. During this interaction, the specific B-cell or T-cell is stimulated to begin proliferation and differentiation. Lymphokines, released from cells involved in the presenting process, further signal the lymphocyte to divide and differentiate (Wright, 1987).

If the antigen is the type that activates a *humoral response,* the first time the body is exposed to the antigen, the B-cell system responds by synthesizing circulating antibody from plasma cells. The first exposure of the body to an antigen is followed by a latent phase, during which time no antibody levels are detected. This latent phase is then followed by a *primary response* when serum antibodies increase rapidly, plateau, and finally decline (Abernathy, 1987).

Because the reaction and production of antibody is not immediate, the antigen has time to spread during the body's first exposure. However, an immunologic memory develops so that when subsequent contact occurs with the same antigen, the antibodies are produced faster and at higher concentrations. This rapid response to a second contact is called the *secondary response* and is the basis for immunization.

The reaction between antibody and antigen activates serum proteins called complement. Complement usually circulates in the bloodstream as a series of inactive proteins produced by mononuclear phagocytes. Once the antigen is "captured" by the antibody, complement proteins receive a signal to activate. When activated, complement breaks down into enzymes that are then capable of destroying antigens. Complement enzymes actually poke holes in the cell membranes of the antigen (many bacteria and some viruses), causing intracellular fluid to leak out and resulting in cell destruction (Abernathy, 1987). With rare exceptions, complement proteins bind only to cells already "labeled" with antibodies so that healthy tissues are protected from the effects of these powerful enzymes.

If the antigens are such that they are physically or structurally inaccessible to attack from antibodies (e.g., viruses, some fungi, bacteria harbored inside cells, and cancer cells), then cell-mediated immunity is the main line of defense in combating these antigens. A cell-mediated reaction begins when an antigen binds with an antigen receptor on the surface of a T-lymphocyte. The antigen is then presented to the lymph node T-cells, and there is proliferation and differentiation of T-cells. Instead of circulatory antibodies, sensitized T-lymphocytes are then released into the circulation and are differentiated into five subsets:

- Helper T-cells (T_h): stimulate production of killer T-cells and in combined response, stimulate B-cell production and differentiation
- Killer T-cells (T_k): activated by helper T-cells directly attack and kill the antigen or cells labeled with the antigen (including cancer cells)
- Lymphokine-producing T-cells: produce mediators such as lymphokines, which further stimulate T-cell production and, in a combined response, stimulate antibody production from B-cells
- Suppressor T-cells (T_s): slow down or stop the activities of both T-cells and B-cells so that the attack can be stopped when the antigen is conquered
- Memory T-cells (T_m): generated during an initial exposure to the antigen, can mount a quick response after re-exposure to the same antigen

Once these differentiated T-lymphocytes are released into the circulation, the activated T-cells seek out the antigen at the site of injection and destroy it. Between 24 and 48 hours is required for the development of inflammation at the site of local invasion.

Chemical examples of cellular immune reactions include:

- Delayed hypersensitivity
- Allograft rejection
- Contact allergies
- Immunity to tumors and intracellular parasites

Most antigens do not cause a purely humoral or purely cell-mediated response, but activate both types of protective mechanisms. The remarkable power of the immune system is best appreciated by the pathologic results that accompany its failure, whether that occurs with the common overreaction of the system known as allergies or the devastating immunodeficient effects of the human immunodeficiency virus (HIV) linked to acquired immunodeficiency syndrome (AIDS) (Page, 1981).

PATHOPHYSIOLOGY OF THE IMMUNE SYSTEM

Immune disorders involve dysfunction of the immune response mechanism, causing over-responsiveness, or blocked, misdirected, or limited responsiveness to antigens. These disorders may result from a developmental defect, infection, malignancy, trauma, metabolic disorder, or drug use. Immunologic disorders may be classified as (Nursing 85, 1985):

- Immunodeficiency
- Hypersensitivity
- Autoimmunity
- Immunoproliferative disorders

When the immune system is underactive or *hypoactive* it is referred to as immunodeficient. When the immune system becomes overactive or *hyperactive,* a state of hypersensitivity exists leading to immunologic diseases such as allergies.

T-cells act as modulators of immune reactions, thus along with clearance of antigen by macrophages, death of antibody-producing plasma cells, and certain humoral factors, the immune response ultimately ceases. Abnormalities in this control system lead to immunodeficiency, autoimmunity, and possibly hematologic diseases, such as aplastic anemia (Reich, 1984).

Autoimmune disorders occur when the immune system fails to distinguish self from nonself and misdirects the immune response against the body's own tissues. The resultant abnormal tissue reaction and tissue damage may cause systemic manifestations varying from minimal localized symptoms to systemic multiorgan involvement with severe impairment of function and life-threatening organ failure (Nursing 85, 1985).

Immunoproliferative disorders occur when abnormal reproduction or multiplication of the cells of the lymphoid system result in leukemia, lymphoma, and other related disorders that have been covered in other parts of this text and are not discussed in this chapter.

Immunodeficiency Disorders

Acquired Immunodeficiency Syndrome

AIDS is a recently recognized condition characterized by a defect in natural immunity against disease. *Acquired* refers to the fact that the disease is not inherited or genetic, but develops as a result of a virus described later. *Immuno* refers to the body's immunologic system and *deficiency* indicates that the immune system is underfunctioning resulting in a group of signs or symptoms that occur together called a *syndrome.* People who have AIDS are vulnerable to serious illnesses (called "opportunistic" infections or diseases because they use the opportunity of lowered resistance to infect and destroy) that would not be a threat to most people whose immune systems function normally. This clinical syndrome consists of both opportunistic infection or neoplasia associated with the unexplained immunodeficiency (Shaw et al, 1988).

AIDS is an infectious disease caused by a specific virus now labeled HIV Type 1. Previously, the AIDS virus was given different names, which may still be seen in the literature: human T-lymphotrophic virus type III (HTLV III) and lymphadenopathy associated virus (LAV). In most literature, including this text, the use of the term "AIDS virus" is used interchangeably with the nomenclature "HIV."

This disease is characterized by a weakened or diminished cell-mediated immunity. A great deal is still unknown about the exact mechanism of HIV, but it is clear that depletion and functional impairment of the T4 lymphocyte helper cells is accompanied by a functional loss of B-cells, T-cells, and monocytes in patients with AIDS. Impaired T-cell–mediated responses have the greatest clinical consequences as the body becomes vulnerable to other infectious organisms (Koenig and Fauci, 1988).

AIDS is a contagious disease, spread through sexual contact, exposure to infected blood or blood components, and perinatally from the mother to the neonate. HIV has been isolated from blood, semen, vaginal secretions, saliva, tears, breast milk, cerebrospinal fluid, amniotic fluid, and urine and is likely to be isolated from other body fluids, secretions, and excretions. However, epidemiologic evidence has implicated only blood, semen, vaginal secretions, and possibly breast milk in transmission (Centers for Disease Control, 1987b). There is no evidence of transmission by "casual contact" through the use of shared food, towels, cups, razors, toothbrushes, or even kissing (Koop, 1986).

AIDS was first observed to occur in homosexuals and intravenous drug abusers, and these still represent the predominant risk groups. However, risk groups now also include bisexual men; blood transfusion, organ transplantation, and dialysis recipients; hemophiliacs; people who have heterosexual contact with partners who are infected by AIDS; and transmission from the mother to the baby. The risk to hemophiliacs is being eliminated by the development of improved processing for the manufacturing of clotting factor concentrates. Transmission from the mother to the child *may* occur by transplacental passage, cesarean section, transmission in utero, and breastfeeding. Studies to substantiate these modes of transmission are currently underway (Shaw et al, 1988).

Health care workers who have contact with patients with AIDS and who follow routine instructions for selfprotection are a very low risk group (see Appendix). The overall incidence of AIDS is rising, and it is estimated that approximately one million individuals in the United States have been exposed to HIV. With an estimated incubation period (the time between exposure and the diagnosis of AIDS) of 2 to 6 years or longer, HIV-related illnesses are likely to increase (Knutsen and Fischer, 1988).

Consistently specific signs and symptoms identifying AIDS cannot be listed as with other autoimmune diseases. Some people remain asymptomatic after infection with the AIDS virus (although these people are still able to pass the virus to others). In some people, the protective immune system may be destroyed by the AIDS virus (HIV) and then "opportunistic diseases" occur as a result of other bacterial and viral invasion. The most common types of these diseases include pneumocystitis pneumonia, tuberculosis, lymphoma, and Kaposi's sarcoma. Kaposi's sarcoma is a cancer of the tissues beneath the skin and the mucous-secreting surfaces of the digestive tract, the lymph nodes, and the lung.

Others infected with HIV may develop a disease that is less serious than AIDS, which is referred to as AIDS related complex (ARC). ARC is a condition caused by the AIDS virus in which the patient tests positive for infection with AIDS and has a specific set of clinical signs and symptoms that are less severe than those with the disease classically referred to as AIDS (Koop, 1986).

CLINICAL SIGNS AND SYMPTOMS OF AIDS RELATED COMPLEX (ARC)

- Loss of appetite
- Weight loss (>10%)
- Intermittent, persistent fever (>100°F for 3 months)
- Night sweats
- Skin rashes
- Chronic diarrhea
- Fatigue
- Lymphadenopathy (persistent, generalized lymph node enlargement present in 2 or more noninguinal sites lasting for more than 3 months)
- Decreased resistance to infection
- Influenzalike symptoms
- Oral thrush (a thick, white coating on the tongue or throat, accompanied by a sore throat)

Most individuals infected with the AIDS virus have no symptoms and feel well. Some people develop symptoms that are similar to many common viral illnesses, such as influenza, bronchitis, and colds. However, with AIDS, the symptoms are generally unexplained, last for a longer period, and tend to recur. The symptoms of ARC can occur over a period of months before specific manifestations of AIDS are diagnosed. These manifestations indicating the progression of the disease from ARC to AIDS include (Centers for Disease Control, 1987a):

- Wasting syndrome
- Central nervous system (CNS) disorders
- Rare skin cancers (Kaposi's sarcoma)
- Opportunistic diseases

CLINICAL SIGNS AND SYMPTOMS OF ACQUIRED IMMUNODEFICIENCY SYNDROME AND THE "OPPORTUNISTIC INFECTIONS" (Koop, 1986):

- Wasting syndrome
  - Extreme fatigue, sometimes accompanied by headache, dizziness, or lightheadedness
  - Unexplained weight loss
  - Progressive dyspnea
- CNS disorder (AIDS dementia):
  - Memory loss, impaired concentration
  - Incoordination, poor balance, frequent falls
  - Unsteady gait, ataxia
  - Weakness of the lower extremities (may progress to upper extremities)
  - Partial paralysis
- Kaposi's sarcoma
  - Multiple purple blotches and bumps on skin
- Opportunistic diseases (e.g., pneumonia, tuberculosis, lymphoma, thrush)
  - Persistent dry cough
  - Fever, night sweats

- Easy bruising
- Thrush (a thick, white coating on the tongue or throat, accompanied by a sore throat)

As the disease progresses, the patient with AIDS develops muscle weakness, atrophy, and neurologic symptoms. The neurologic complications of HIV infection are both common and varied and contribute to the patient's morbidity and mortality. Both the CNS and the peripheral nervous system (PNS) are affected as early as the period of acute HIV infection, although most occur as the infection progresses to its terminal stages (Brew et al, 1988).

Diagnosis. The diagnosis is usually made on the basis of the clinical manifestations associated with AIDS or ARC. Supportive serologic tests to isolate HIV or antibodies to HIV can be used, but these tests still have many limitations associated with them. Prognosis is poor for those in whom HIV infection leads to AIDS; in such cases, AIDS remains virtually 100% fatal with pneumonia as the predominant opportunistic infection causing death in the majority of patients (DeVita et al, 1988).

Prognosis and Treatment. Survival time after diagnosis depends on the length of time that the patient has had the syndrome and what specific opportunistic diseases have occurred. At present, with the exception of any breakthroughs in treatment, at least 50% of patients with AIDS can be expected to die within 18 months of diagnosis and approximately 80% can be expected to die within 36 months of diagnosis, with the prognosis slightly better in those who have only Kaposi's sarcoma (Centers for Disease Control, 1987a).

Treatment is usually supportive because there is no known cure for AIDS. Prevention is considered to be the primary method of treatment. Treatment can be given for the various diseases and infections that affect patients with AIDS. However, because the immune system's normal operating capacity has been damaged, a person with AIDS continues to be at risk for the development of other serious infections and cancers.

Physical therapy may be used for symptomatic relief of pain and pain control, restoration of function, energy conservation to manage chronic fatigue, and an endurance program per patient tolerance to maintain daily work and living activities.

Hypersensitivity Disorders

Allergies

Allergy refers to the abnormal hypersensitivity that takes place when a foreign substance (allergen) is introduced into the body of a person likely to have allergies. The body fights these invaders by producing the special antibody immunoglobulin E (IgE). This antibody (now a vital diagnostic sign of many allergies), when released into the blood, breaks down mast cells, which contain chemical mediators such as histamine that cause dilation of blood vessels and the characteristic symptoms of allergy. *Atopy* differs from allergy because it refers to people who have a genetic predisposition to produce large quantities of IgE causing this state of clinical hypersensitivity or allergy. The reaction between the allergen and the susceptible person (i.e., allergy-prone host) results in the development of a number of typical signs and symptoms usually involving the gastrointestinal tract, respiratory tract, or skin.

Clinical signs and symptoms vary from one patient to another according to the allergies present. Using the *Family/Personal History* form, each patient should be asked what known allergies are present and what the specific reaction to the allergen would be for that particular patient. The physical therapist can then be alert to any of these warning signs during treatment and can take necessary measures, whether that means grading exercise to the patient's tolerance, controlling the room temperature, or appropriately using medications prescribed.

Treatment may include desensitization, the regular injection of small quantities of allergen to help immunize the person against the offending allergies. Steady exposure builds up high quantities of IgG antibodies in the bloodstream and creates competition between two classes of antibodies for the same antigen. Allergens that bind to IgG antibodies do not reach the IgE antibodies coating mast cells. Without the interaction of IgE antibodies, allergens, and mast cells, smaller amounts of histamine enter the body making the allergic response less severe (Page, 1981).

Anaphylaxis

Anaphylaxis, the most dramatic and devastating form of atopic disease, is the systemic manifestation of immediate hypersensitivity. The implicated antigen is often introduced parenterally, such as by injection of penicillin or a bee sting. The activation and breakdown of mast cells systemically, with massive mediator release, results in the clinical picture of bronchospasms, urticaria (wheals or hives), and anaphylactic shock (Saxon, 1988).

Clinical signs and symptoms of anaphylaxis are listed by system in Table 11-3. Patients with previous anaphylactic reactions (and the specific signs and symptoms of that individual's reaction) should be identified by using the *Family/Personal History* form. Identification information should be worn at all times by patients who have had previous anaphylactic reactions. For identified and unidentified patients, immediate action is required when the patient has a severe reaction. In such situations, the physical therapist is advised to call for emergency assistance.

Table 11-3. CLINICAL ASPECTS OF ANAPHYLAXIS BY TARGET ORGAN*

System	Signs and Symptoms
General	Malaise, weakness Sense of illness
Dermal	Hives, erythema
Mucosal	Periorbital edema Nasal congestion and pruritus Flushing or pallor, cyanosis
Respiratory	Sneezing Rhinorrhea Dyspnea
Upper airway	Hoarseness, stridor Tongue and pharyngeal edema
Lower airway	Dyspnea Acute emphysema Air trapping: asthma, bronchospasm
Gastrointestinal	Increased peristalsis Vomiting Dysphagia Nausea Abdominal cramps Diarrhea (occasionally with blood)
Cardiovascular	Tachycardia Palpitations Hypotension Cardiac arrest
Central nervous system	Anxiety, seizures

* Adapted from Lawlor, G.J., and Rosenblatt, H.M.: Anaphylaxis. *In* Lawlor, G.J., and Fischer, T.J. (eds): Manual of Allergy and Immunology: Diagnosis and Therapy, 2nd ed. Boston, Little, Brown, 1988, p. 228.

Neurologic Disorders

Some neurologic disorders encountered by the physical therapist display features that suggest an immunologic basis for the disorder. Such diseases include myasthenia gravis, Guillain-Barré syndrome, and multiple sclerosis. Other dysfunctions, such as amyotrophic lateral sclerosis (ALS) and acute disseminated encephalomyelitis, also associated with immunologic dysfunction, but seen less often by the physical therapist, are not discussed.

Myasthenia Gravis

Myasthenia gravis (MG) is a disease of unknown cause in which there is motor weakness due to a disorder of neuromuscular transmission. The largest proportion of the group of disorders known as MG has an immunologic basis with autoimmune mechanisms causing a block or destruction of the acetylcholine receptor (Daube, 1983). In MG, an autoaggressive antibody response directed against acetylcholine receptor protein at the myoneural junction is involved directly in disease pathogenesis (Hoffman and Panitch, 1987). This deactivation of acetylcholine receptor sites, necessary for normal impulse transmission to muscles, occurs when antibodies to acetylcholine receptors block and remove the receptor sites from the postsynaptic membrane. Without acetylcholine, the nerve impulses fail to pass across the neuromuscular junction and stimulate contraction of the muscles.

These antibodies may also activate the complement system, leading to further damage at the myoneural junction (Nursing 85, 1985). In MG, there are often other autoantibodies present and other associated diseases, such as thyroiditis, systemic lupus erythematosus, and rheumatoid arthritis. In most cases, an association with a pathologic thymus gland (either thymic hyperplasia or a thymoma) occurs, necessitating the removal of the thymus gland (Rodnan and Schumacher, 1983).

This disease affects young adults, primarily women between 20 and 40 years of age with an incidence of between 2 and 10 per 100,000 (Daube, 1983). When men are affected, this occurs most often in the sixth or seventh decade. Remission may occur spontaneously in 25% of the cases within the first 2 years (Hoffman and Panitch, 1987).

Symptoms show fluctuations in intensity and are more severe late in the day or after prolonged activity. Skeletal muscle weakness is often the first symptom noted, especially affecting the extraocular muscles and producing ptosis and diplopia. The weakness is due primarily to postactivation exhaustion and lasts for 10 to 30 minutes. This weakness fluctuates with superimposed illness, menses, and air temperature (worsening with warming) (Daube, 1983). Proximal muscles are affected more than distal muscles, and difficulty in climbing stairs, rising from chairs, combing the hair, or even holding up the head occur. Cranial muscles, neck, respiratory muscles, and muscles of the proximal limbs are the primary areas of muscular involvement. Neurologic findings are normal except for muscle weakness (Hoffman and Panitch, 1987).

The muscular weakness is believed to be caused by the presence of circulating antibodies that are directed against the postsynaptic acetylcholine receptors at the neuromuscular junction. It is not clear what events initiate the formation of these antibodies. There is no muscular atrophy or loss of sensation. Muscular weakness ranges from mild to being life-threatening (when involving respiratory muscles) (Miller and Keane, 1987).

CLINICAL SIGNS AND SYMPTOMS OF MYASTHENIA GRAVIS

- Muscle fatigability and proximal muscle weakness, aggravated by exertion
- Respiratory failure from progressive involvement of respiratory muscles
- Ptosis (extraocular muscle weakness resulting in drooping of the upper eyelid)
- Diplopia (double vision)
- Dysarthria (speech disturbance)
- Severe quadriparesis
- Bulbar involvement
  - Alteration in voice quality
  - Dysphagia (speech impairment)
  - Nasal regurgitation
  - Choking, difficulty in chewing

Diagnosis. Diagnosis is difficult because laboratory tests for immune-related neurologic disorders rarely prove to be conclusive. Physicians must rely on the patient's history and clinical findings in association with supportive information from electrodiagnostic tests involving the injection of anticholinesterase drugs. Injection of these drugs elicits a sudden, although short-lasting improvement in muscle function (which is measured by improvement in the loss of amplitude of the evoked motor potential) of the patient with MG; the same injection worsens the symptoms of a cholinergic patient.

Prognosis and Treatment. Prognosis has improved with improved medical treatment. Improvement and remission within 5 years occurs in up to 90% of patients undergoing medical treatment. Serious exacerbations of the illness, including respiratory involvement (especially in the elderly population suffering from other complicating diseases) account for most deaths from MG (Hoffman and Panitch, 1987).

Medical treatment may include the use of anticholinesterase, immunosuppressive and corticosteroid drugs, thymectomy (removal of the thymus implicated in this disorder), and plasmapheresis (plasma exchange to remove the circulating autoantibodies is used for the severely ill patient who has not responded to other treatments). Physical therapy may be indicated as supportive care in MG to assist the patient in recovering motor skills.

Guillain-Barré Syndrome (Acute Idiopathic Polyneuritis)

Guillain-Barré syndrome is a demyelinative disease that affects the PNS (especially spinal nerves) and is characterized by an abrupt onset of paralysis. The exact cause of the disease is unknown but it frequently occurs after an infectious illness. Upper respiratory infections, vaccinations, viral infections such as measles, hepatitis, or mononucleosis commonly precede acute idiopathic polyneuritis by 1 to 3 weeks (Hoffman and Panitch, 1987).

Like MG, acute idiopathic polyneuritis may be an autoimmune disease which, after surgery, a viral infection, or immunization, occurs as a result of a viral antigen triggering an autoimmune reaction to myelin. Evidence of cell-mediated immune response includes serum specimens containing antinerve and antimyelin antibodies, presence of lymphocytes infiltrating the peripheral nerve sheaths, and low levels of immune complexes and complement components (Nursing 85, 1985).

The disease affects all age groups, and incidence is not related to race or sex. The onset of acute idiopathic polyneuritis is generally characterized by a rapidly progressing weakness for a period of 3 to 7 days. It is usually symmetric first of the lower extremities, then the upper extremities, and then the respiratory musculature. Weakness and paralysis are frequently preceded by paresthesias and numbness of the limbs, but actual objective sensory loss is usually mild and transient. Cranial nerves, most commonly the facial nerve, can be involved. The tendon reflexes are decreased or lost early in the course of the illness (Hoffman and Panitch, 1987).

CLINICAL SIGNS AND SYMPTOMS OF GUILLAIN-BARRÉ SYNDROME (OR ACUTE IDIOPATHIC POLYNEURITIS)

- Muscular weakness (bilateral progressing from the legs to the arms to the chest and the neck)
- Diminished deep tendon reflexes
- Paresthesias (without loss of sensation)
- Fever, malaise
- Nausea

Although muscular weakness is usually described as bilateral, progressing from the legs upward toward the arms, this syndrome may be missed when the patient presents with unilateral symptoms that do not progress proximally. Muscular weakness of the chest may present early in this disease process as respiratory compromise. Respiratory involvement as such may go unnoticed until the patient develops more severe symptoms associated with Guillain-Barré syndrome.

Diagnosis. Medical diagnosis is based usually on the history and presenting clinical signs and symptoms associated with this syndrome. Laboratory studies may be used to support the diagnosis, but are not usually required in typical cases.

Prognosis and Treatment. The progression of paralysis varies from one patient to another, often with full recovery from the paralysis. Usually symptoms develop over a period of 1 to 3 weeks, and progression of paralysis may stop at any point. Once the weakness reaches a maximum (usually during the second week), the patient's condition plateaus for days or even weeks before spontaneous improvement and eventual recovery begin extending over a period of 6 to 9 months. Prognosis is favorable with decreased mortality due to improved medical technology to provide advanced respiratory care for patients with compromised pulmonary status. Incidence of residual neurologic deficits is higher than was previously recognized and may occur in as many as 50% of all cases (Hoffman and Panitch, 1987).

There is no immediate cure for this disease, but medical support is vital during the progression of symptoms, particularly in the acute phase when respiratory function may be compromised. Physical therapy is initiated at an early stage to maintain joint range of motion within the patient's pain tolerance and to monitor muscle strength until active exercises can be initiated. Usual precautions for patients immobilized in bed are required to prevent complications during the acute phase. A major precaution is to provide active exercise at a level consistent with the patient's muscle strength. Overstretching and overuse of painful muscles may result in prolonged recovery or a lack of recovery.

Multiple Sclerosis (O'Sullivan and Schmitz, 1988)

Multiple sclerosis (MS) is a demyelinating disease of the CNS. The disease is characterized by demyelinating (destructive removal or loss) lesions known as plaques that are scattered throughout the CNS white matter. The myelin membrane (which serves as an insulator and speeds up the conduction along nerve fibers) breaks down with relative sparing of the axons themselves. Demyelinization impairs neural transmission and causes nerves to fatigue rapidly. The myelin sheath is replaced ultimately by fibrous scarring produced by glial cells (gliosis).

The exact etiology of MS is still unknown. Proposed theories include:

- Immune-mediated pathogenesis
- Infectious origin (slow or latent virus)
- Disorder of immune regulation characterized by a deficiency in suppressor T-cells

Marked infiltration of mononuclear cells, consisting mainly of T-cells and macrophages, has been found in the plaques, supporting an immunologically mediated pathogenesis. Epidemiologic studies and the identification of increased immunoglobulin G (IgG) in the cerebrospinal fluid (CSF) support an infectious origin. Suppressor T-cell levels are known to decline just before an MS attack. This change, or perhaps an MS antigen present on suppressor T-cells, allows a latent autoimmune reaction to occur (Nursing 85, 1985). Multiple agents may be implicated as research continues. Genetic predisposition and familial tendency have also been identified. Susceptibility to MS appears to depend on the genetically linked antigen system.

Evidence of active immune responses in immunoglobulin production in the CNS serum and in CSF is abundant. Activated T-cells have been found in the blood and CSF of patients with MS in both clinically active and inactive stages of the disease. The exact role of these immune-control mechanisms is unclear. They have been suggested as being the direct cause of the demyelination or as the result of the disease process itself. Perhaps a viral infection is the initial causative factor in triggering an autoimmune response that produces demyelination. Inflammatory reactions and the production of antibodies then occur as the body reacts to the primary infection.

The onset of symptoms occurs usually between 10 and 40 years, with peak onset at age 30 and onset being rare in children or in adults over the age of 50. Men and women are affected equally. Environmental factors may affect onset as MS is more common in temperate climates than in tropical areas.

Clinically, MS is characterized by multiple signs and symptoms and by fluctuating periods of remissions and exacerbations. The symptoms vary greatly, and the course of the disease is unpredictable. In the early stages, a relatively complete remission of initial symptoms may occur; however, as the disease progresses, the remissions become less complete and neurologic dysfunction increases. Symptoms may vary considerably in character, intensity, and duration. The onset of symptoms can develop rapidly over a course of minutes or hours; less frequently, the onset may be insidious, occurring during a period of weeks or months. Symptoms depend on the location of lesions, and early symptoms often demonstrate involvement of the sensory, pyramidal, cerebellar, and visual pathways or disruption of cranial nerves and their linkage to the brain stem.

CLINICAL SIGNS AND SYMPTOMS OF MULTIPLE SCLEROSIS

- Fatigue
- Spasticity
- Visual disturbances (nystagmus, diplopia, scotomas)
- Decreased motor function
- Increased deep tendon reflexes
- Positive Babinski's sign and clonus
- Incoordination
- Bowel and bladder dysfunctions
  - Frequency
  - Urgency
  - Incontinence
  - Retention
  - Hesitancy
- Intention tremor
- Ataxia
- Paresthesias
- Speech impairment (slow, slurred speech)
- Vertigo (sensation of rotation of self or surroundings)

Diagnosis. The diagnosis of MS is difficult because of the wide variety of possible clinical manifestations and the resemblance that they bear to other neurologic disorders, hysteria, and alcohol intoxication. There is no definitive diagnostic test for MS, rather the physician relies on objectively measured CNS abnormalities, history of episodic exacerbations, and remissions of symptoms with progressive worsening of symptoms over time (Miller and Keane, 1987).

Prognosis and Treatment. Prognosis is difficult to predict and depends on several factors including the age and intensity of onset, the neurologic status at 5 years after the onset, and the course of exacerbations-remissions. The survival rate after the onset of symptoms is at least 25 years, and the cause of death typically results from either respiratory or urinary infection. Medical treatment is directed at the overall disease process and the specific symptoms as these emerge. There is no known cure or prevention for MS. Physical therapy is one of many disciplines used in the ongoing management of MS.

Autoimmune Disorders

(Nursing 85, 1985)

Autoimmunity results from an inability to distinguish self from nonself, causing the immune system to direct immune responses against normal self tissue. The body begins to manufacture antibodies directed against the body's own cellular components or specific organs. These antibodies are known as autoantibodies, and the diseases that they produce are called autoimmune diseases (National Institutes of Health, 1985).

Autoimmune disorders may be classified as organ-specific diseases and generalized (systemic) diseases. Organ-specific diseases involve autoimmune reactions limited to one organ (e.g., thyroiditis). Generalized autoimmune diseases involve reactions in various body organs and tissues (e.g., systemic lupus erythematosus [SLE]).

Autoimmune disorders involve disruption of the immunoregulatory mechanism, causing normal cell-mediated and humoral immune responses to turn self-destructive, which results in tissue damage. Autoimmune disorders may be related to disorders of T-cell subsets or defective recognition of antigens (Nursing 85, 1985). The exact cause of autoimmune diseases is not understood, but factors implicated in the development of autoimmune immunologic abnormalities may include (Theofilopoulos, 1987):

- Genetics (familial tendency)
- Sex hormones (women are affected more often than men by autoimmune diseases)
- Viruses
- Stress

- Environment (e.g., exposure to sunlight, drugs that may destroy suppressor T-cells)

Organ-specific autoimmune diseases include thyroiditis, Addison's disease, Graves' disease, chronic active hepatitis, pernicious anemia, ulcerative colitis, and insulin-dependent diabetes (Theofilopoulos, 1987). These diseases have been discussed in the text appropriate to the organ involved and are not covered further in this chapter.

Systemic autoimmune diseases lead to a sequence of abnormal tissue reaction and damage to tissue that may result in diffuse systemic manifestations. These diseases fall into two categories:

- Diffuse connective tissue diseases (previously known as collagen-vascular diseases)
- Spondyloarthropathies (arthritis associated with spondylitis)

Diffuse connective tissue diseases are more common in women and have a strong potential for multiorgan involvement in addition to arthritis and skin manifestations. Disorders that follow this pattern include:

- Rheumatoid arthritis (RA)
- Systemic lupus erythematosus (SLE)
- Scleroderma (progressive systemic sclerosis)
- Polymyositis/dermatomyositis
- Mixed connective tissue disease (MCTD)

Spondyloarthropathies represent a group of noninfected, inflammatory, erosive, rheumatic diseases that target the sacroiliac joints, the bony insertions of the annuli fibrosi of the intervertebral disks, and the facet or apophyseal joints (Hadler, 1987). Spondyloarthropathies are more common in men who share a familial tendency and overlapping clinical features now associated with the genetic marker human leukocyte antigen (HLA-B27). The exact role of HLA in these disorders is still unknown. This group includes:

- Ankylosing spondylitis
- Reiter's syndrome
- Psoriatic arthritis
- Arthritis associated with chronic inflammatory bowel disease (see the discussion in Chapter 6)

For most affected individuals, backache is the principal symptom of illness with a corresponding history similar to the following list (Hadler, 1987).

- Insidious onset of each episode of backache
- First episode of backache before 30 years of age
- Each episode lasts for months
- Pain intensifies after rest
- Pain lessens with movement
- Family history of a spondyloarthropathy

Radiographic evidence of sacroiliitis is confirmatory, but years can pass before it is apparent (Hadler, 1987).

Rheumatoid Arthritis

RA is a chronic, systemic disease, inflammatory disorder of unknown etiology, characterized mainly by the manner in which it involves the joints (Zvaifler, 1988). There are more than 100 rheumatic diseases affecting joints, muscles, and extra-articular systems of the body. Extra-articular features, such as rheumatoid nodules, arteritis, neuropathy, scleritis, pericarditis, lymphadenopathy, and splenomegaly occur with considerable frequency. Once thought to be complications of RA, they are now recognized as being integral parts of the disease and serve to emphasize its systemic nature (Zvaifler, 1988). The potential for renal, pulmonary, vascular, and cardiac involvement also contributes to RA being included as a systemic disease. Although RA is a major subclassification within the category of diffuse connective tissue diseases, in this text, rheumatic disease is discussed from an immunogenetic basis as an autoimmune disease.

Not all of the immunologic mechanisms of RA are fully understood, but it is known that rheumatoid factor (antibody to IgG) is present in 60 to 80% of adults and approximately 20% of children with RA. This factor is thought to participate in the pathogenesis of RA by forming an immune complex with human gamma globulin. This complex then activates the complement system, and complement in turn causes neutrophils to be attracted to the immune complex (chemotaxis), particularly in the joint. The neutrophils then phagocytize the immune complex and, in the process of doing so, release toxic enzymes in the surrounding tissue. These proteases, collagenases, and cathepsins cause the synovium to proliferate and become inflamed. They also cause cartilage and bone destruction by invasion called pannus. Simultaneously, the immune complexes are stored in articular cartilage and synovium, causing a chronic inflammatory response (Gall, 1988).

The cellular immune response is also active in RA. T-cells become activated and release lymphokines (humoral inflammatory substances). Helper T-cells cluster around macrophages in the synovium. As a phagocytic cell, the macrophage processes antigen for presentation to the T-cells and the activated T-helper cells induce B-cells to form immunoglobulin (e.g., rheumatoid factors). Macrophages are also activated to produce IL-1, angiogenesis factors (causing proliferation of capillaries), and toxic enzymes. All of these agents cause further inflammation and destruction (Gall, 1988).

The etiologic factor or trigger for this process is as yet unknown. A multifactorial etiology is proposed, including bacterial or viral agents as possible triggering agents. The genetic factor of susceptibility to RA has been substantiated as demonstrated by the presence of HLA-DR4 antibody, which has been shown to be present in more than 70% of patients with RA (Stasney, 1978). This suggests that a linked gene causes patients to be susceptible to RA. This may be added to the fact that women manifest RA two to four times more commonly than men and that certain populations have a very high incidence of the disease (Gall, 1988).

CLINICAL SIGNS AND SYMPTOMS OF RHEUMATOID ARTHRITIS

- Morning stiffness
- Anorexia
- Weight loss
- Fatigue, malaise
- Joint involvement (one or more joints)
    - Immobility and inflammation (pain, redness, swelling, heat)
- Muscle atrophy
- Subcutaneous nodules (consisting of fibrotic tissue)

In most patients, the symptoms begin gradually during a period of weeks or months. Frequently malaise and fatigue prevail during this period, sometimes accompanied by diffuse musculoskeletal pain. Subsequently, specific joints exhibit pain, tenderness, swelling, and redness. A symmetric pattern is characteristic, commonly involves the joints of the hands, wrists, elbows, and shoulders, usually sparing the distal interphalangeal (DIP) joints (Bennett, 1988).

Inactivity, such as sleep or prolonged sitting, is commonly followed by stiffness. Morning stiffness lasting more than 30 minutes may occur upon arising in the morning or after prolonged inactivity. The duration of morning stiffness is an accepted measure of the severity of the condition. Pain and stiffness increase gradually as RA progresses and may limit a person's ability to walk, climb stairs, open doors, or perform other activities of daily living (ADLs). Weight loss, depression, and low-grade fever can accompany this process (Bennett, 1988).

Subcutaneous nodules, present in approximately 25 to 35% of patients with RA, occur most commonly in the subcutaneous or deeper connective tissues in areas subjected to repeated mechanical pressure, such as the olecranon bursae, the extensor surfaces of the forearms, the elbows, and the Achilles tendons (Guccione, 1988).

Diagnosis. The clinical diagnosis of RA is based on careful consideration of three factors: the clinical presentation of the patient, which is elucidated through history taking and physical examination, the corroborating evidence gathered through laboratory tests and radiography, and the exclusion of other possible diagnoses (Guccione, 1988). The physical presence of rheumatoid nodules and the presence of rheumatoid factor measured by laboratory studies are two indicators of RA, although some patients with actual rheumatoid factors are missed by commonly available methodology. This may account for the 20% of patients with RA who are seronegative (Gall, 1988).

There are four classifications of RA: classical, definite, probable, and possible. The criteria for diagnosis by classification include a combination of signs, symptoms, and laboratory findings that have persisted for a specified period of time (Guccione, 1988). Classification is difficult in the early course of the disease, when articular symptoms are accompanied only by constitutional symptoms such as fatigue and loss of appetite, which are common to a number of chronic diseases. A full array of clinical signs and symptoms may not manifest itself for 1 to 2 years.

A diagnosis of *classical* RA is established on the presentation of 7 of the 11 listed (Table 11–4) criteria with a duration of joint signs and symptoms for at least 6 weeks. A diagnosis of *definite* RA is made after observation of five of these criteria with a similar duration of joint complaints. *Probable* RA is defined as the presentation of any three criteria with continuing joint signs and symptoms for 6 weeks (Guccione, 1988). A diagnosis of *possible* RA is made in the case in which an individual presents with two of the following criteria lasting for 3 weeks:

- Morning stiffness
- History of pain or joint swelling
- Subcutaneous nodules
- Elevated sedimentation rate
- C-reactive protein

Prognosis and Treatment. Although RA is a systemic disease involving the connective tissues of other than the musculoskeletal system (e.g., lungs, heart, blood vessels, pleura), RA itself is not usually the cause of death. More likely, this disease creates a progressive func-

Table 11–4. AMERICAN RHEUMATISM ASSOCIATION CRITERIA FOR THE CLASSIFICATION OF RHEUMATOID ARTHRITIS*

Classic RA: 7 criteria needed
Definite RA: 5 criteria needed
Probable RA: 3 criteria needed

To meet criteria 1 to 5, signs or symptoms must be present for at least 6 weeks. Criteria 2 to 6 must be observed by a physician

Criteria

1. Morning stiffness
2. Pain on motion or tenderness in at least one joint
3. Swelling of one joint, representing soft tissue or fluid
4. Swelling of at least one other joint (soft tissue or fluid) with an interval free of symptoms no longer than 3 months
5. Symmetric joint swelling (simultaneous involvement of the same joint, right and left)
6. Subcutaneous nodules over bone prominences, extensor surfaces, or near joints
7. Typical x-ray changes that must include demineralization in periarticular bone as an index of inflammation; degenerative changes do not exclude diagnosis of RA
8. Positive test for rheumatoid factor in serum
9. Synovial fluid: A poor mucin clot formation on adding synovial fluid to dilute acetic acid
10. Synovial histology consistent with RA
    - Marked villous hypertrophy
    - Proliferation of synovial cells
    - Lymphocyte/plasma cell infiltration in subsynovium
    - Fibrin deposition within or upon microvilli
11. Characteristic histopathology of rheumatoid nodules biopsied from any site

* Adapted from Harris, E.D., Jr.: The clinical features of rheumatoid arthritis. *In* Kelley, W.N., Harris, E.D., Ruddy, S., and Sledge, C.B.: Textbook of Rheumatology, 3rd ed. Philadelphia, W.B. Saunders Company, 1989.

tional disability that can lead to a loss of income and work capacity. Medical management with medication is geared toward the control of inflammation augmented by rest, minimizing emotional stress, preventing or correcting deformities, maintaining muscle performance, and maintaining cardiovascular endurance to provide the patient with as independent a level of function as possible. Physical therapy in conjunction with occupational therapy assists in meeting this goal through various treatment techniques.

Systemic Lupus Erythematosus

Systemic lupus erythematosus (SLE) belongs to the family of rheumatic diseases. It is known to be a chronic systemic inflammatory disease characterized by injury to the skin, joints, kidneys, heart and blood-forming organs, nervous system, and mucous membranes. There are actually two common forms of lupus: discoid and systemic. Discoid lupus is a limited form of the disease confined to the skin. Discoid lupus rarely develops into systemic lupus (Christian, 1986). The course of SLE or lupus is one of alternating exacerbations and remissions. Multiple organ system involvement occurs during periods of disease activity.

The exact cause of SLE is unknown, although it appears to result from an immunoregulatory disturbance brought about by the interplay of genetic, hormonal, and environmental factors (Alarcon-Segovia, 1988). The disease affects women predominantly (4:1 over men) of childbearing age (onset can range from 2 to 90 years). The incidence is higher among nonwhites (particularly blacks) than whites (Fye and Sack, 1987).

As with other autoimmune diseases, antibodies exist without any invading organisms and attack the body's own healthy tissues. Antinuclear antibody (ANA) is an unusual type of antibody that is found in the blood of almost all people with lupus (Christian, 1986). ANA often includes anti-DNA antibodies during the active phase of the disease. Antigen-antibody complexes accumulate throughout the body and are destroyed along with surrounding tissues, as well as interfering with normal organ functions. As a result there can be damage to the joints, lymph nodes, spleen, liver, lungs, and gastrointestinal tract, and internal bleeding of the kidneys and heart (Weiner, 1986).

What triggers the chain of events that leads to this abnormal autoimmune reaction in lupus is unknown. It is known that B-cells are hyperactive whereas suppressor cells are underactive, although it is unclear which defect comes first (National Institutes of Health, 1985). Scientists are exploring the possibility of heredity as a possible factor; others postulate that a virus may trigger the genetic tendency (Christian, 1986). Environmental factors, such as sunlight and thermal burns, may contribute to the development of SLE (Alarcon-Segovia, 1988). This disease often has its onset after an episode of stress, especially in the loss of a significant relationship or fear of the loss of love. Lupus is often associated with depression and with an unusual need for activity and independence (Solomon, 1981).

Clinical signs and symptoms of systemic lupus erythematosus follow no single characteristic pattern. Patients may differ dramatically in the relative severity and pattern of organ involvement; two patients with this diagnosis may have no symptoms in common (Ashman, 1988). The onset can be acute or insidious. Every organ system may become involved (Table 11–5). Although these symptoms may not be present at disease onset, most patients soon develop manifestations of multisystem disease (Hollister, 1988). Either glomerulonephritis (usually mild) or cardiovascular manifestations are found in about one half of the patients with SLE (Miller and Keane, 1987).

Distal sensory polyneuropathy has been reported in 5 to 7% of patients with SLE. This may evolve subacutely or may pursue an insidious, progressive course, starting in the lower extremities and spreading to the distal upper extremities. Numbness on the tip of the tongue and inside the mouth is a frequent complaint. Touch, vibration, and position sense are most prominently affected, and the distal limb reflexes are depressed (Layzer, 1985).

Table 11–5. CLINICAL FEATURES OF SYSTEMIC LUPUS ERYTHEMATOSUS*

Clinical manifestations of systemic lupus erythematosus (SLE) are diverse due to the involvement of connective tissue throughout the body and may include the following:

- Skin
  - Rash of areas of the body exposed to ultraviolet light
  - Vasculitis (inflammation of cutaneous blood vessels)
  - Alopecia (loss of hair; baldness)
  - Raynaud's phenomenon
  - Subcutaneous nodules and thickening of the skin
- Joints and Muscles
  - Symmetric polyarthralgia or arthritis
  - Avascular necrosis of bone
  - Myalgias
- Polyserositis (inflammation of serous membranes with effusion)
  - Pleurisy
  - Pleuritic chest pain
  - Shortness of breath
  - Peritonitis with abdominal pain, anorexia, nausea, and vomiting
- Lungs
  - Pulmonary hypertension
  - Pneumothorax
  - Alveolar hemorrhage
  - Vasculitis
- Cardiovascular
  - Coronary artery disease
  - Myocarditis, usually without clinical signs
  - Pericarditis
  - Endocarditis
  - Stocking-glove peripheral neuropathy due to small-vessel vasculitis
  - Vasculitis
    - Distal leg ulcers
    - Involution and scarring of the fingertips and nail beds
    - Gangrene of the fingertips
    - Alopecia (baldness or loss of hair)
- Kidney
  - Nephritis
  - Glomerulonephritis
  - Renal failure
  - Systemic hypertension contributing to renal dysfunction
- Central Nervous System
  - Disturbances of mentation (psychosis, depression)
  - Diplopia (double vision)
  - Convulsions
  - Cranial nerve palsies
  - Migraine headaches
  - Peripheral neuritis
  - Cerebrovascular accidents

* Adapted from Fye, K.H., and Sack, K.E.: Rheumatic diseases. *In* Stites, D.P., Stobo, J.D., and Wells, J.Y.: Basic and Clinical Immunology, 6th ed. Norwalk, CT, Appleton & Lange, 1987.

CLINICAL SIGNS AND SYMPTOMS OF EARLY STAGES OF SYSTEMIC LUPUS ERYTHEMATOSUS

- Continuous or intermittent fever
- Weight loss
- Malaise and lethargy
- Arthralgias: joint pain and swelling (hands, wrists, elbows, knees, or ankles)
- Skin rash on the face, neck, or arms, often a characteristic "butterfly" erythema (involves the nose and cheeks)
- Raynaud's phenomenon
- Muscle weakness
- Myalgia
- Nausea and vomiting
- Lack of appetite

Diagnosis. Tests for autoantibodies, ANA and DNA binding, are the major diagnostic tests in SLE. The American Rheumatism Association has proposed that patients meeting four of the 14 criteria present in Table 11–6 be considered to have SLE (Ashman, 1988).

Table 11–6. SYSTEMIC LUPUS ERYTHEMATOSUS (SLE)*
(American Rheumatism Association Preliminary Criteria)†

1. Arthritis without deformity
2. Lupus erythematosus (LE) cells
3. Facial erythema
4. Alopecia
5. Pleurisy or pericarditis
6. Hemolytic anemia, leukopenia, or thrombocytopenia
7. Photosensitivity
8. Cellular casts in urine
9. Raynaud's phenomenon
10. Discoid LE
11. Oral or nasopharyngeal ulcers
12. Proteinuria (3.5 g/24 hr)
13. Psychosis or seizures
14. False-positive test for syphilis for 6 months

* From Lawlor, G.J., and Fischer, T.J.: Manual of Allergy and Immunology: Diagnosis and Therapy, 2nd ed. Boston, Little, Brown, 1988, p. 304.

† Criteria are listed in approximate order of incidence. If four or more criteria are present, SLE is the presumptive clinical diagnosis, but the ANA should also be positive.

Prognosis and Treatment. SLE may run a very mild course confined to one or a few organs, or it may be a fatal disease. Although the prognosis has improved greatly in the last three decades, a significant mortality remains (Hollister, 1988). Renal failure and CNS involvement were the leading causes of death until corticosteroids and cytotoxic agents came into widespread use. Since then, the complications of therapy, including atherosclerosis, infection, and cancer have become common causes of death. The 5-year survival rate with SLE has improved greatly during the past decade and now approaches 80 to 90% (Fye and Sack, 1987).

Medical treatment is supportive for the underlying pathologies of SLE, because there is no specific treatment for SLE itself. Supportive measures are aimed at preventing or minimizing acute relapses and exacerbations of symptoms. Active disease is treated with topical steroids, salicylates for fever and joint pain, corticosteroids, and immunosuppressive agents (Miller and Keane, 1987). Physical therapy for muscle weakness and prevention of orthopedic deformities is often indicated.

Scleroderma (Progressive Systemic Sclerosis)

Scleroderma, one of the lesser known chronic disorders in the family of rheumatic diseases, affects joints, muscles, and connective tissue of the body. The word scleroderma means "hard skin" (Leroy, 1983). Scleroderma is a disease of unknown cause affecting the connective tissue found in many parts of the body, including the skin, blood vessels, synovium, skeletal muscle, and certain internal organs, including the kidneys, lungs, heart, and gastrointestinal tract (Leroy, 1983; Medsger, 1988).

Although there are eight classifications of scleroderma, physical therapists most often come in contact with patients who fall in one of two classifications:

- Localized or limited scleroderma
- Systemic or generalized scleroderma

Localized Scleroderma. In localized scleroderma, changes occur only in limited parts of the body, such as the skin, muscles, or bones, without the typical serologic and visceral manifestations of systemic sclerosis. This condition should not be confused with limited cutaneous scleroderma, which is a form of systemic rather than localized disease (Medsger, 1988). Localized scleroderma creates cosmetic disfigurement and difficult mobility (Layzer, 1985). This type of scleroderma may also be referred to as morphea, a condition in which there is connective tissue replacement of the skin and sometimes of the subcutaneous tissue, marked by the formation of ivory white or pink patches, bands, or lines that are sometimes bordered by a purple areola. The lesions are firm, but not hard, and are usually depressed (Miller and Keane, 1987). Localized scleroderma primarily affects children and young (usually female) adults (Medsger, 1988).

Systemic Sclerosis. Systemic sclerosis may be classified according to the degree and extent of skin thickening (scleroderma). It may affect the skin as well as internal organs, including the blood vessels, digestive system (esophagus, stomach, and bowel), the lungs, heart, kidneys, muscles, and joints. Patients with rapidly progressive, widespread skin thickening *(diffuse cutaneous scleroderma)* that affects the distal and often proximal extremities and trunk are at greater risk for developing early serious visceral involvement. In contrast, individuals with *limited cutaneous scleroderma,* frequently confined to the distal extremities or fingers and face, may have a protracted interval of one or more decades before the appearance of characteristic visceral involvement (Medsger, 1988).

The full manifestation of sytemic scleroderma characterized by internal organ involvement has been described by the mnemonic: *CREST syndrome:*

- **C**alcinosis (abnormal deposition of calcium salts in the tissues; usually on the fingertips and over bone prominences)
- **R**aynaud's phenomenon
- **E**sophageal dysmotility

- **S**clerodactyly (chronic hardening and shrinking of the fingers and toes)
- **T**elangiectasia (vascular lesion formed by dilation of a group of small blood vessels; occurs most commonly on the fingers, face, lips, and tongue)

There are three stages in the clinical evolution of scleroderma:

- Edematous stage
- Sclerotic stage
- Atrophic stage

In the *edematous stage,* bilateral nonpitting edema is present in the fingers and hands and, rarely, in the feet. The edema can progress to the forearms, arms, upper anterior chest, abdomen, back, and face. After a few weeks to several months, edema is replaced by thick, hard skin.

The replacement of edema takes place in the *sclerotic stage,* when the skin becomes tight, smooth, and waxy and seems bound down to underlying structures. Accompanying changes include a loss of normal skin folds and skin hyperpigmentation and hypopigmentation. The face appears to be stretched and masklike with thin lips and a "pinched" nose. In diffuse cutaneous scleroderma, skin thickness spreads rapidly in a central direction and within months may affect the forearms, upper arms, face, and finally the trunk, particularly the anterior chest and abdomen. Distal thickening is always more severe than proximal involvement. However, patients with limited cutaneous scleroderma most often have these changes only in the fingers or face and fingers, although sometimes hand and forearm involvement is found (Medsger, 1988).

The skin changes may stabilize for prolonged periods (years) and may then either progress to the third *(atrophic) stage* or soften and return to normal. Actual atrophy of skin may occur, particularly over joints at sites of flexion contractures, such as the proximal interphalangeal joints and the elbows. Such thinning of the skin contributes to the development of ulcerations at these sites. Improvement of the skin (actual softening and return to normal) may occur to some extent in most patients. Improvement typically begins centrally so that the last areas to become clinically involved are the first to show regression (Medsger, 1988).

Not all patients pass through all the stages. Subcutaneous calcification (calcinosis) is a late-developing complication that is considerably more frequent in limited cutaneous scleroderma. Sites of trauma are often affected, such as the fingers, forearms, elbows, and knees. These calcifications vary in size from tiny deposits to large masses (Fye and Sack, 1987; Medsger, 1988).

Articular complaints are very common in progressive systemic sclerosis and may begin at any time during the course of the disease. The arthralgias, stiffness, and frank arthritis seen may be difficult to distinguish from those of RA, particularly in the early stages of the disease. Involved joints include the metacarpophalangeals, proximal interphalangeals, wrists, elbows, knees, ankles, and small joints of the feet. Flexion contractures, due to changes in the skin or joints, are common. Muscle involvement is usually mild with weakness, tenderness, and pain of proximal muscles of the upper and lower extremities (Fye and Sack, 1987).

The exact cause of scleroderma is as yet unknown. It is known that the connective tissue cells of people who have scleroderma produce too much of the protein called collagen. This excess of collagen is deposited in the skin and body organs causing thickening and hardening of the skin (induration). Estimates with regard to how many people in the United States have scleroderma range from 100,000 to 250,000. Women are affected two to three times more often than men. The disease usually affects young people between the ages of 20 and 40, although it is seen in children and the elderly.

CLINICAL SIGNS AND SYMPTOMS OF SCLERODERMA

- Raynaud's phenomenon (occurs in 90% of the cases)

- Swelling in the hands and feet
- Skin becomes shiny and skin creases disappear
- Thickening and hardening of the skin, especially on the hands, arms, and face
- Ulcerations of the fingers secondary to constriction of small blood vessels
- Calcinosis (small, white calcium deposits on the fingers)
- Polyarthralgia (joint pain affecting both large and small joints with inflammation, stiffness, swelling, warmth, tenderness)
- Muscle weakness
- Flexion contractures of large and small joints

The disease may affect only the connective tissue of the digestive system or some other organ system, leaving the skin and joints intact. Esophageal involvement is the most common visceral manifestation of scleroderma and is often the only one. The gastrointestinal system and the lungs may also be involved.

CLINICAL SIGNS AND SYMPTOMS OF ESOPHAGEAL INVOLVEMENT

- Muscle weakness of esophagus
- Dysphagia (difficulty in swallowing liquids or solids)
- Heartburn

CLINICAL SIGNS AND SYMPTOMS OF GASTROINTESTINAL INVOLVEMENT

- Bloating
- Cramps
- Diarrhea or constipation

CLINICAL SIGNS AND SYMPTOMS OF LUNG INVOLVEMENT

- Dyspnea on exertion (usually the first symptom)
- Chronic cough
- Pleurisy

Kidney involvement is the most common cause of death in scleroderma. The renal lesion involves intimal proliferation in small renal arteries leading to excess renin production and malignant hypertension. Once renal involvement has begun to produce renal insufficiency, life expectancy is only a few months unless the associated hypertension is treated successfully. Clinical evidence of *heart* disease (left ventricular dysfunction) is uncommon but may be manifested by congestive heart failure and various atrial and ventricular arrhythmias (Medsger, 1988).

Diagnosis. There is no specific test to confirm the diagnosis of scleroderma. Various medical tests including x-rays, skin biopsies, tests for antinuclear antibodies, gamma globulin, and others may be used to diagnose scleroderma. The symptoms of scleroderma often mimic those of other diseases, such as bursitis, osteoarthritis, RA, and other connective tissue diseases that makes medical diagnosis difficult (Miller and Keane, 1987).

Prognosis and Treatment. The prognosis for systemic scleroderma (more serious form) varies and depends on the extent of visceral involvement; prognosis is poor if cardiac, pulmonary, or renal systems are affected at the time of diagnosis. The 10-year survival rate after first diagnosis for systemic sclerosis is approximately 65% (Medsger, 1988).

Medical treatment involves the use of agents that inhibit excessive collagen production in addition to supportive and symptomatic measures (Medsger, 1988). Physical therapy is essential in assisting patients with skin, joint, and muscle involvement to maintain range of motion, to prevent contractures, to increase the nutritional blood supply to the tissues, and to protect the joints through positioning, splinting, and modified ADLs. Evaluation of the effectiveness of intervention in systemic sclerosis is difficult because of its slowly progressive nature, the frequent tendency toward spontaneous improvement, limitations in objective criteria for determining improvement or deterioration, and the influence of psychologic factors on many symptoms (Medsger, 1988).

Polymyositis/Dermatomyositis

Polymyositis and dermatomyositis are related illnesses belonging to the family of rheumatic diseases resulting in damage to connective tissue primarily in muscles and skin. The major result of these diseases is weakness (Pearson, 1983). There are actually five categories of inflammatory muscle disease that are distinguished under myositis (Ashman, 1988):

- Polymyositis
- Dermatomyositis
- Myositis with malignancy
- Childhood dermatomyositis
- Polymyositis associated with other inflammatory diseases (Sjögren's syndrome, MCTD, RA)

Polymyositis (PM) literally means "many muscles inflamed." It is a subacute or chronic generalized disorder of skeletal muscle and skin characterized clinically by progressive muscular weakness and pathologically by scattered muscle fiber necrosis and inflammation, without a known infectious cause. PM is an uncommon disease and has an annual incidence of one per 200,000. It occurs at all ages, and young women are affected about twice as often as young men. About 40% of all patients have cutaneous features of dermatomyositis, which is an acute, subacute, or chronic disease marked by inflammation of the skin, subcutaneous tissue, and muscles (Layzer, 1985).

CLINICAL SIGNS AND SYMPTOMS OF POLYMYOSITIS/DERMATOMYOSITIS

- Proximal muscle weakness (shoulder and pelvic girdles)
- Distal muscle weakness (less common than proximal weakness)
- Respiratory muscle weakness
- Myalgias
- Dysphagia
- Low-grade fever
- Weight loss
- Raynaud's phenomenon (rare)

Additional clinical signs and symptoms of dermatomyositis usually include:

- Red, scaly thickening of the skin over bony prominences of extensor surfaces (e.g., elbows, knees, knuckles)
- Patchy, red skin rash on the face and around the eyes
- Periorbital edema (puffy eyelids)

The onset of this connective tissue disorder is almost always gradual. The muscle weakness increases during a period of weeks or months before diagnosis. Usually muscle weakness is noticed first in the proximal limb muscles (usually lower extremities first) and trunk, but facial muscles and distal muscles are not spared. Patients may have difficulty in lifting body parts, such as the head from a pillow or arms overhead, and similar difficulty is encountered when trying to rise from a chair or climb stairs.

Muscle aches or tenderness occur in about half of the patients. Initially, the muscles may be slightly swollen, but as the disease progresses, muscular atrophy and induration (hardening) become more noticeable, reflecting the deposition of fibrous tissue. Musculotendinous contractures are a common complication and may begin to appear within the first 2 or 3 weeks. Muscle stretch reflexes are often depressed in the affected muscles. Pharyngeal weakness produces a nasal voice, nasal regurgitation of liquids, and difficulty in swallowing with a tendency to aspirate liquids. Eventually, respiratory muscle weakness may occur, and, together with pharyngeal weakness, this disposes the patient to pulmonary infections, which constitute the principal cause of death (except for complications of treatment) (Layzer, 1985).

A small minority of patients with polymyositis-dermatomyositis have a concomitant malignant tumor. This tumor is more likely to occur in people over 40 or 50 years of age. Tumors are more likely to occur in people with dermatomyositis than in those with polymyositis. The most common places for such tumors are in the lungs, ovaries, breasts, and stomach, but they may occur in or spread to other areas of the body (Pearson, 1983). Other features of this disorder may include a mild transitory arthritis and Raynaud's phenomenon. Interstitial pneumonia and pulmonary fibrosis may occur in patients with severe muscle disease (Fye and Sack, 1987).

Diagnosis. Various tests may be used in conjunction with the presence of a characteristic skin rash and proximal muscle weakness by the physician to determine the diagnosis. These tests may include muscle biopsy, serum enzyme levels (elevated muscle enzymes), and electromyogram (EMG) studies (Pearson, 1983).

Prognosis and Treatment. The prognosis depends on accompanying complications, such as malignant tumors, cardiac, or pulmonary involvement in which polymyositis tends to be more severe. Long remissions and even recovery in children have been observed, but death in adults can occur after severe and progressive muscle weakness and dysphagia with aspiration and subsequent aspiration pneumonia. As with other autoimmune disorders, medical treatment is symptomatically supportive.

The specific treatment for myositis varies from one person to another, but usually includes medication (corticosteroids, immunosuppressants), exercise, and rest. Physical therapy to improve muscle strength should not be initiated until the drug treatment takes effect. In the early stages of treating myositis, the muscle fibers are fragile and could be damaged further by exercises and other forms of physical therapy. The physical therapist treating a patient with myositis should keep in close contact with the physician who will be using physical examination and laboratory tests to determine the most opportune time for an exercise program (Pearson, 1983).

Mixed Connective Tissue Disease
(Ashman, 1988)

MCTD, a rheumatic disease syndrome, combines the clinical features of scleroderma, RA, polymyositis/dermatomyositis, and SLE. In most patients, the greatest clinical resemblance is to scleroderma. The prevalence of MCTD is unknown, but it appears to be more common than polymyositis and is less frequent than SLE. Eighty per cent of the patients are female, and any age group can be affected (Rodnan and Schumacher, 1983).

CLINICAL SIGNS AND SYMPTOMS OF MIXED CONNECTIVE TISSUE DISEASE
(in decreasing order of incidence)

- Polyarthritis or polyarthralgias
- Swollen hands (sausagelike appearance of fingers)
- Raynaud's phenomenon
- Abnormal esophageal motility
- Myositis (inflammation of a voluntary muscle)
- Proximal muscle weakness (with or without tenderness)
- Lymphadenopathy (disease of the lymph nodes)
- Sensory polyneuropathy (occurs in about 10% of all cases) (Layzer, 1985)

Raynaud's phenomenon, present in approximately 85% of patients, may precede other disease manifestations by months or years (Rodnan and Schumacher, 1983). Skin changes, such as lupuslike rashes, erythematous patches over the knuckles, alopecia, and telangiectasia over the hands and face, may occur. Esophageal abnormalities, lung and cardiac involvement are not uncommon. Renal disease is unusual, although death has occurred secondary to progressive renal failure in some patients. Other findings in patients diagnosed with MCTD may include fever, lymphadenopathy, splenomegaly, hepatomegaly, persistent hoarseness, and intestinal involvement similar to that seen in scleroderma.

Diagnosis. When classic skin changes and Raynaud's phenomenon are associated with characteristic visceral complaints, the medical diagnosis is easier to determine than in patients presenting with visceral or arthritic complaints without skin changes. In many cases, only the presence or absence of certain ANAs makes it possible to differentiate scleroderma from MCTD (Fye and Sack, 1987). Treatment varies with the presenting symptoms, combining the measures appropriate for each component disease.

Ankylosing Spondylitis (Ashman, 1988; Fye and Sack, 1987)

Ankylosing spondylitis (AS) is a chronic, progressive inflammatory disorder involving the sacroiliac joints, spine, and large peripheral joints. AS is actually more an inflammation of fibrous tissue than of synovium affecting men in 90% of all cases. Traditionally, the incidence has been reported as approximately 6 per 1,000 adult males with the usual onset of age during the second or third decade of life. Studies now suggest that the disease has a more uniform sex distribution, but it may be milder in women, because they are less likely than men to have progressive spinal disease. Women tend to have more peripheral joint manifestations, thus leading to an inappropriate diagnosis of seronegative RA (Calin, 1988).

The pathogenesis of AS is unknown. Patients are seronegative for rheumatoid factor, and antinuclear antibodies are not seen. There may be a genetic predisposition to ankylosing spondylitis. Ninety per cent of patients have HLA-B27; the gene that determines this specific cell surface antigen may be linked to other genes that determine pathologic autoimmune phenomena or that lead to an increased susceptibility to infectious or environmental agents. As yet, there are no other data to confirm an autoimmune pathogenetic mechanism.

For 80% of patients with AS, the disease begins with the insidious onset of low back pain and stiffness, which is usually worse in the morning. Most patients present with sacroiliitis as the earliest feature seen on x-ray before clinical involvement extends to the lumbar spine. Twenty per cent of the population with AS may present with sharp, jolting pain in the buttocks or hips, which is often exacerbated by coughing. Paravertebral muscle spasm, aching, and stiffness are common, but some patients may have slow progressive limitation of motion with no pain at all. The disease typically involves ligamentous insertions, fibrocartilage, and the intervertebral disks.

Peripheral joint involvement occurs in 25% of patients, usually (but not always) after involvement of the spine. Typical extraspinal sites include manubriosternal joint, the symphysis pubis, shoulder, and hip joints. Diminished chest expansion (less than 2 cm) occurs as a result of decreased rib movement secondary to vertebral and costovertebral fusion caused by syndesmophytes (ossification of cartilagenous structures, see Fig. 11–4).

CLINICAL SIGNS AND SYMPTOMS OF ANKYLOSING SPONDYLITIS

Early stages:

- Intermittent, low-grade fever
- Fatigue
- Anorexia, weight loss
- Anemia
- Sacroiliitis (inflammation, pain, and tenderness in the sacroiliac joints)
- Spasm of the paravertebral muscles
- Intermittent low back pain (nontraumatic, insidious onset)

Advanced stages:

- Constant low back pain
- Ankylosis (immobility and consolidation or fusion) of the sacroiliac joints and spine
- Muscle wasting in shoulder and pelvic girdles
- Loss of lumbar lordosis
- Marked dorsocervical kyphosis
- Decreased chest expansion
- Arthritis involving the peripheral joints (hips and knees)
- Iritis or iridocyclitis (inflammation of the iris; occurs in 25% of all cases)
- Carditis (10% occurrence)

- Pericarditis and pulmonary fibrosis (rare)
- Fatigue and weight loss
- Low-grade fever

Diagnosis. After 3 months of low back pain and stiffness of insidious onset, which is unrelieved by rest, the disease is usually diagnosed by demonstration of the appropriate features on physical examination and x-ray studies. X-rays of the sacroiliac joints reveal osteoporosis and erosions early in the disease and sclerosis with fusion in advanced disease. Calcification of the anterior longitudinal ligament of the spine and squaring of the vertebrae are seen on lateral x-rays of the spine. Ossification of the outer margins of the intervertebral disk (syndesmophyte formation) may lead to fusion of the spine (Fig. 11–4).

Prognosis and Treatment. Prognosis is good with treatment to minimize deformity or disability. Treatment is with medication (anti-inflammatory agents to decrease acute inflammation and relieve pain) and physical therapy to maintain muscle strength and flexibility. Patient education toward preserving body posture and mechanics, and work modification as indicated, may also be augmented by breathing exercises and the use of modalities for symptomatic comfort.

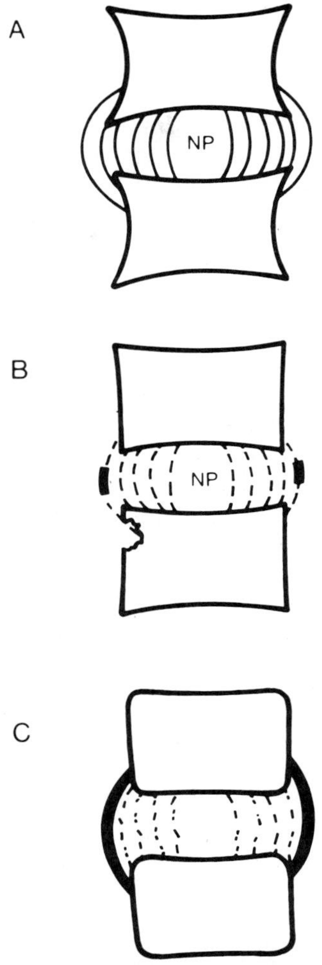

Figure 11–4. The pathogenesis of the syndesmophyte. The syndesmophyte, along with destruction of the sacroiliac joint, is the hallmark of the inflammatory spondyloarthropathies, such as ankylosing spondylitis. It should be distinguished from the osteophyte, which is characteristic of degenerative spondylosis. *A*, This depicts the normal intervertebral disk. The inner fibers of the annulus fibrosis are next to the nucleus pulposus (NP). The outer fibers insert into the periosteum of the vertebral body at least one third the distance toward the next end-plate. *B*, With early inflammation, the corners of the bodies are reabsorbed and appear to be square or even eroded. Fine deposits of amorphous apatite (calcium phosphate, a mineral constituent of bone) appear on radiographs at first as thin delicate calcification in the outer fibers of the midannulus. *C*, The process progresses to bridging calcification, the syndesmophyte, extending from one midbody to the next; thus the spine takes on its "bamboo" appearance on radiographs. (From Hadler, N.M.: Medical Management of the Regional Musculoskeletal Diseases. Orlando, FL, Grune & Stratton, 1984, p. 5.)

Reiter's Syndrome (Ashman, 1988)

The triad of arthritis, conjunctivitis, and nonspecific urethritis defines Reiter's syndrome, although some patients develop only two of the three symptoms. Reiter's syndrome occurs mainly in young adult males between the ages of 20 and 40, although women and children can be affected. Two forms have been identified: cases that have been associated with dysentery and a sexually transmitted form most often implicated with veneral infection. When it occurs in a woman, HLA-B27 is found in almost 100% of the cases, which supports a genetic predisposition for the development of this syndrome after being exposed to certain enteric bacterial infections or after sexual contact. Having HLA-B27 does not necessarily mean that the person will develop this syndrome, but indicates that the person will have a greater chance of developing it than do people without this marker (Ford, 1983).

CLINICAL SIGNS AND SYMPTOMS OF REITER'S SYNDROME

- Low-grade fever
- Urethritis (when present, precedes other symptoms by 1 to 2 weeks)
- Conjunctivitis and iritis, bilaterally
- Polyarthritis (occurs several days or weeks after symptoms of infection appear)
- Sacroiliac joint changes
- Low back pain
- Small joint involvement, especially the feet: heel pain
- Plantar fasciitis
- Skin involvement: inflammatory hyperkeratotic lesions of the toes, nails, and soles of the feet resembling psoriasis
- May be preceded by bowel infection: diarrhea, nausea, vomiting
- Anorexia and weight loss

Arthritis usually occurs suddenly as the second or third symptom to appear, but the dominant feature in this syndrome typically begins in the weight-bearing joints, especially of the lower extremities. This pattern is asymmetric and generally continues for weeks to months. It may vary in severity from absence to extreme joint destruction. Involvement of the feet and spine are most common and are associated with HLA-B27 positivity. Affected joints are usually swollen and warm. Although the joints usually begin to improve after 2 or 3 weeks, many people continue to have pain, especially in the heels and back, even after the other symptoms have resolved (Ford, 1983).

One third of the patients with Reiter's syndrome have sacroiliac x-ray changes that may be asymmetric and are similar to those in ankylosing spondylitis. Small-joint involvement, especially in the feet, is more common in Reiter's syndrome than in ankylosing spondylitis and is often asymmetric. Reiter's syndrome can be differentiated from ankylosing spondylitis by the presence of urethritis and conjunctivitis, the prominent involvement of distal joints, and the presence of asymmetric radiologic changes in the sacroiliac joints and spine (Fye and Sack, 1987). Inflammation at tendinous insertions into bone is common in Reiter's syndrome and causes plantar fasciitis, digital periostitis, or Archilles tendinitis.

Diagnosis. Diagnosis is based on the overall pattern of symptoms and on results of a physical examination. Diagnosis of Reiter's syndrome requires peripheral arthritis occurring in association with urethritis, lasting more than 3 or 4 weeks. Although there are no blood or urine tests that will confirm Reiter's syndrome, these tests can be used to rule out other similar diseases and to indicate evidence of infection. Testing for the HLA-B27 genetic marker may also assist in confirming the diagnosis, but is not an absolute finding to indicate Reiter's syndrome (Ford, 1983).

Prognosis and Treatment. This syndrome demonstrates a selflimited (for 3 to 4 months) but relapsing course of events (sometimes recurring for 2 to 3 years). Joint deformity, ankylosis, and inflammation of the sacroiliac joint may occur with chronic or recurrent Reiter's syndrome. Heel pain is a particularly ominous predictor of eventual disability. Medical treatment is primarily with medication. Physical therapy during the recovery phase can offer the patient symptomatic relief and can provide the patient with preventive and selfcare measures to reduce joint trauma.

Psoriatic Arthritis (Ashman, 1988; Fye and Sack, 1987)

Psoriatic arthritis is a chronic, recurrent, erosive form of polyarthritis associated with the skin disease psoriasis; the arthritis occurs in 5 to 7% of patients with psoriasis. Women are more likely to develop this condition, and although it occurs usually between the ages of 20 and 30, it can occur at any age. The onset of the arthritis may be acute or insidious and is usually preceded by the skin disease.

About 50% of patients with psoriatic arthritis have a distal distribution of arthritis, which is distinguished from RA by the early and more severe involvement of the distal interphalangeal joints (fingers and toes) before involvement of the metacarpophalangeal joints. Other distinguishing features may include typical nail changes (pitting or onycholysis, a loosening or separation of a nail from its bed) associated with psoriatic arthritis; rheumatoid nodules are not present. Psoriatic arthritis is often asymmetric throughout its course and, compared with Reiter's syndrome, psoriatic arthritis characteristically involves the upper extremities earlier and more severely than the lower extremities.

Severe erosive disease may lead to marked deformity of the hands and feet (arthritis mutilans), and marked vertebral involvement can result in ankylosis of the spine. This differs from ankylosing spondylitis in a number of respects, most notably in the tendency for many of the syndesmophytes to arise not at the margins of the vertebral bodies, but from the lateral and anterior surfaces of the bodies (McEwan, 1971). Sacroiliac changes, including erosions, sclerosis, and ankylosis similar to that in Reiter's syndrome, occur in 10 to 30% of patients.

The cause of psoriasis and psoriatic arthritis is unknown. Genetic factors appear to play a role in the development of this disease, because psoriasis and rheumatic diseases are found in other family members. The presence of HLA-B27 and other HLA antigens is not uncommon and they occur in patients with peripheral arthritis and spondylitis. The presence of these genetic markers may be associated with an increased susceptibility to unknown infectious or environmental agents or to primary abnormal autoimmune phenomena. As yet, no known immunologic pathogenetic mechanism has been demonstrated.

CLINICAL SIGNS AND SYMPTOMS OF PSORIATIC ARTHRITIS

- Fever
- Fatigue
- Polyarthritis
- Psoriasis
- Sore fingers (sometimes sausage-like swelling)

Diagnosis and Treatment. Diagnosis is difficult in the absence of skin involvement. There are no specific laboratory tests for psoriasis or the arthritis associated with it. Treatment is the same as that described for AS and Reiter's syndrome. Skin and arthritic manifestations require medical treatment and the physical therapy treatment for arthritis is similar to that for RA.

SUMMARY

This chapter on immunology and immunologic disorders has presented a simplified presentation of the physiology and pathophysiology of the immune system including:

- Organs of the immune system
- Cells of the immune system
- Normal immune response
- Disorders of the immune system
    - Immunodeficiency disorders
    - Hypersensitivity disorders
    - Neurologic disorders
    - Autoimmune disorders

Of particular interest to physical therapists are the systemic autoimmune diseases and immune-related neurologic disorders. Systemic autoimmune diseases were represented by two categories: diffuse connective tissue diseases and spondyloarthropathies (arthritis associated with spondylitis), including these distinct disorders:

- RA
- SLE
- Scleroderma (progressive systemic sclerosis)
- Polymyositis/dermatomyositis
- MCTD
- AS

- Reiter's syndrome
- Psoriatic arthritis

Immune-related neurologic disorders discussed include:

- MG
- Guillain-Barré syndrome
- Multiple sclerosis

CLINICAL SIGNS AND SYMPTOMS REQUIRING PHYSICIAN REFERRAL

Anaphylactic reaction
Ataxia
Bowel/bladder dysfunction
Calcinosis
Change in voice
Choking, difficulty in chewing
Chronic diarrhea
Dysarthria
Dysphagia
Dyspnea on exertion
Easy bruising
Enlarged lymph nodes
Fatigue
Fever, malaise
Finger ulceration
Heartburn
Hoarseness
Incoordination
Increased deep tendon reflexes
Joint inflammation
Loss of appetite
Morning stiffness
Muscle fatigue with exertion
Myalgia
Myositis (inflamed muscle)
Nausea, vomiting
Night sweats
Paresthesias
Persistent, dry cough
Polyarthralgia
Positive Babinski/clonus
Progressive dyspnea
Proximal muscle weakness
Ptosis
Raynaud's phenomenon
Recurrent influenza-like symptoms
Skin rash or thickening
Spasticity
Speech impairment
Subcutaneous nodules
Thrush in the mouth/tongue
Vertigo
Visual disturbances (diplopia, nystagmus, scotomas)
Weight loss
Wheals

SUBJECTIVE EXAMINATION

Special Questions to Ask

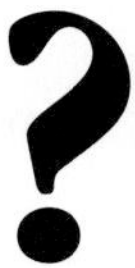

Signs and symptoms of immune disorders can appear in any body system. A thorough review of the *Family/Personal History* form, subjective interview, and appropriate follow-up questions will help the physical therapist to identify signs and symptoms that are not part of a musculoskeletal pattern. Special attention should be given to the question on the *Family/Personal History* form concerning general health. Patients with immune disorders often have poor general health or recurrent infections.

- □ Have you ever been told that you had/have an immune disorder, autoimmune disease, or cancer? (Predisposes the patient to other diseases)
- □ Have you ever received radiation treatment? (Diminishes blood cell production, predisposes to infection)
- □ Have you ever had an organ transplant (especially kidney) or removal of your thymus? **(Myasthenia gravis)**
- □ Do you have difficulty with combing your hair, raising your arms, getting out of a bathtub, bed, or chair, or climbing stairs? **(Polymyositis, dermatomyositis, myasthenia gravis)**
- □ Do you have difficulty when raising your head from the pillow when you are lying down on your back? **(Polymyositis, dermatomyositis, myasthenia gravis)**
- □ Do you have difficulty with swallowing or have you noticed any changes in your voice? **(Polymyositis, dermatomyositis, myasthenia gravis)**
- □ Do you have any trouble taking a deep breath? **(Weak chest muscles secondary to polymyositis, dermatomyositis, myasthenia gravis)**
- □ Have you noticed any changes in your skin texture or pigmentation? Do you have any skin rashes? **(Scleroderma, allergic reactions, SLE, RA, dermatomyositis, psoriatic arthritis, AIDS)**

  Have you noticed any association between the development of the skin rash and pain or swelling in any of your joints (or other symptoms)?

  Do these other symptoms go away when the skin rash clears up?
- □ Have you had any recent vision problems? **(Multiple sclerosis, SLE)**
- □ Have you had any difficulties with urination, for example, a change in appearance of urine, accidents, increased frequency? **(Multiple sclerosis, myasthenia gravis)**

For the patient with known allergies (check the *Family/Personal History* form):

Subjective Exam

Special Questions to Ask

What are the usual symptoms that you experience in association with your allergies?

Describe a typical allergic reaction for you.

Do the symptoms relate to physical changes (e.g., cold, heat, or dampness)?

Do the symptoms occur in association with activities (e.g., exercise)?

Do you take medications for your allergies?

For the patient complaining of fatigue and weakness:

□ Do you feel tired all of the time or only after exertion?

□ Do you get short of breath after mild exercise or at rest?

□ How much sleep do you get at night?

□ Do you take naps during the day?

□ Have you ever been told by a physician that you are anemic?

□ How long have you had this weakness?

□ Does it come and go or is it persistent (there all the time)?

□ Are you able to perform your usual daily activities without stopping to rest or nap?

For the patient with fever (fevers recurring every few days, fevers that rise and fall within 24 hours and fevers that recur frequently should be documented and reported to the patient's physician):

□ When did you first notice this fever?

□ Is it constant or does it come and go?

□ Does your temperature fluctuate?

If yes, over what period of time does this occur?

PHYSICIAN REFERRAL

In the case of most immunologic disorders, physicians must rely on the patient's history and clinical findings in association with supportive information from diagnostic tests to make a differential diagnosis. Often, there are no definitive diagnostic tests, such as in the case of multiple sclerosis. The physician relies instead on objectively measured CNS abnormalities, a history of episodic exacerbations, and remissions of symptoms with progressive worsening of symptoms over time (Miller and Keane, 1987). In other situations, such as with dermatomyositis, various tests may be used by the physician in conjunction with the presence of the characteristic skin rash and proximal muscle weakness to determine the diagnosis.

In the early stages of treating disorders such as multiple sclerosis, Guillain-Barré syndrome, and myositis, factors such as the effect of fatigue on the patient's progress and fragile muscle fibers necessitate that the physical therapist keep close contact with the physician, who will use a physical examination and laboratory tests to determine the most opportune time for an exercise program. While the physician is monitoring serum enzyme levels and the overall medical status of the patient, the physical therapist will continue to provide the physician with essential feedback regarding objective findings, such as muscle tenderness, muscle strength, and overall physical endurance.

A careful history and close clinical observations may elicit indications that the patient is demonstrating signs and symptoms unrelated to a musculoskeletal disorder. Because the immune system can implicate many of the body systems, the physical therapist should not hesitate to report to the physician any unusual findings reported or observed.

CASE STUDY

Referral

A 28-year-old Mexican-American has come to you for an evaluation without a medical referral. He has seen no medical practitioner for his current symptoms that consist of an unusual gait pattern and weakness of the lower extremities, which he noticed during the last 2 days. He speaks English with a heavy accent, making it difficult to obtain a clear medical history, but the *Personal/Family History* form indicates no previous or current health or medical problems of any kind. He does note that he has had influenza in the last 3 weeks, but that he is fully recovered now.

What further questions would be appropriate for your physical therapy interview with this patient?

Using the format outlined in the chapter on *The Physical Therapy Interview,* begin with an open-ended question and follow up with additional appropriate questions incorporating the following:

Current Symptoms

Tell me why you are here (open-ended question) . . . or you may prefer to say, "I notice from your intake form that you have had some weakness in your legs and a change in the way you walk. What can you tell me about this?"

When did you first notice these changes?

What did you notice that made you think that something was happening?

Just before the development of these symptoms, did you injure yourself in any way that you can remember?

Did you have a car accident, fall down, or twist your trunk or hips in any unusual way?

Do you have any pain in your back, hips, or legs?

If yes, follow the outline in *The Physical Therapy Interview* to elicit a further description.

Associated Symptoms

Have you had any numbness or tingling in your back, buttocks, hips, or down your legs?

CASE STUDY

Have you had any other changes in sensation in these areas, such as a burning or prickling feeling?

Have you had the "flu," a cold, an upper respiratory infection, or other infection recently?

Have you had a fever or elevated temperature in the last 48 hours?

Do you think that you have a temperature right now?

Have you noticed any other symptoms that I should know about?

Give the patient time to answer the question. Prompt him if you need to with various suggestions (include any others that seem appropriate to the information and responses already given by the patient), such as:

Nausea or dizziness

Diarrhea or constipation

Unusual fatigue

Recent headaches

Choking, difficulty with chewing

Shortness of breath with mild exertion (e.g., walking to the car or even at rest)

Vomiting

Cold sweats during the day or night

Changes in vision or speech

Skin rashes

Joint pains

Have you noticed any other respiratory, lung, or breathing problems?

Final Question

Is there anything else you think that I should know about your current condition or general health that I have not asked yet?

What test procedures will you carry out during the first session?

Given the patient's report of lower extremity weakness and antalgic gait of sudden onset without precipitating cause, the following possible problems should be ruled out during the objective assessment:

Neurologic disease or disorder (immunologically based or otherwise) such as:

- Discogenic lesion
- Tumor
- Myasthenia gravis (unlikely due to the patient's age)
- Guillain-Barré syndrome
- Multiple sclerosis

Other possible immunologic disorders

- AIDS dementia (unlikely from the way that the history was presented)

Psychogenic disorder (e.g., hysteria, anxiety, alcoholism, or drug addiction)

CASE STUDY

Observation/Inspection

- Take the patient's vital signs
- Note any obvious changes, such as muscle atrophy, difficulty with breathing or swallowing, facial paralysis, intention tremor
- Describe the gait pattern: Observe for ataxia, incoordination, positive Trendelenburg position, balance, patterns of muscular weakness or imbalance, other gait deviations

Neurologic Screen

- All deep tendon reflexes
- Manual muscle testing of proximal-to-distal large muscle groups looking for a pattern of weakness
- Babinski sign and clonus
- Gross sensory screen looking for any differences in perceived sensation from one side to the other
- Test for dysmetria, balance, and coordination

Orthopedic Assessment

- Lower extremity range of motion (ROM): active and passive
- Back, lower quadrant evaluation protocol (Magee, 1987)

Testing Results

In the case of this patient, the interview revealed very little additional information, because the patient denied any other associated (systemic) signs or symptoms, denied bowel/bladder dysfunction, precipitating injury or trauma, or neurologic indications such as numbness, tingling, or paresthesias. Although he was difficult to understand, the physical therapist thought that the patient had understood the questions and had answered them truthfully. Subjectively, he did not appear to be a malingerer or a hysterical/anxious individual.

His gait pattern could best be described as ataxic. His lower extremities would not support him fully, and he frequently lost his balance and fell down, although he denied any pain or warning that he was about to fall.

Objective findings revealed inconsistent results of muscle testing: The proximal muscles were more involved than the distal muscles (difference of one grade: proximal muscles = fair grade; distal muscles = good grade), but repeated tests elicited alternatively strong, weak, or cogwheel responses, as if the muscles were moving in a ratching motion against resistance through the ROM.

The only other positive findings were slightly diminished deep tendon reflexes of the lower extremities compared with the upper extremities, but again these findings were inconsistent when tested over time.

CASE STUDY

Final Results

Because the subjective and objective examinations were so inconsistent and puzzling, the therapist asked another therapist to briefly examine this patient. In turn, they decided either to ask the patient to either return at the end of the day or for the first appointment of the next day to re-examine the patient for any changes in the pattern of his symptoms. It was more convenient for him to return the next day and he did.

At that time, it became clear that the therapist's difficulty in understanding the patient had less to do with his use of English as a second language and had more to do with an increasingly slurred speech pattern. His gait remained unchanged, but the muscle strength of the proximal pelvic muscles was consistently weak over several trials spread out during the therapy session, which lasted for 1 hour. This time, the therapist checked the muscles of his upper extremities and found that the scapular muscles were also unable to move against any manual resistance. Deep tendon reflexes of the upper extremities were inconsistently diminished, and reflexes of the lower extremities were now consistently diminished.

The patient was referred to a physician for further follow-up and was not treated at the physical therapy clinic that day. He was examined by his family physician, who referred him to a neurologist. A diagnosis of Guillain-Barré syndrome was confirmed when the patient's symptoms progressed dramatically, requiring hospitalization.

References

Abernathy, E.: How the immune system works. Am. J. Nurs. *87*:4 and 456, 1987.

Acquired Immune Deficiency Syndrome: Information and procedural guidelines for providing services to persons with AIDS/HIV. Helena, MT, Department of Health and Environmental Sciences, Feb. 1987.

Alarcon-Segovia, D.: Systemic lupus erythematosus: Pathology and pathogenesis. *In* Schumacher, H.R. (ed): Primer on the Rheumatic Diseases, 9th ed. Atlanta, GA, Arthritis Foundation, 1988, pp. 96–99.

Ashman, R.F.: Rheumatic diseases. *In* Lawlor, G.J. and Fischer, T.J. (eds): Manual of Allergy and Immunology: Diagnosis and Therapy, 2nd ed. Boston, Little, Brown, 1988, pp. 284–323.

Bennett, J.C.: Rheumatoid arthritis: Clinical features. *In* Schumacher, H.R. (ed): Primer on the Rheumatic Diseases, 9th ed. Atlanta, GA, Arthritis Foundation, 1988, pp. 87–92.

Brew, B., Rosenblum, M., and Price, R.W.: Central and peripheral nervous system complications of HIV infection and AIDS. *In* DeVita, V.T., Hellman, S., and Rosenberg, S.A. (eds): AIDS: Etiology, Diagnosis, Treatment and Prevention, 2nd ed. Philadelphia, J.B. Lippincott, 1988, pp. 185–197.

Calin, A.: Ankylosing spondylitis and the spondyloarthropathies. *In* Schumacher, H.R. (ed): Primer on the Rheumatic Diseases, 9th ed. Atlanta, GA, Arthritis Foundation, 1988, pp. 142–147.

Centers for Disease Control: Human Immunodeficiency Virus Infection in the United States: A Review of Current Knowledge. U.S. Department of Health and Human Services, AIDS Program. Vol. 36, No. S-6, Dec. 18, 1987a.

Centers for Disease Control: Recommendations for Prevention of HIV Transmission in Health-Care Settings. U.S. Department of Health and Human Services, AIDS Program, Atlanta, GA, Vol. 36, No. 2–6, Aug. 21, 1987b.

Centers for Disease Control: Update: Universal Precautions for Prevention of Transmission of Human Immunodeficiency Virus, Hepatitis B Virus, and Other Bloodborne Pathogens in Health Care Settings. U.S. Department of Health and Human Services, Public Health Service, Vol. 37, No. 24, June 24, 1988, pp. 377–382, 387–388.

Christian, C.L.: Systemic Lupus Erythematosus, 2nd ed. Atlanta, GA, Arthritis Foundation, 1986.

Daube, J.R.: Disorders of neuromuscular transmission: A review. Arch. Phys. Med. Rehabil., *64*:195, 1983.

DeVita, V.T., Hellman, S., and Rosenberg, S.A. (eds): AIDS: Etiology, Diagnosis, Treatment and Prevention, 2nd ed. Philadelphia, J.B. Lippincott, 1988.

Ford, D.K.: Reiter's Syndrome. Atlanta, GA, Arthritis Foundation, 1983.

Fye, K.H., and Sack, K.E.: Rheumatic diseases. *In* Stites, D.P., Stobo, J.D., and Wells, J.V.: Basic and Clinical Immunology, 6th ed. Norwalk, CT, Appleton & Lange, 1987, pp. 356–385.

Gall, E.P.: Pathophysiology of rheumatic disease. *In* Physical Therapy Management of Arthritis. New York, Churchill Livingstone, 1988, pp. 1–15.

Guccione, A.A.: Rheumatoid arthritis. *In* O'Sullivan, S.B., and Schmitz, T.J.: Physical Rehabilitation: Assessment and Treatment, 2nd ed. Philadelphia, F.A. Davis, 1988, pp. 435–453.

Hadler, N.M.: The patient with low back pain. Hosp. Pract., Oct. 30, 1987, pp. 17–22.

Hess, C.E.: The immune system: structure, development, and function. *In* Thorup, O.A.: Leavell and Thorup's Fundamentals of Clinical Hematology, 5th ed. Philadelphia, W.B. Saunders Company, 1987, pp. 23–63.

Hoffman, P.M. and Panitch, H.S.: Neurologic diseases. *In* Stites, D.P., Stobo, J.D., and Wells, J.V.: Basic and Clinical Immunology, 6th ed. Norwalk, CT, Appleton & Lange, 1987, pp. 598–609.

Hollister, R.: Collagen vascular disease. *In* Bierman, C.W., and Pearlman, D.S. (eds): Allergic Diseases from Infancy to Adulthood, 2nd ed. Philadelphia, W.B. Saunders Company, 1988, pp. 779–787.

Jaret, P.: Our immune system: The wars within. National Geographic, *169*:702, 1986.

Koenig, S., and Fauci, A.S.: AIDS: Immunopathogenesis and immune response to the human immunodeficiency virus: *In* DeVita, V.T., Hellman, S., and Rosenberg, S.A. (eds): AIDS: Etiology, Diagnosis, Treatment and Prevention, 2nd ed. Philadelphia, J.B. Lippincott, 1988, pp. 61–77.

Knutsen, A.P., and Fischer, T.J.: Immunodeficiency diseases. *In* Lawlor, G.J., and Fischer, T.J., (eds): Manual of Allergy and Immunology: Diagnosis and Therapy, 2nd ed. Boston, Little, Brown, 1988, pp. 356–379.

Koop, C.E.: Surgeon general's report on: Acquired immune deficiency syndrome. Bethesda, MD, U.S. Department of Health and Human Services, Oct. 22, 1986.

Layzer, R.B.: Neuromuscular Manifestations of Systemic Disease. Philadelphia, F.A. Davis, 1985.

Leroy, E.C.: Scleroderma. Atlanta, GA, Arthritis Foundation, 1983.

Magee, D.J.: Orthopedic Physical Assessment. Philadelphia, W.B. Saunders Company, 1987.

McEwan, C. (ed): Ankylosing spondylitis and spondylitis accompanying ulcerative colitis, regional enteritis, psoriasis and Reiter's disease: A comparative study, Arthritis Rheum., *14*:291, 1971.

Medsger, T.A.: Systemic sclerosis and localized scleroderma. *In* Schumacher, H.R. (ed): Primer on the Rheumatic Diseases, 9th ed. Atlanta, GA, Arthritis Foundation, 1988, pp. 111–117.

Miller, B.F., and Keane, C.B.: Encyclopedia and Dictionary of Medicine, Nursing and Allied Health, 4th ed. Philadelphia, W.B. Saunders Company, 1987.

National Institutes of Health: Understanding the immune system. U.S. Department of Health and Human Services, Public Health Service, National Institutes of Health, Bethesda, MD, Publication No. 85-529, July 1985.

Nursing 85: Immune Disorders. Springhouse, PA, Springhouse Corporation, 1985.

O'Sullivan, S.B., and Schmitz, T.J.: Physical Rehabilitation: Assessment and Treatment, 2nd ed. Philadelphia, F.A. Davis, 1988.

Page, J.: Blood: The River of Life. Washington, DC, U.S. News Books, 1981.

Pearson, C.M.: Polymyositis and dermatomyositis. Atlanta, GA, Arthritis Foundation, 1983.

Purtilo, D.T., and Purtilo, R.B.: A Survey of Human Diseases, 2nd ed. Boston, Little, Brown, 1989.)

Reich, P.R.: Hematology: Physiopathologic Basis for Clinical Practice, 2nd ed. Boston, Little, Brown, 1984.

Rodnan, G.P., and Schumacher, H.R. (eds): Primer on Rheumatic Diseases, 8th ed. Atlanta, GA, Arthritis Foundation, 1983.

Saxon, A.: Immediate hypersensitivity: Approach to diagnosis. *In* Lawlor, G.J., and Fischer, T.J. (eds): Manual of Allergy and Immunology: Diagnosis and Therapy, 2nd ed. Boston, Little, Brown, 1988, pp. 15–35.

Shaw, G.M., Wong-Staal, F., and Gallo, R.C.: Etiology of AIDS: Virology, molecular biology, and evolution of human immunodeficiency viruses. *In* DeVita, V.T., Hellman, S., and Rosenberg, S.A. (eds): AIDS: Etiology, Diagnosis, Treatment and Prevention, 2nd ed. Philadelphia, J.B. Lippincott, 1988, pp. 11–32.

Solomon, G.F.: Emotional and personality factors in the onset and course of autoimmune disease, particularly rheumatoid arthritis. *In* Ader, R. (ed): Psychoneuroimmunology. New York, Academic Press, 1981.

Stasney, P.: Association of B cell antigen DR4 with rheumatoid arthritis. N. Engl. J. Med. *298*:869, 1978.

Theofilopoulos, A.N.: Autoimmunity. *In* Stites, D.P., Stobo, J.D., and Wells, J.V.: Basic and Clinical Immunology, 6th ed. Norwalk, CT, Appleton & Lange, 1987, pp. 128–158.

Weiner, M.A.: Maximum Immunity. Boston, Houghton Mifflin Company, 1986.

Wright, R.: Biologic defense mechanisms. *In* Phipps, W., Long, B., and Woods, N.: Medical-Surgical Nursing: Concepts and Clinical Practice. St. Louis, C.V. Mosby, 1987, pp. 1883–1909.

Zvaifler, N.J.: Rheumatoid arthritis. *In* Schumacher, H.R. (ed): Primer on the Rheumatic Diseases, 9th ed. Atlanta, GA, Arthritis Foundation, 1988, pp. 83–87.

Bibliography

Alarcon, G.S.: Arthritis: Where are we now? Arthritis Today: The University of Alabama at Birmingham Multipurpose Arthritis Center, No. 32, Winter 1988, pp. 1–2.

Alexander, J.W., and Good, R.: Fundamentals of Clinical Immunology. Philadelphia, W.B. Saunders Company, 1977.

Ball, G.V.: Clinical Rheumatology. Philadelphia, W.B. Saunders Company, 1986.

Banwell, B.F., and Gall, V. (eds): Physical Therapy Management of Arthritis. New York, Churchill Livingstone, 1988.

Bellanti, J.A.: Immunology: Basic Processes, 2nd ed. Philadelphia, W.B. Saunders Company, 1985.

Berczi, I.: Pituitary Function and Immunity. Boca Raton, FL, CRC Press, 1986.

Bierman, C.W., and Pearlman, D.S. (eds): Allergic Diseases from Infancy to Adulthood, 2nd ed. Philadelphia, W.B. Saunders Company, 1988.

Brewer, E.J., Gianni, E.H., and Person, D.A.: Juvenile Rheumatoid Arthritis, 2nd ed. Philadelphia, W.B. Saunders Company, 1982.

Brower, A.C.: Arthritis in Black and White. Philadelphia, W.B. Saunders Company, 1988.

Burnet, F.M.: Immunology, Aging and Cancer: Medical Aspects of Mutation and Selection. San Francisco, W.H. Freeman, 1976.

Centers for Disease Control: AIDS: Information and Procedural Guidelines for Providing Services to Persons with AIDS/HIV. Centers for Disease Control, Feb. 1987.

Centers for Disease Control: Update: Universal precautions for prevention of transmission of HIV, HBV, and other bloodborne pathogens in health-care settings. MMWR, *37*:24, 1988.

Ebbesen, P., Biggar, R.J., and Melbye, M.: AIDS: A Basic Guide for Clinicians. Philadelphia, W.B. Saunders Company, 1984.

Kelley, W.N., Harris, E.D., Ruddy, S., and Sledge, C.B.: Textbook of Rheumatology, Vols. 1 and 2, 3rd ed. Philadelphia, W.B. Saunders Company, 1988.

Lockey, R.F., and Bukantz, S.C.: Fundamentals of Immunology and Allergy. Philadelphia, W.B. Saunders Company, 1987.

Myrvik, Q.N., and Weiser, R.S.: Fundamentals of Immunology, 2nd ed. Philadelphia, Lea & Febiger, 1984.

Purtilo, D.T.: Immune Deficiency and Cancer: Epstein-Barr Virus and Lymphoproliferative Malignancies. Plenum Publications, 1984.

Steinberg, J.: Guillain-Barré Syndrome: An Overview for the Layperson, 4th ed. Wynewood, PA, Guillain-Barré Syndrome Support Group International, 1987.

Stites, D.P., Stobo, J.D., and Wells, J.V.: Basic and Clinical Immunology, 6th ed. Norwalk, CT, Appleton & Lange, 1987.

Thorup, O.A.: Leavell and Thorup's Fundamentals of Clinical Hematology, 5th ed. Philadelphia, W.B. Saunders Company, 1987.

Weiss, L.: The Cells and Tissues of the Immune System: Structure, Functions, Interactions. Englewood Cliffs, NJ, Prentice-Hall, 1972.

Wilson, G., and Dick, H.M. (eds): Topley and Wilson's Principles of Bacteriology, Virology and Immunity, Vols. 1 to 4, 7th ed. Baltimore, Williams & Wilkins, 1984.

Youmans, G.P., Paterson, P.Y., and Sommers, H.M.: The Biologic and Clinical Basis of Infectious Diseases, 3rd ed. Philadelphia, W.B. Saunders Company, 1985.

Chapter 12

Systemic Origins of Musculoskeletal Pain: Associated Signs and Symptoms

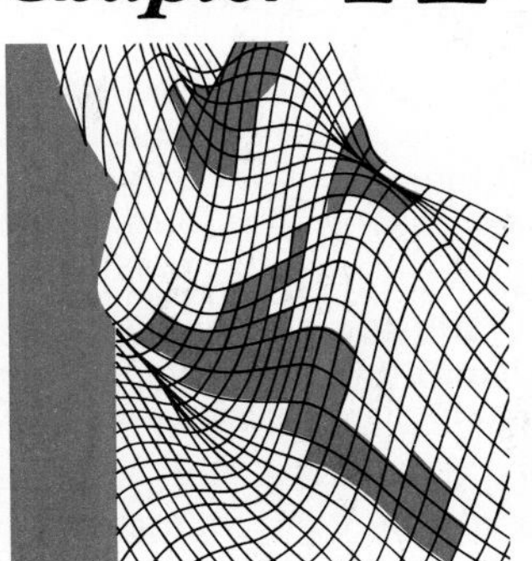

☐ ***Clinical Signs and Symptoms of:***

- Systemic Pain
- Musculoskeletal Pain
- Gynecologic Disorders
- Tietze's Syndrome or Costochondritis
- Neoplasm
- Hip Avascular Necrosis
- Hip Hemarthrosis

The potential for referral of pain from systemic diseases to specific muscles and joints is well documented in the medical literature. These referral patterns most often affect the back and shoulder, but may also present in the chest, thorax, hip, groin, or sacroiliac (SI) joint. In this chapter, we have attempted to provide an overview of systemic diseases that can refer pain or symptoms to the aforementioned musculoskeletal areas. Unless otherwise stated, in each section of this chapter, it is assumed that the text pertains to systemic origins of symptoms for specific joints or areas of the body.

Up until this point, the text has focused on each organ system and the pain or symptoms referred from organs to musculoskeletal sites. In this chapter, we have turned the focus around so that the reader can quickly refer to the site of presenting pain or symptoms and determine possible systemic involvement. The physical therapist may then question the patient, as suggested, and determine the possible need for a medical referral. For an indepth discussion of the specific systemic causes of musculoskeletal signs or symptoms, the reader is referred to the individual chapters within this text.

It is essential that the physical therapist conduct a thorough interview and correlate the subjective findings with the objective findings in order to recognize presenting conditions that require medical follow-up. Accordingly, the physical therapist will want to obtain the patient's history, conduct a systems review, and remain familiar with types of pain, pain patterns, and signs and symptoms that may suggest systemic origins of problems presenting in the musculoskeletal system. A brief review of each of these parameters has been included in this chapter for the clinician who is using this text as a quick reference guide.

These guidelines for collecting and correlating subjective and objective information are suggested for all patients who develop musculoskeletal symptoms insidiously (i.e., without a traumatic origin or known precipitating cause) as well as for the patient being treated by a physical therapist for any reason. Even with a history of trauma or injury, the physical therapist should keep in mind that trauma has been related to symptoms in 10% of patients with neoplasm, compared with 10 to 30% or more in patients with discogenic pain. In most cases, an injury associated with a neoplasm is precipitated by a neurologic deficit that is caused by cord or root compression due to the tumor (Hedler, 1987).

Finally, trauma does not solely imply some external force creating injury. Trauma may be intrinsic, resulting from internal derangement of either muscle (e.g., ruptures of the tendinous insertion) or joint (e.g., meniscal injury or joint dysfunction). Intrinsic trauma is associated with an unguarded movement occurring during the performance of a normal functional activity. If the episode producing the pain is the result of extrinsic trauma, the history of onset is usually quite clear. However, extrinsic trauma to one part of the musculoskeletal system may be associated with intrinsic trauma of another part (Zohn, 1988).

For example, a direct injury to the cervical spine during an automobile accident may also result in an intrinsic injury to the lumbar spine, which goes unnoticed at the time of the more severe and obvious injury (Zohn, 1988). These cases point out the need to question the patient carefully regarding previous trauma, because the patient may not realize the potential importance of such information.

PATIENT HISTORY

A carefully taken, detailed medical history is the most important single element in the evaluation of a patient presenting with musculoskeletal pain of unknown origin or etiology. It is essential for the recognition of systemic disease that may be causing muscle or joint symptoms (Rodnan and Schumacher, 1983). Symptoms are likely to appear some time before striking physical signs of disease are evident and before laboratory tests are useful to the physician in detecting disordered physiology. Thus, an accurate and sufficiently detailed history provides historical clues that can be significant in determining when the patient should be referred to a physician (Blacklow, 1983).

It is important to know the patient's age, occupation, and previous illnesses and injuries. The age is important because some musculoskeletal or systemic problems are likely to affect people during specific decades of life. Occupation is important because well-defined problems occur in people who engage in different occupational activities, including exposure to occupational gases or chemicals (Zohn, 1988).

Other important information may include recent travel (hepatitis, tropical diseases associated with arthralgias), ingestion of raw cow or goat's milk (tuberculosis), or whether undercooked meat or fish has been eaten (hepatitis). If the patient indicates that illness occurred while traveling abroad, it should be remembered that amebiasis (infections with amebas), fungal infections, and some rare tropical diseases may manifest themselves as joint pain in their chronic course (Mennell,

1964). A forgotten accident or childhood disease or illness may contribute important information.

The past history of a patient with joint pain must be examined, because there may be a clue to the true nature of the pathologic cause of the pain. A previous history of heart disease in childhood, chorea, or St. Vitus' dance suggests that the cause of pain may be acute rheumatic fever. Migraine or allergic conditions, such as asthma or hay fever, suggest a diagnosis of nonspecific intermittent hydrarthrosis (fluid in a joint). A chronic cough, loss of weight, unexplained fever, undue sweating, and the drinking of raw milk in the past suggest that the underlying cause of the joint symptoms may be tuberculosis or brucellosis, whereas fleeting pains in the small joints of the extremities are suggestive of rheumatoid arthritis. Joint pain after dietary extravagance may suggest gout, and the history of recent injection of antitoxin or the administration of a new drug might suggest an allergic basis for the joint symptoms (Mennell, 1964).

Acute pain in joints may have a sudden onset at rest. In this event, systemic disease should be suspected. It is more often the case that the history will reveal a gradual onset, starting with aching and progressing with time to a point of severe discomfort or even acute pain (Zohn, 1988).

A previous history of cancer, either personal or family, is always a reason to question the patient further regarding the onset and the pattern of current symptoms. This is especially true for women with a previous personal or family history of breast cancer or cancer of the reproductive system, who now present with shoulder, chest, back, hip, or SI pain of unknown etiology. Likewise, any patient with back problems should be questioned both with regard to the previous history of cancer and to the presence of any other pain or symptoms felt before the onset of back pain. Pain that begins in one anatomic location and then migrates to the back may not be associated by the patient as being caused by the same phenomenon, and thus a good history taking is important.

If pain has commenced for no apparent reason and is gradually and insidiously increasing, serious pathology should be suspected, particularly if the patient feels or looks unwell. A careful evaluation of the patient's information regarding the onset of the symptoms is important. The patient may think that the pain began for no apparent reason, whereas the alert therapist may recognize a causative factor. Alternately, the patient may wrongfully relate the onset to certain activities in an attempt to find a cause for the pain that really appeared for very different reasons (McKenzie, 1981). When the symptoms seem out of proportion to the injury, or if they persist beyond the expected time for the nature of the injury, the presence of a tumor may be suspected (D'Ambrosia, 1986).

If, during the examination, no position or movement can be found that reduces the presenting pain, the existence of serious pathology should be considered. This is especially true when the patient states that there has been no apparent reason for the onset of symptoms or that the symptoms have been present for weeks or months and have been increasing in intensity over time. There is usually no loss of function or postural deformity (McKenzie, 1981).

Women with back pain who have an unusual menstrual history should be questioned in greater detail regarding gynecologic function in order to rule out any relationship between the reproductive system and the back pain. Any suspicious findings should be reported to the physician for further consideration in making a medical diagnosis. Both men and women with back pain should be questioned regarding the potential for urologic conditions causing back pain.

It is the associated signs and symptoms that are most often warning signs for the therapist to indicate the possibility of systemic origin of presenting musculoskeletal problems. Because the patient may not associate such symptoms with the current joint, muscular, or skeletal pain, the therapist must know the possible systemic causes of musculoskeletal pain and the appropriate questions to ask to elicit the presence of associated symptoms in the patient's history.

For example, more obvious examples of related gastrointestinal (GI) complaints include a history of nausea and vomiting of recently ingested food, significant weight loss without effort, a change in the bowel habits or the character of the stool, increase or decrease of musculoskeletal symptoms with ingestion of food are all important associated features of back, thoracic, or scapular pain (Aach, 1983). Such a history, even in the presence of objective musculoskeletal findings, requires careful interpretation of subjective and objective results and consultation with the physician. This principle is even more important when the patient does not present with significant objective findings to support a primary musculoskeletal lesion.

TYPES OF PAIN (Engel, 1983; Kirkaldy-Willis, 1983)

Body activities and physiologic processes serve to modify pain by increasing or decreasing afferent activity. These relationships are helpful in identifying the site and nature (i.e., musculoskeletal or potentially systemic) of the pathologic process responsible for the pain.

For example, muscular pain is intensified by the use of the muscle as well as by mechanical forces, such as pressure or stretch. The sudden movements of coughing, sneezing, or laughing will increase pain coming from abdominal or trunk musculature. When pain is due to ischemia, which is characteristic of intermittent claudication, there is a direct relationship between the degree of circulatory insufficiency and muscle work. The interval between the beginning of muscle contraction and the onset of pain depends on how long it takes for hypoxic products of muscle metabolism to accumulate and exceed the threshold of receptor response. Therefore, pain from an ischemic muscle builds up with the use of the muscle and subsides with rest. Movable skeletal parts including bones, joints, bursae, and tendons, give rise to pain when the structure is used and to relief when rested (Engel, 1983).

Heart pain, a consequence of muscle ischemia, correlates with metabolic demand. With coronary insufficiency (angina pectoris), pain may develop when the work of the heart increases, such as with exertion, cold, or emotion, and subsides with rest and relaxation. Pain from the mediastinum may be influenced by the activity of neighboring moving parts: esophagus (swallowing), musculoskeletal structures (movement), or aorta (increased systolic thrust).

Pain arising from arteries, such as with arteritis (inflammation of an artery), migraine, and vascular headaches, increases with systolic impulse so that any process associated with increased systolic pressure, such as exercise, fever, alcohol, or bending over, may intensify the already throbbing pain. Pain from pleura, as well as from the trachea, correlates with respiratory movements.

Pain arising from the GI tract tends to increase with peristaltic activity, particularly if there is any obstruction to forward progress. The pain increases with ingestion and may lessen with fasting or after emptying the involved segment (vomiting or bowel movement). When hollow viscera, such as the liver, kidneys, spleen, and pancreas, are distended, body positions or movements that increase intra-abdominal pressure may intensify the pain, whereas positions that reduce pressure or support the structure may ease the pain (Engel, 1983).

For example, the patient with an acutely distended gallbladder may slightly flex his or her trunk. With pain arising from a tense, swollen kidney (or distended renal pelvis), the patient flexes the trunk and tilts toward the involved side; with pancreatic pain, the patient may sit up and lean forward or lie down with the knees drawn up to the chest. Pain may occur secondary to the effect of gastric acid on the esophagus, stomach, or duodenum. This pain is relieved by the presence of food or by other neutralizing material in the stomach, and the pain is intensified when the stomach is empty and secreting acid (Engel, 1983). In these cases, it is important to ask the patient about the effect of eating on musculoskeletal pain:

whether the pain increases, decreases, or stays the same after eating.

Referred Pain

Referred pain is pain that is experienced at a site other than the actual site that is stimulated, but in tissues supplied by the same or adjacent neural segments. It does not follow normal anatomic pathways and is perceived by the patient in an area far removed from the site of the lesion, because the sensory pathways are distorted. The borders of the area of referred pain are not sharply demarcated. There is local tenderness in the tissues of the referred pain area, but there is no objective sensory deficit (Zohn, 1988).

There are numerous theories regarding the mechanism by which referred pain develops. However it occurs, it is known that continuous irritation of pain receptor systems in a particular tissue (e.g., posterior joint capsule) creates a state of hyperexcitability in related nerve cells in the dorsal horn of the spinal cord. After this, afferent input from receptors in other segmentally related tissues gives rise to pain in these tissues. Referred pain is often associated with muscle hypertonus over the referred area of pain.

Radicular Pain

Radicular (radiating) pain is experienced in the musculoskeletal system in a dermatome, sclerotome, or myotome because of direct irritation or involvement of a spinal nerve. In systemic disease, radiating pain occurs because of dysfunction of the autonomic innervation of the body (see Fig. 6–3). Radicular pain of the viscera (organs) is generally within the segmental innervation of the affected organ. For example, cardiac pain may be described as beginning retrosternally (behind the sternum) and radiating to the left shoulder and down the inner side of the left arm; gallbladder pain may be felt to originate in the right upper abdomen and to radiate to the angle of the scapula (Engel, 1983). This second type of radicular pain may be characterized by a detectable sensory, motor, or reflex deficit.

Diffuse Pain

Diffuse pain that characterizes some diseases of the nervous system and viscera may be difficult to distinguish from the equally diffuse pains so often caused by lesions of the moving parts. Most patients in this category are patients with obscure pain in the trunk, especially when the symptoms are felt anteriorly only (Cyriax, 1982). The distinction between visceral pain and pain caused by lesions of the vertebral column may be difficult to make and will require a medical diagnosis.

Pain at Rest

Pain at rest may arise from ischemia of a wide variety of tissue (e.g., vascular disease or tumor growth). The acute onset of severe unilateral extremity involvement accompanied by the "five Ps" of pain, pallor, pulselessness, paresthesia, and paralysis signifies the onset of acute arterial occlusion (peripheral vascular disease [PVD]). Pain in this case is usually described by the patient as burning or shooting and may be accompanied by paresthesia. Restless legs are an early manifestation of arterial insufficiency. Ischemia of the skin and subcutaneous tissues is characterized by the patient as burning and boring. All of these chronic causes of pain are usually worse at night and are relieved to some degree by dangling the leg over the side of the bed and by frequent massaging of the extremity (Zohn, 1988; Zohn and Mennell, 1988).

Although neoplasms are highly vascularized, the host organ's vascular supply and nutrients may be compromised simultaneously causing ischemia of the local tissue. Pain at rest secondary to neoplasm occurs usually at night. The pain awakens the patient from sleep and prevents the person from going back to sleep, despite all efforts to do so. The patient may describe pain on weight-bearing or bone pain that may be mild and intermittent in the initial stages, becoming progressively more severe and more constant.

Activity Pain

Activity pain, such as cramping pain from intermittent claudication, may occur as a symptom due to ischemia secondary to peripheral or spinal vascular disease. The patient complains that a certain distance walked or a fixed amount of usage of the upper extremity brings on the pain. Rest promptly relieves the pain. The location of the pain depends on the location of the vascular pathology. Activity pain differs from the pain of spinal stenosis, for example, which may be relieved temporarily by activity (walking).

Joint Pain

Joint pain that awakens the patient at night is often due to bone disease or neoplasm. The pain of systemic joint disease is most often deep, aching, and throbbing; it may be reduced by pressure. This type of pain may be constant or occur in waves or spasms, and it may be sharp or dull. On the other hand, the pain of joint dysfunction is invariably sharp; it usually ceases immediately when the stressful action that produces it ceases; it is invariably relieved or is at least greatly improved by rest and is aggravated by activity. The patient's answers to questions regarding what aggravates and what improves the pain may be very significant (Mennell, 1964).

When joint dysfunction is the primary cause of joint pain, the clues in the patient's history are that the symptom of pain was sudden in onset, occurred after some unguarded joint movement, and was unassociated with marked swelling or warmth. The pain is limited to one joint, is reduced by rest (which is not followed by stiffness), and is aggravated by activity (Mennell, 1964).

The development of characteristic features of systemic involvement, such as jaundice in cases of infectious hepatitis, migratory nature of the pain (moves from joint to joint), presence of skin rash, fatigue, weight loss, low-grade fever, muscular weakness, or cyclical, progressive nature of symptoms should help the physical therapist to identify joint pain of a systemic nature.

Chronic Pain

Chronic pain is defined as pain lasting for more than 6 months without a known cause, although there are cases in which a diagnosis is finally made and appropriate treatment eradicates the pain. A constellation of life changes that produce altered behavior in the individual and that may persist even after the cause of the pain has been eradicated, are what make up the chronic pain syndrome (Zohn, 1988).

In acute pain, the pain is proportional and appropriate to the problem, whereas, in the chronic pain syndrome, the pain may be both intractable and inappropriate (i.e., exaggerated) to the existing problem. The syndrome is characterized by multiple complaints, excessive preoccupation with pain, and frequently, excessive drug use. The patient may live in a socially narrow world and exhibit altered behavior patterns, such as depression, neurosis, and anxiety. Secondary gain may be a factor in perpetuating the problem. This may be primarily financial, but social and family benefits, such as increased attention, avoidance of sex, and avoidance of unpleasant work situations may all enter into the situation (Zohn, 1988).

SYSTEMS REVIEW

Musculoskeletal symptoms accompany many systemic diseases. By using the interview format, a complete review of a patient's visceral systems should be undertaken, because cutaneous (skin) manifestations and joint pain may be the presenting feature of systemic disease such as systemic lupus erythematosus (SLE), scleroderma, dermatomyositis, Reiter's disease, progressive systemic sclerosis (PSS), and psoriatic arthritis. Symptoms of joint pain may be associated with and draw attention to acromegaly, pulmonary disease, and kidney diseases (Mennell, 1964).

Arthralgia (joint pain) may be associated with ulcerative colitis and Crohn's disease (regional enteritis). These diseases primarily involving the GI tract may begin with a disturbance of peripheral joints or spine (Rodnan and Schumacher, 1983).

General questions about fevers, excessive weight gain or loss, and appetite loss should be followed by questions related to specific organ systems. Questions about *rheumatologic* problems focus on the presence and location of joint swelling, muscle pains and weakness, skin rashes, reaction to sunlight, and Raynaud's phenomenon. Appropriate questions about *neurologic* problems deal with headaches, vision changes, vertigo, paresthesias, weakness, atrophy, and radicular pains. *Vascular* problems are identified by questions about claudication (limping), coldness of extremities, discoloration, and the patient's response to cold. *Psychologic* problems are elicited by questions about sleeping patterns, stress levels, and changes in personal habits. Questions about *GI* problems deal with abdominal pain, indigestion, nausea and vomiting, change in bowel habits, and rectal bleeding. *Genitourinary* problems are identified by questions about bleeding, burning, frequency, hesitation, nocturia (excessive urination at night), and dysuria (painful or difficult urination). *Endocrine* disturbances are discovered by questions about hair and nail changes, temperature intolerance, cramps, unexplained weakness, and edema. Questions about *pulmonary* problems might center on the presence of cough, sputum, and night sweats. *Gynecologic* problems are identified by questions about irregularity of menses, pain with menses, vaginal discharge, surgical procedures, birth histories, spotting, or bleeding (Zohn, 1988).

Vital signs, including blood pressure, temperature, and pulse must be taken to avoid overlooking a problem of systemic origin. In assessing pulses, a comparison should be made of their force on both sides of the body, as well as in various positions. Differences in the blood pressure between the limbs of each side may be a clue of vascular disease (Zohn, 1988). A difference of 10 mm Hg (increase or decrease) of the diastolic or systolic blood pressure with a position change should be considered suspect of systemic problems, especially when accompanied by associated symptoms, such as dizziness, headache, nausea, vomiting, diaphoresis (perspiration), heart palpitations, and increased primary pain or symptoms.

CLINICAL SIGNS AND SYMPTOMS OF SYSTEMIC PAIN

Onset:

- Recent, sudden
- Does not present as chronically observed for several years intermittently

Description:

- Knifelike quality stabbing from the inside out, boring, deep aching
- Cutting, gnawing
- Throbbing
- Bone pain
- Unilateral or bilateral

Intensity: Intensity is related to the degree of noxious stimuli

- Dull to severe
- Mild to severe

Duration:

- Constant, no change, awakens the patient at night

Pattern:

- Although constant, may come in waves
- Gradually progressive, cyclical
- Night pain, especially night pain relieved by aspirin* (characteristic of osteoid osteoma)

* Relief with aspirin in these cases demonstrates a greater effect than expected (i.e., the relief is out of proportion with the severity of pain felt by the patient).

- Symptoms unrelieved by rest or change in position
- Migratory arthralgias: pain/symptoms last for 1 week in one joint, then resolve and appear in another joint

Aggravating Factors:

- Depends on the organ involved (see individual chapters)

Relieving Factors:

- Usually none, but also depends on the specific problem
- If rest relieves the pain, there is usually a cyclical progression of increasing frequency, intensity, or duration of pain until rest is no longer a relieving factor

Associated Signs and Symptoms:

- Fever, chills
- Night sweats
- Unusual vital signs
- Warning signs of cancer (see Chapter 10)
- GI symptoms: nausea, vomiting, anorexia, unexplained weight loss, diarrhea, constipation
- Early satiety (feeling full after eating)
- Bilateral symptoms (e.g., paresthesias [abnormal sensation], weakness)
- Painless weakness of muscles: more often proximal, but may occur distally
- Dyspnea (breathlessness at rest or after mild exertion)
- Diaphoresis (excessive perspiration)
- Headaches, dizziness, fainting
- Visual disturbances
- Skin lesions, rashes, or itching that the patient may not associate with the musculoskeletal symptoms
- Bowel/bladder symptoms
    - Hematuria (blood in the urine)
    - Nocturia
    - Urgency (sudden need to urinate)
    - Frequency
    - Melena (blood in feces)
    - Fecal or urinary incontinence (inability to control bowels or urine)
    - Bowel smears

CLINICAL SIGNS AND SYMPTOMS OF MUSCULOSKELETAL PAIN
(Kirkaldy-Willis, 1983):

Onset: May be sudden or gradual depending on the history

- Sudden: Usually associated with acute overload stress, traumatic event, repetitive motion
- Gradual: Secondary to chronic overload of the affected part
  May be present off and on for a period of years

Description:

- Local tenderness to pressure is present
- Achy, cramping pain
- Stiff after rest
- Usually unilateral

Intensity:

- May be mild to severe
- May depend on the patient's anxiety level—if fearful of a "serious" condition, the level of pain may increase and often decreases with medical reassurance that the condition is not life-threatening

Duration:

- May be constant, but is more likely to be intermittent, depending on the activity or the position

Pattern:

- Restriction of active/passive/accessory movement observed

- One or more particular movements "catch" the patient and aggravate the pain

Aggravating Factors:

- Pain may become worse by movement (some myalgia decreases with movement)

Relieving Factors:

- Pain is relieved by short periods of rest without resulting stiffness
- Stretching

Associated Signs and Symptoms:

- Usually none, although stimulation of trigger points may cause sweating, nausea, blanching

Muscles may be responsible for pain in the areas that may also be focal points for pain of a systemic origin. The muscles most likely to refer pain to a given area are shown in Table 12–1 (Travell and Simons, 1983). For more specific information regarding examination of these muscles, the reader is referred to Travell and Simons listed in the references.

Table 12–1. TRIGGER POINT PAIN GUIDE*

Location	Potential Muscles Involved
Chest pain	Pectoralis major
	Pectoralis minor
	Scaleni
	Sternocleidomastoid (sternal)
	Sternalis
	Iliocostalis cervicis
	Subclavius
	External abdominal oblique
Side of chest pain	Serratus anterior
	Lattissimus
Low thoracic back pain	Iliocostalis thoracis
	Multifidi
	Serratus posterior inferior
	Rectus abdominis
	Lattissimus dorsi
Lumbar pain	Longissimus thoracis
	Iliocostalis lumborum
	Iliocostalis thoracis
	Multifidi
	Rectus abdominis
Sacral and gluteal pain	Longissimus thoracis
	Iliocostalis lumborum
	Multifidi
Abdominal pain	Rectus abdominis
	Abdominal obliques
	Transversus abdominis
	Iliocostalis thoracis
	Multifidi
	Pyramidalis

* Adapted from Travell, J.G., and Simons, D.G.: Myofascial Pain and Dysfunction: The Trigger Point Manual. Baltimore, Williams & Wilkins, 1983, p. 574.

BACK PAIN

Patients with complaints of back pain can be divided into two categories: patients whose back pain is a manifestation of an underlying systemic disorder (including those with a spondyloarthropathy, a disease of the joints of the spine) and those who would be entirely well if it were not for their back pain. The latter patient has a regional backache. Most episodes of backache are caused by regional (i.e., nonsystemic) disease (Hadler, 1984).

One clue to systemic back pain is that it is not relieved by recumbency. The bone pain of metastasis or myeloma tends to be more continuous, progressive, and prominent when recumbent. Systemic back pain may get worse at night with any of the following problems (Hadler, 1987):

- Vertebral osteomyelitis (inflammation of bone)
- Septic diskitis (inflammation of an intervertebral disk with toxins in the blood)
- Cushing's disease
- Osteomalacia (softening of the bones)
- Primary and metastatic cancer
- Paget's disease

Beware of the patient with an acute backache who refuses to lie still, because almost all patients with a regional backache seek the most comfortable position (usually recumbency) and stay in that position. In contrast, patients with systemic backache move. In particular, visceral diseases, such as pancreatic neoplasm, pancreatitis, and posterior penetrating ulcers, often present with a systemic backache that causes the patient to try to curl up. In cases of pancreatitis, the patient often takes a curled-up sitting position. Primary tumors of the spinal cord or its roots (notably cauda equina tumor) may also present as low back pain. Patients with these lesions try to sleep in a chair and often pace the floor at night. Some patients with systemic backache writhe; they may have had a vascular catastrophe, such as an abdominal aortic dissection or rupture of an abdominal aortic aneurysm (sac formed by dilatation of blood vessel) (Hadler, 1987).

If a patient has had a low backache for years, progressive, serious disease is unlikely. However, a month or two of increasing backache, often in an elderly patient, may be a signal of lumbar metastases. When back pain is accompanied by severe or chronic pain and fever, referral to a physician is necessary. Other possible associated symptoms may include fatigue, dyspnea, and sweating after only minor exertion, and GI symptoms (Cyriax, 1982). Clues suggesting systemic backache follow.*

- Age over 45 years
- Nocturnal back pain
- Back pain that causes writhing, prompts the patient to move about or curl up in the sitting position
- Back pain with constitutional symptoms: nausea, fatigue, vomiting, diarrhea, fever
- Back pain that is insidious in onset and progression
- Previous history of cancer
- Back and abdominal pain at the same level
- Sacral pain in the absence of history of trauma or overuse
- Elevated body temperature, night sweats, febrile chills
- Back pain that is unrelieved by recumbency
- Back pain that does not vary with exertion or activity
- Severe, persistent back pain with full and painless movement of the spine
- Severe back and lower extremity weakness without pain
- Back pain associated with meals

The therapist must be aware that many different diseases can present as low back pain.

The clues about the quality of pain, the age of the patient, and the presence of systemic complaints indicate the need to investigate further before determining that the patient is complaining of pain or symptoms associated with regional musculoskeletal back disease. The history and physical examination provide essential clues in determining the need for referral to a physician (Hadler, 1987).

Classifications of Back Pain

Visceral

Visceral back pain (Tables 12–2 and 12–3) is more likely to result from visceral disease in the abdomen and pelvis than from intrathoracic disease (Hall, 1983). Visceral back pain is not very often confused with pain originating in the spine, because usually sufficient specific symptoms and signs are present to localize the problem correctly. For example, pancreatic carcinoma can cause severe and persistent back pain. However, this lesion causes other problems that turn attention away from the spine. When pain is referred to the back from an intra-abdominal or pelvic viscus (organs in the pelvis and abdomen), the outstanding finding is a full and painless range of movement at the lumbar spine. This finding focuses attention on the nonmoving parts of the body: the kidney, colon, ovary, uterus, and rectum.

Back pain associated with perforation of organs, gynecologic conditions, or gastroenterologic disease seldom mimics "typical back pain" because of the history, associated symptoms, and lack of accompanying objective findings to support a musculoskeletal origin of

* This list is compiled based on Hadler, NM: The patient with low back pain. Hosp. Pract., Oct. 30, 1987, and Mennell, J.M.: Handout provided during his course, May 1986.

Table 12–2. VISCEROGENIC CAUSES OF NECK AND BACK PAIN

Cervical	Thoracic/Scapula	Lumbar	Sacroiliac (SI)/Sacrum
Tracheobronchial irritation	Pleuropulmonary disorders	Metastatic lesions	Prostatitis/cancer
Primary bone tumors (benign or malignant)	Peptic ulcer	Kidney disorders	Gynecologic disorders
Cervical cord tumors	Pancreatic cancer	Pyelonephritis	
Spinal metastases	Pancreatitis	Perinephric abscess	
	Gallbladder	Nephrolithiasis	
	Cholecystitis	UTI	
	Biliary colic	Prostatitis/cancer	
	Pyelonephritis	Abdominal aortic aneurysm	
	Kidney disease	Acute pancreatitis	
	Mediastinal tumors	Small intestine	
	Aortic aneurysm	Obstruction(neoplasm)	
	Esophagitis (severe)	Irritable bowel syndrome	
	Myocardial infarct	Crohn's disease (regional enteritis)	
		Gynecologic disorders	
		Tuberculosis	

pain. For example, low back pain of mechanical spondylitic origin is normally relieved by rest, whereas lesions in solid or hollow viscera are not relieved in this way (Cyriax, 1982; Wedge, 1983).

Neurogenic

Neurogenic back pain is not as easily differentiated. A serious delay in diagnosis can result from failure to appreciate the fact that neoplasms of the cord and cauda equina can mimic spondylogenic pain. Diabetic neuropathy can cause nerve root irritation. A clinical picture that is indistinguishable from sciatica can result, and this similarity may lead to long and serious delays in diagnosis (Wedge, 1983). Such a situation may require persistence upon the part of the therapist and patient in requesting further medical follow-up.

Vasculogenic

The symptoms of vasculogenic back pain may be mistaken for those of a wide variety of musculoskeletal, neurologic, and arthritic dis-

Table 12–3. SYSTEMIC CAUSES OF THORACIC/SCAPULAR PAIN

Systemic Origin	Location
Gallbladder disease	Midback between scapula
Acute cholecystitis	Right subscapular area
Peptic ulcer: stomach/duodenal ulcers	5th–10th thoracic vertebrae
Pleuropulmonary disorders	
Basilar pneumonia	Right upper back
Empyema	Scapula
Pleurisy	Scapula
Spontaneous pneumothorax	Ipsilateral scapula
Pancreatic carcinoma	Middle thoracic or lumbar spine
Acute pyelonephritis	Costovertebral angle (posteriorly)
Esophagitis	Midback between scapula
Myocardial infarct	Midthoracic spine
Biliary colic	Right upper back; midback between scapula; right interscapular or subscapular areas

orders. Conversely, the diagnosed presence of vascular impairment of a minor degree may direct attention away from a primary disorder that originates elsewhere. Such disorders include low back pain of musculoskeletal origin, nerve root compression, spinal cord tumor, arthritis of the hip, or peripheral neuritis (Zohn and Mennell, 1988).

The location of vasculogenic pain depends on the location of the vascular pathology (Zohn and Mennell, 1988). Gradual *obstruction of the aortic bifurcation* produces:

- Bilateral buttock and leg pain
- Weakness and fatigue of the lower extremities
- Atrophy of the leg musculature
- Absent femoral pulses
- Color and temperature changes in the lower extremities

When the pathology is in the *iliac artery* symptoms may include:

- Pain in the low back, buttock, and leg of the affected side
- Numbness

Involvement of the *femoral artery,* along its course or at the femoropopliteal junction, produces:

- Thigh and calf pain
- Pulses absent below femoral pulse

Obstruction of the *popliteal artery* or its branches produces:

- Pain in the calf, ankle, or foot

PVD with claudication can be confused with neurogenic claudication and spinal stenosis (narrowing of the vertebral canal) (Table 12–4). The major difference in the clinical features is the response of pain to rest and the position of the spine. The medical diagnosis is difficult to make, because vascular and neurogenic claudication occur in approximately the same age group and can coexist. Vascular studies and myelography may be required to help determine which problem dominates (Zohn, 1988).

Although spinal stenosis is not a vasculogenic cause of back pain, it is included to assist the reader in comparing back pain and symptoms caused by vasculogenic causes versus neurogenic causes versus spinal stenosis. Spinal stenosis is caused by a narrowing of the spinal canal, nerve root canals, or intervertebral foramina. The canal tends to be narrow at the lumbosacral junction, and any combination of degenerative changes, such as disk protrusion, osteophyte formation, or ligamentous thickening, reduces the space needed for the spinal cord and its nerve roots (Hall, 1983).

Psychogenic

Psychogenic back pain is observed in the hysterical patient or in patients who have extreme anxiety that increases the person's perception of pain. The hysterical patient has severe pain as a product of inadequate defense mechanisms or severe anxiety. The anxiety leads to muscle tension, more anxiety, and then to muscle spasm. In either situation, look for bizarre signs such as:

- Paraplegia with only stocking glove anesthesia
- Reflexes inconsistent with the presenting problem or other symptoms present
- Cogwheel motion of muscles for weakness
- Straight leg raising (SLR) in the sitting versus the supine position (patient is unable to complete SLR in supine, but can easily perform an SLR in a sitting position)
- SLR supine with plantar flexion instead of dorsiflexion reproduces symptoms

Spondylogenic

Spondylogenic back pain (or the symptoms produced by bone lesions) is relatively limited in nature and quality, although the conditions producing these symptoms are numerous. The age of the patient, character of the pain, weight loss, fever, deformity, and bone tenderness are most helpful to the physician in making the correct diagnosis. *Multiple myeloma* is the most common malignant primary bone tumor, and early in its course it can easily be overlooked as the cause of back pain. The

Table 12–4. SYMPTOMS AND DIFFERENTIATION OF CLAUDICATION

Vascular Claudication	Neurogenic Claudication	Spinal Stenosis
Pain* is usually bilateral	Pain is usually bilateral, but may be unilateral	Usually bilateral pain
Occurs in the calf (foot, thigh, hip, or buttocks)	Occurs in back, buttocks, thighs, calves, feet	Occurs in back, buttocks, thighs, calves, feet
Pain consistent in all spinal positions	Pain decreased in spinal flexion Pain increased in spinal extension	Pain decreased in spinal flexion Pain increased in spinal extension
Pain brought on by physical exertion (e.g., walking)	Pain increased with walking	Pain increased with walking
Pain relieved promptly by rest (1–5 min)	Pain decreased by recumbency	Pain relieved with prolonged rest (may persist hours after resting)
Pain increased by walking uphill		Pain decreased when walking uphill
No burning or dysesthesia	Burning and dysesthesia from the back to the buttocks and leg(s)	Burning and numbness present in lower extremities
Decreased or absent pulses in lower extremities	Normal pulses	Normal pulses
Color and skin changes in feet Cold, numb, dry, or scaly skin Poor nail and hair growth	Good skin nutrition	Good skin nutrition
Affects ages from 40 to over 60	Affects ages from 40 to over 60	Peaks in seventh decade Affects men primarily

* "Pain" associated with vascular claudication may also be described as an "aching," "cramping," or "tired" feeling.

complaints may be nonspecific, but the general lack of well-being is an indicator of the need for medical referral.

Secondary Cancer

Secondary cancer from the breast, thyroid, lung, kidney, and prostate can present as back pain. The first suggestion of malignant disease lies in the history, which is not of pain varying with exertion but of steady aggravation irrespective of activity. This distinguishing feature is one of unrelenting, intense, and progressive nature of the back pain (Wedge, 1983).

A short period of increasing central backache in the elderly is always suspect. The pain then spreads down both lower limbs in a distribution that does not correspond with any one root. Bilateral sciatica then appears, and the backache becomes worse. Severe weakness without pain is very suggestive of spinal metastases. Gross muscle weakness with a full range of SLR and without a history of recent acute sciatica at the upper two lumbar levels is also suggestive of *spinal metastases* (Cyriax, 1982).

Neoplasm (whether primary or secondary) may interfere with the sympathetic nerves; if so, the foot on the affected side is warmer than the foot on the unaffected side. It is more difficult to detect sacral neoplasm than lower lumbar metastasis, because the spinal joints retain a full and painless range of movement. The patient complains of sacral pain, sometimes of coccygodynia (pain in the coccyx) only. Paresis of the gross muscles of one or both feet in the absence of root pain suggests a tumor. The patient looks anxious and fatigued and is often desperate for relief. Back pain due to degenerative joint disease is seldom, if ever, unrelenting and usually responds to bed rest. The patient's past medical history regarding previous cancer must be obtained. Removal of a breast due to primary cancer may seem so remote from the present symptoms that the patient may not volunteer this essential information (Cyriax, 1982; Wedge, 1983).

Osteoid osteoma (benign blood-filled tumor of cortical bone; osteoblastoma) of the spine may not present with the characteristic history of night pain relieved by aspirin. Hamstring spasm with marked limitation of SLR is often found with osteoid osteoma of the lumbar spine, causing further confusion.

Osteoporosis (decreased mass of bone) can result in compression fractures. The acute pain of a compression fracture superimposed on chronic discomfort, often in the absence of a history of trauma, may be the only presenting symptom. The patient may recall a "snap" associated with mild back pain that occurred when bending over to pick up a small object. More intense pain may not develop for hours or until the next day (Wedge, 1983).

Vertebral osteomyelitis (bone infection) as a cause of low back pain may occur in diabetics, drug addicts, alcoholics, patients on corticosteroid drugs, and otherwise debilitated patients. There may be no rise in temperature or abnormality in white blood cell count, although an elevated erythrocyte sedimentation rate is likely. The most constant clinical finding is marked tenderness over the spinous process of the involved vertebrae.

Rheumatic diseases, such as ankylosing spondylitis, Reiter's syndrome, psoriatic arthritis, or arthritis associated with chronic inflammatory bowel disease, may present with back and sacroiliac joint pain. Each of these clinical entities has been discussed in detail in Chapter 11. The most significant finding in ankylosing spondylitis is that the patient presents with night (back) pain and morning stiffness as the two major complaints, but asymmetric sacroiliac involvement with radiation into the buttock and thigh can occur (Wedge, 1983). In addition to back pain, these rheumatic diseases usually include a constellation of associated signs and symptoms, such as fever, skin lesions, anorexia, and weight loss to alert the physical therapist to the presence of systemic disease.

Cushing's syndrome occurs as a result of large doses of cortisol in some patients. Patients with Cushing's syndrome of long duration will almost always demonstrate demineralization of bone. In severe cases, this may lead to pathologic fractures, but more commonly results in wedging of the vertebrae, kyphosis, bone pain, and back pain (secondary to bone loss).

Cervical (D'Ambrosia, 1986)

Tracheobronchial pain can be referred to sites in the neck or anterior chest at the same levels as the points of irritation in the air passages (see Fig. 4–6). This irritation may be caused by inflammatory lesions, irritating foreign materials, or cancerous tumors (Bauwens and Paine, 1983).

Tumors of the adult cervical spine may be primary, arising from the bone, or secondary (i.e., metastatic from a distant primary site) (see Table 12–2). Tumors of the cervical cord may cause neck pain. These tumors may be primary, metastatic, extramedullary, or intramedullary. Pain of insidious onset, with or without neurologic signs and symptoms (e.g., progressive leg weakness, bladder paralysis, and sensory loss), may occur.

The presenting symptom of metastatic tumor to the cervical spine is pain that is constant, persistent through the night, and usually not relieved by rest. There may be a palpable external mass and pain on motion of the cervical spine. With progressive vertebral body collapse, bone may protrude into the spinal canal, compressing the anterior spinal cord surface and producing paralysis.

Primary tumors of the cervical spine may be benign or malignant. The most common benign tumors of adults are osteochondromas, osteoblastomas, aneurysmal bone cysts, chondromes, osteoid osteoma, and hemangiomas (benign blood-filled tumor). The most common malignant tumors are osteogenic sarcoma, giant cell tumor, and chordoma.

Thoracic (D'Ambrosia, 1986)

Systemic origins of musculoskeletal pain in the thoracic spine (see Table 12–2) are usually accompanied by constitutional symptoms (affecting the whole body, systemic) and other associated symptoms that the patient may not relate to the back pain, and, therefore, may fail to mention to the physical therapist. Such additional symptoms should be discovered during the subjective examination by the careful interviewer. When the patient (or the objective examination) indicates the presence of a fever (or night sweats), a referral to a physician is indicated.

The close proximity of the thoracic spine to the chest and respiratory organs may result in a correlation between respiratory movements and increased thoracic symptoms. This situation requires careful screening of *pleuropulmonary* (involving the pleura and the lungs) symptoms. When screening the patient through the physical therapy interview, the physical therapist should remember that symptoms of pleural, intercostal muscular, costal, and dural origin all increase on coughing or deep inspiration; thus, only pain of a cardiac origin is ruled out when symptoms increase in association with respiratory movements (Cyriax, 1982).

Peptic Ulcer

The pain of peptic ulcer occasionally occurs only in the back between the eighth and tenth thoracic vertebrae. Duodenal ulcers may refer pain from the fifth to tenth thoracic vertebrae, either at the midline or just to one side of the spine (may be either side). This localization may accompany penetration through the viscera (organs). The patient usually describes a typical history of ulcers with periodic symptoms, relief with antacids, and the relationship of pain to certain foods and the timing of meals. For example, the patient may have relief from pain after eating initially, but the pain then returns and increases 1 to 2 hours after eating when the stomach is emptied. When questioned further, the patient may indicate that blood is present in the feces.

Pancreatic Carcinoma

In pancreatic carcinoma, the most frequent symptom is pain. It can be first noted as a paroxysmal or steady dull pain radiating from the epigastrium into the back. The pain is usually slowly progressive, is worse at night, and is unrelated to digestive activities. Other signs and symptoms may include jaundice, anorexia, severe weight loss, and GI difficulties but unrelated to meals. This disease is predominantly found in men (3 : 1) and occurs in the sixth and seventh decades.

Acute Cholecystitis

Acute cholecystitis (gallbladder infection) may refer intense, sudden, paroxysmal (sudden, recurrent or intensifying) pain to the right upper quadrant of the back with muscle guarding. This muscle guarding causes tenderness, pain, and biomechanical disturbances that further increase the patient's pain. Fever and chills are common associated symptoms.

Biliary Colic

The pain of biliary colic (bile duct obstruction that may be caused by various disorders, including stones, stricture, pancreatic carcinoma, and primary biliary cirrhosis) refers pain to the right upper quadrant, posteriorly with pain in the right shoulder. There may be back pain between the scapulae with referred pain to the right side in the interscapular or subscapular area. Occasionally, the pain beneath the right costal margin may be confused with the shoulder girdle pain secondary to intracostal nerve compression.

Acute Pyelonephritis

Acute pyelonephritis (inflammation of the kidney and renal pelvis) and other kidney conditions present with aching pain at one or several costovertebral areas, posteriorly with radiation to the pelvic crest or groin possible. The patient may describe febrile chills, frequent urination, hematuria, and shoulder pain (if the diaphragm is irritated). Percussion to the flank areas reveals tenderness.

Mediastinal Tumors

Mediastinal tumors or an aortic aneurysm may refer pain to the thoracic spine, but the pain is agonizing and is disproportionate to any musculoskeletal problem. In the case of neoplasm, the patient may report symptoms typical of cancer (see Chapter 10); with aortic aneurysms, there may be a history of cardiac involvement. Tumors occur most often in the thoracic spine because of its length, the proximity to the mediastinum, and the proximity to direct metastatic extension from lymph nodes involved with lymphoma, breast, or lung cancer.

Severe Esophagitis

Severe esophagitis may refer pain to the thoracic spine. This referred pain is always accompanied by epigastric pain and heartburn. The patient may be an alcoholic and have esophageal varices (distention of veins in lower esophagus) in association with the esophagitis.

Myocardial Infarction

The pain of an acute myocardial infarction ("heart attack") may radiate into the thoracic spine area. It is accompanied usually by a crushing, compressing pain or a sensation across the chest with an associated cold sweat, weak blood pressure, and thready pulse.

Scapula (see Table 12–3)

Most causes of scapular pain occur along the vertebral border and result from various primary musculoskeletal lesions. However, any respiratory viral infection or pulmonary disorders, such as empyema (pus in the pleural cavity), pleurisy (inflammation of the pleura), or spontaneous pneumothorax (air in the pleural cavity) can cause scapular pain. Patients with these pulmonary or respiratory origins of pain usually also show signs of general malaise and associated symptoms related to the pulmonary system. Gallbladder disease and biliary colic from other causes may also refer pain to the interscapular or subscapular areas. Specific questions should be asked to rule out potential pulmonary or GI problems because the patient may not associate such signs and symptoms with scapular pain.

Patients presenting with a pneumothorax develop acute pleuritic chest pain localized to the side of the pneumothorax. This pain may be referred to the ipsilateral scapula or shoulder, across the chest, or over the abdomen (see Fig. 4–5); associated symptoms may include dyspnea, cough, hemoptysis (blood in sputum), tachycardia (increased heart rate), tachypnea (rapid respirations), and cyanosis (blue lips and skin due to a lack of oxygen). The patient may have severe pain in the upper and lateral thoracic wall, which is aggravated by any movement and by the cough and dyspnea that accompany it (Bauwens and Paine, 1983). The patient may be most comfortable sitting in an upright position.

Lumbar (Low Back Pain) (see Table 12–2)

Metastatic Lesions

Metastatic lesions affecting the lumbar spine occur most commonly from the ovary, breast, kidney, lung, or prostate gland. Cancer of the prostate is the second most common site of cancer among men and is often diagnosed when the man seeks medical assistance because of symptoms of urinary obstruction or sciatica. The sciatic (low back, hip and leg) pain is caused by metastasis of the cancer to the bones of the pelvis, lumbar spine, or femur.

Kidney Disorders

Kidney disorders, such as acute pyelonephritis or perinephric abscess of the kidney, may be confused with a back condition. Most renal and urologic conditions present with a combination of systemic signs and symptoms accompanied by either pelvic, flank, or low back pain. The patient may have a history of recent trauma or a past medical history of urinary tract infections (UTIs) to alert the clinician to possible systemic origin of symptoms. In *pyelonephritis,* an aching pain is noted in one or both costovertebral areas. The patient usually has a fever and shaking chills. The flank areas are tender to percussion.

Nephrolithiasis (kidney stones) may present as back pain radiating to the flank or to the iliac crest. These stones are subsequently passed through the ureters to the bladder and then through the urethra. They are usually due to the precipitation of calcium salts, but can be urate salts, cystine (amino acid), or rarely xanthine (purine compound). The calcium-containing variety most often occurs with diseases associated with hypercalcemia (excess calcium in the blood), such as hyperparathyroidism, metastatic carcinoma, multiple myeloma, senile osteoporosis, specific renal tubular disease, hyperthyroidism, and Cushing's disease. Other conditions associated with calculus formation are infection, urinary stasis, dehydration, and excessive ingestion or absorption of calcium. Urate crystals are associated with gouty conditions and hyperuricemia (excess uric acid in blood)(D'Ambrosia, 1986). The focal symptoms of nephrolithiasis are characterized by back pain radiating to the flank or iliac crest (see Fig. 7–3).

Ureteral colic caused by passage of a calculus (kidney stone) presents as an excruciating pain that radiates down the course of the ureter into the urethra or groin area. These attacks are intermittent and can be accompanied by nausea, vomiting, sweating, and tachycardia. The urine usually contains erythrocytes or is grossly bloody (D'Ambrosia, 1986).

UTI affecting the lower urinary tract is related directly to irritation of the bladder and urethra. The intensity of symptoms depends on the severity of the infection, and although low back pain may be the patient's chief complaint, further questioning usually elicits additional urologic symptoms, such as urinary frequency, urinary urgency, dysuria, or hematuria. Patients can be asymptomatic with regard to urologic symptoms and a medical work-up will be necessary for making the diagnosis.

Prostatitis

Prostatitis or prostate cancer can cause low back, pelvic, and sciatic pain. Associated symptoms include melena (blood in stool), sudden moderate-to-high fever, chills, and changes in bowel function. Men from the fifth decade on are most commonly affected.

Abdominal Aortic Aneurysm

On occasion, an abdominal aortic aneurysm can cause severe back pain. Prompt medical attention is imperative because rupture can result in death. The patients are usually men in the sixth or seventh decade of life who present with a deep, boring pain in the midlumbar region. Other historical clues of coronary disease or intermittent claudication of the lower extremities may be present. An objective examination may reveal a pulsing abdominal mass. Peripheral pulses may be diminished or absent (D'Ambrosia, 1986).

Acute Pancreatitis

The pain of acute pancreatitis may radiate into the midback to low back. Usually the pain originates in the epigastrium; it is sudden, severe, and widespread. Associated symptoms are related primarily to the GI system, including diarrhea, pain after a meal, anorexia, and unexplained weight loss. The pain is relieved initially by heat, which decreases muscular tension and may be relieved by leaning forward, sitting up, or lying still and motionless (D'Ambrosia, 1986).

Diseases of the Small Intestine

Diseases of the small intestine, such as Crohn's disease (regional enteritis), irritable bowel syndrome, or obstruction (neoplasm) usually produce abdominal pain, but the pain may be referred to the back if the stimulus is sufficiently intense or if the individual's pain threshold is low. There will almost always be accompanying GI symptoms to alert the careful examiner.

Gynecologic Disorders

Gynecologic disorders can cause midpelvic or low back discomfort. These conditions can include:

- Retroversion (tipping back) of the uterus
- Ovarian cysts
- Uterine fibroids (fibrous connective tissue)
- Endometriosis (uterine lining attaches to pelvic cavity and organs therein)
- Pelvic inflammatory disease (PID)
- Cystocele (herniation of the urinary bladder into the vagina)
- Rectocele (hernial protrusion of part of the rectum into the vagina)

The woman may have sharp, bilateral, and cramping pain in the lower quadrants. These conditions are most common in women aged 20 to 45 years. A diagnosis of pelvic disorders in the woman is made by careful pelvic examination by the physician and should be included in all complete back work-ups, because these conditions can be confused with ruptured appendix, ectopic pregnancy (fertilized ovum implants outside the uterus), or perforation of GI abscesses. The physical therapist is encouraged to ask appropriate questions to determine the need for a gynecologic evaluation (see *Special Questions for Women* in this chapter), especially in the absence of objective musculoskeletal findings (D'Ambrosia, 1986).

ASSOCIATED SYMPTOMS OF GYNECOLOGIC DISORDERS

- Missed menses, irregular menses, history of menstrual disturbances
- Tender breasts
- Nausea, vomiting
- Chronic constipation (with laxative and enema dependency)
- Pain on defecation
- Fever, night sweats, chills
- History of vaginal discharge
- Abnormal uterine bleeding
  - Late menstrual periods with persistent bleeding
  - Irregular, longer, heavier menstrual periods, no specific pattern

The patient may reveal rectum and lower sacral or coccygeal pain that can be referred menstrual pain. There may be a history of sexually transmitted disease, ectopic pregnancy, use of an intrauterine device (IUD), dysuria, or a recent abortion. With a cystocele or a rectocele, there may be a history of multiparity (woman who has had two or more pregnancies resulting in viable offspring), prolonged labor, instrument delivery, chronic cough, or lifting heavy objects.

Tumors, masses, and even endometriosis may involve the sacral plexus or its branches, causing severe, burning pain that is sciatic in nature. Multiple roots are usually involved, and the pain is of a severe, burning nature (D'Ambrosia, 1986).

Tuberculosis

Tuberculosis most commonly affects the lower thoracic vertebrae at the level of the kidney. There may be a history of previous lymph or pulmonary infection or a positive family history for tuberculosis. The tuberculosis bacilli spread through the bloodstream with the following musculoskeletal findings (D'Ambrosia, 1986).

- Kyphosis secondary to the destruction of vertebral bodies (especially the thoracolumbar junction)
- Spasticity or paraplegia may occur if abscess or bone impingement puts pressure on the cord
- Low-grade fever, pallor
- Local back pain aggravated by movement
- Listlessness, muscle atrophy
- Night pain

Sacroiliac Joint/Sacrum

The most typical pain referral patterns of systemic disease to the sacrum and sacroiliac joint include *prostatitis, prostate cancer,* and *gynecologic disorders.* These specific disorders also refer pain to the lumbar spine and have already been discussed in that section. Disorders of the large intestine and colon, such as ulcerative colitis, Crohn's disease (regional enteritis), carcinoma of the colon, and the irritable bowel syndrome can refer pain to the sacrum when the rectum is stimulated.

Most commonly, unless pain causes muscle spasm, splinting, and subsequent biomechanical changes, these patients demonstrate a remarkable lack of objective findings to implicate the sacroiliac or sacrum as the causative factor in the symptoms presented. Mennell (see Table 12–2) suggests that sacral pain in the absence of history of trauma or overuse is a clue to the presentation of systemic backache. Pain elicited by pressing on the sacrum with the patient in a prone position suggests sacroiliitis (inflammation of the sacroiliac joint) (Hadler, 1987).

Spondyloarthropathies

Spondyloarthropathies, representing a group of noninfected, inflammatory, erosive rheumatic diseases, target the sacroiliac joints. Sacroiliac and back pain are present in patients who have ankylosing spondylitis, Reiter's syndrome, psoriatic arthritis, or arthritis associated with chronic inflammatory bowel disease. Each of these disorders is characterized by additional systemic signs and symptoms fully discussed in this text, which should be discovered by the careful interviewer. Such findings will assist the physical therapist in determining the need for further medical follow-up.

Paget's Disease

Paget's disease (osteitis deformans) is a metabolic bone disorder characterized by slowly progressive enlargement and deformity of multiple bones associated with unexplained acceleration of both deposition and resorption of bone that causes the bones to become spongelike, weakened, and deformed. The bones most commonly involved are the pelvis, lumbar spine, and sacrum. Although this disorder is often asymptomatic, when symptoms do occur, they occur insidiously and may include deep, aching bone pain, nocturnal pain, joint stiffness, fatigue, headaches, and dizziness, increased temperature over the long bones, and periosteal tenderness.

SUBJECTIVE EXAMINATION

Special Questions to Ask: Back

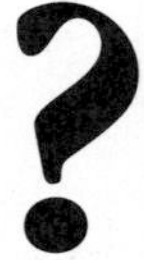

- ☐ When did the pain or symptoms start?
- ☐ Did it start gradually or suddenly? **(Vascular versus trauma problem)**
- ☐ Was there an illness or injury before the onset of pain?
- ☐ Have you noticed any changes in your symptoms since they first started up to the present time?
- ☐ Is the pain aggravated or relieved by coughing or sneezing? **(Nerve root involvement, muscular)**
- ☐ Is the pain aggravated or relieved by activity?
- ☐ Are there any particular positions (sitting, lying, standing) that aggravate or relieve the pain?
- ☐ Does the pain radiate down the leg? If so, where?
- ☐ Have you noticed any muscular weakness?
- ☐ Have you had a fever, chills, or burning with urination during the last 3 to 4 weeks?
- ☐ Have you been treated previously for back disorders?
- ☐ How has your general health been both before the beginning of your back problem and now today?
- ☐ How does rest affect the pain or symptoms?
- ☐ Do you feel worse in the morning or evening . . . **OR** . . . what difference do you notice in your symptoms from the morning when you first wake up, until the evening when you go to bed?
- ☐ Do you ever have swollen feet or ankles? If yes, are they swollen when you get up in the morning? **(Edema/congestive heart failure)**
- ☐ Do you ever get cramps in your legs if you walk for several blocks? **(Intermittent claudication)**

General Systemic

Most of these questions may be asked of patients with pain or symptoms anywhere in the musculoskeletal system.

- ☐ Have you ever been told that you have osteoporosis or brittle bones, fractures, back problems? **(Wasting of bone matrix in Cushing's syndrome)**
- ☐ Have you ever been diagnosed or treated for cancer in any part of your body?
- ☐ Do you ever notice sweating, nausea, or chest pains when your current symptoms occur?

Subjective Exam

Special Questions to Ask

□ What other symptoms have you had with this problem? For example, state whether you have had any:

Numbness
Burning, tingling
Nausea, vomiting
Loss of appetite
Unexpected (significant = 10 or 15 lb) weight gain or loss
Diarrhea, constipation, blood in your stool or urine
Difficulty in starting the flow of urine or incontinence (inability to hold your urine)
Hoarseness or difficulty in swallowing
Heart palpitations or fluttering
Difficulty in breathing while just sitting or resting or with mild effort (e.g., when walking from the car to the house)
Unexplained sweating or perspiration
Night sweats, fever, chills
Changes in vision: blurred vision, black spots, double vision, temporary blindness
Fatigue, weakness, sudden paralysis of one side of your body, arm, or leg **(TIA)**
Headaches
Dizziness or fainting spells

Gastrointestinal

□ Have you noticed any association between when you eat and when your symptoms increase or decrease?

Do you notice any change in your symptoms 1 to 3 hours after you eat?

Do you notice any epigastric (beneath the breastbone) or subscapular (just beneath the wing bone) pain 1 to 2 hours after eating?

□ Do you have a feeling of fullness after only one or two bites of food?

□ Is your back pain relieved after having a bowel movement? **(GI obstruction)**

□ Do you have rectal, low back, or sacroiliac pain when passing stool or having a bowel movement?

□ Do you have frequent heartburn or take antacids to relieve heartburn or acid indigestion?

Urology

□ Have you noticed any changes in your bowel movement or in the flow of urine since your back/groin pain started?

Subjective Exam

Special Questions to Ask

If no, it may be necessary to provide prompts or examples of what changes you are referring to (e.g., difficulty in starting or stopping the flow of urine, numbness, or tingling in the groin or pelvis)

□ Have you had burning with urination during the last 3 to 4 weeks?

□ Do you ever have blood in your stool or notice blood in the toilet after having a bowel movement? **(Hemorrhoids, prostate problems, cancer)**

□ Do you have any problems with your kidneys or bladder? If so, please describe.

□ Have you ever had kidney or bladder stones? If so, how were these stones treated?

□ Have you ever had an injury to your bladder or to your kidneys? If so, how was this treated?

□ Have you had any infections of the bladder, and how were these infections treated?

Were they related to any specific circumstances (e.g., pregnancy, intercourse)?

□ Have you had any kidney infections, and how were these treated?

Were they related to any specific circumstances (e.g., pregnancy, after bladder infections, a strep throat, or strep skin infections)?

□ Do you ever have a pain, discomfort, or a burning sensation when you urinate? **(Lower urinary tract irritation)**

□ Have you noticed any blood in your urine?

Special Questions for Women (experiencing low back, hip, groin, or SI pain/symptoms):

□ Since your back/SI, or other type of pain or symptoms started, have you seen a gynecologist to rule out any gynecologic cause of this problem?

□ Are you pregnant or have you recently terminated a pregnancy either by miscarriage or abortion?

□ Have you ever been pregnant?

If yes, how many pregnancies have you had?

Were these vaginally or by cesarian (C) section?

Did you have any significant medical problems during your pregnancy or delivery?

□ When was your last menstrual period?

□ Is the backache associated with your menstrual cycle either around the 14th day (ovulation) or at the onset of menses?

□ Where were you in your menstrual cycle when your injury or illness occurred?

Subjective Exam

Special Questions to Ask

□ Are you taking birth control pills?

If yes, how long have you been taking these pills?

□ Do you use an IUD?

□ Do you have any unusual discharge from your vagina?

If yes, do you know what is causing this discharge?

How long have you had this problem?

What color is this discharge?

How often do you notice this discharge (constant versus intermittent)?

□ Do you have any premenstrual symptoms (e.g., water retention, mood changes including depression, headaches, food cravings, painful or tender breasts)?

If yes, describe:

□ State whether you have ever been told that you have:

Retroversion of the uterus (tipped back)
Ovarian cysts
Fibroids or tumors
Endometriosis
Pelvic inflammatory disease
Cystocele (sagging bladder)
Rectocele (sagging rectum)

Special Questions for Men (experiencing low back, hip, groin, or SI pain/symptoms):

□ Do you ever have difficulty with urination (e.g., difficulty with starting or continuing flow/slow flow)?

□ Do you ever have blood in your urine?

□ Do you ever have pain on urination?

□ Have you ever been treated for a prostate problem? If so, how long ago and what was the treatment?

□ Have you ever been told that you have a hernia, or do you think that you have a hernia?

Special Questions to Ask: Sacroiliac/Sacrum

Follow the same format as for *Special Questions for Back Patients* with particular emphasis on gynecologic (for women) and urologic questions for both men and women.

CHEST PAIN (Rodnan and Schumacher, 1983; Strauss, 1984)

Musculoskeletal causes of chest (wall) pain must be differentiated from pain of cardiac, pulmonary, epigastric, and breast origins (Table 12–5) before physical therapy treatment begins. Tietze's syndrome, costochondritis, the hypersensitive xiphoid, and the syndrome of the slipping rib must be differentiated from problems involving the thoracic viscera, particularly those of the heart, great vessels, mediastinum as well as from illness originating in the head, neck, or abdomen.

Table 12–5. CAUSES OF CHEST PAIN

Systemic Causes	Musculoskeletal Causes
Pulmonary	Tietze's syndrome
Pulmonary embolism	Costochondritis
Spontaneous pneumothorax	Hypersensitive xiphoid
	Slipping rib syndrome
	Trigger points
Cardiac	Myalgia
Myocardial ischemia (angina)	Thoracic outlet syndrome
	Rib fracture
Pericarditis	
Myocardial infarct	
Dissecting aortic aneurysm	
Epigastric/Upper Gastrointestinal	
Esophagitis	
Upper GI ulcer	
Breast	
Breast tumor	
Abscess	
Mastitis	
Lactation problems	
Other	
Rheumatic disease	

Because of the potentially confusing nature of chest pain, this is the only section in which musculoskeletal causes of pain are discussed. Whereas the musculoskeletal causes of back, scapula, hip, shoulder, and sacrum/sacroiliac are well addressed in other texts, it has been our experience that this information (as it relates to the chest) is not readily available. Understanding both the systemic and musculoskeletal causes of chest pain or symptoms is essential when determining the need for medical referral.

Musculoskeletal Causes (Rodnan and Schumacher, 1983)

Tietze's Syndrome

According to Zohn (1988), medical literature overstresses the importance of a condition called *Tietze's syndrome* in discussion of anterior chest wall pain. The symptoms are localized to the second, third, and fourth costochondral junctions, and the syndrome is associated with increased blood pressure, increased heart rate, and pain radiating down the left arm. This syndrome's symptoms are very similar to those of a heart attack, except for the raised blood pressure (Zohn, 1988).

The terms Tietze's syndrome and costochondritis are often used interchangeably. Although both disorders are characterized by inflammation of one or more costal cartilages, Tietze's syndrome is associated with notable local swelling, whereas costochondritis is not. *Costochondritis* can be similar to muscular pain and is elicited by pressure over the costochondral junctions. Costochondritis is more common than Tietze's syndrome. In most cases, the cause of Tietze's syndrome is unknown and occurs in all age groups, including children, with a predilection for the second and third decades.

Approximately 80% of patients have only single sites of involvement, most commonly the second or third costal cartilage. Costochondritis (inflammation of rib and its cartilage; costal chondritis), also known as the anterior chest wall syndrome, the costosternal syndrome, and parasternal chondrodynia (pain in a cartilage), is characterized by pain of the anterior chest wall that may radiate widely, thus simulating intrathoracic or intra-abdominal disease. Costochondritis may follow trauma or may be associated with systemic rheumatic disease. Palpation of the affected portion of the thoracic cage elicits tenderness. Inflammation of upper costal cartilages may cause annoying chest pain, whereas inflammation of lower costal cartilages may cause abdominal discomfort.

CLINICAL MANIFESTATIONS OF TIETZE'S SYNDROME OR COSTOCHONDRITIS

- Sudden or gradual onset of upper anterior chest pain
- Bulbous swelling of the involved costal cartilage (Tietze's syndrome)
- Mild-to-severe chest pain that may radiate to the shoulder and arm
- Pain is aggravated by sneezing, coughing, inspiration, bending, recumbency, or exertion

The *hypersensitive xiphoid* is tender to palpation, and local pressure may cause nausea and vomiting. This syndrome is manifested as

- Epigastric pain
- Nausea
- Vomiting

In the syndrome of the *slipping rib* (usually the tenth), the involved cartilage moves upwards and overrides the cartilage above it, thus causing pain.

Trigger Points

Trigger points (hypersensitivity) in the thoracic paravertebral muscles refer pain to the chest, as do trigger points in the pectoralis major, pectoralis minor, and scalenus anterior muscles (Zohn, 1988) (see Table 12–1). Posterior chest wall pain may also be caused by irritable trigger points. One of the most extensive patterns of pain from irritable trigger points is the complex one from the anterior scalene muscle. This may produce ipsilateral sternal pain, anterior chest wall pain, or breast pain and vertebral border of the scapula, shoulder, shawl, and arm pain radiating to the thumb and index finger (Zohn, 1988). Trigger points in the pectoral muscles can also cause anterior chest wall pain.

Myalgia

Myalgia (muscular pain) in the respiratory muscles is well localized, reproducible by palpation, and exacerbated by manipulations of the chest wall. The discomfort of myalgia is almost always described as aching and may range from mild to intense. Diaphragmatic irritation may be referred to the ipsilateral neck and shoulder or to the lower thorax and upper abdomen.

Thoracic Outlet Syndrome

Thoracic outlet syndrome refers to a compression of the neural and vascular structures that leave, or pass over, the superior rim of the thoracic cage. The compressive forces associated with this neurovascular problem can be caused by musculoskeletal forces and can result in chest pain. Thoracic outlet syndrome usually affects the upper extremity in the distribution of the ulnar nerve with possible radiation to the neck, shoulder, scapula, or axilla, but the pain may occur primarily in the anterior chest wall, mimicking coronary heart disease.

Rib Fractures

Periosteal (bone) pain is usually described as being intense and can be well localized, whereas chronic disease, often affecting the bone marrow and endosteum, may result in poorly localized pain of varying degrees of severity (Bauwens and Paine, 1983). Occult (hidden) rib fractures may occur, especially in patients with a chronic cough or who have had an explosive sneeze. Rib fractures must be confirmed by x-ray diagnosis. Rib pain without fracture may indicate bone tumor or disease affecting bone, such as multiple myeloma (Zohn, 1988).

Systemic Causes (Strauss, 1984)

Pulmonary Causes

Parietal Pain. Parietal (somatic) pain refers to pain generating from the wall of any cavity, such as the chest or pelvic cavities. Whereas the visceral pleura is insensitive to pain, the parietal pleura is well supplied with pain nerve endings. Parietal pain may present as unilateral chest pain (rather than midline only) because at any given point, the parietal peritoneum obtains innervation from only one side of the nervous system. Parietal chest pain is usually localized more precisely to the site of the lesion than visceral pain. When pain is referred, the pattern is usually along the costal margins or into the upper abdominal quadrants.

Pleural Pain

This type of pain is a common chest discomfort usually associated with infectious diseases, but is also seen in spontaneous pneumothorax, rib fractures, and pulmonary embolism (blood clot) with infarction (death of tissue due to occlusion of the blood supply). The pleural pain is characteristically close to the chest wall, sharp in character, and exacerbated by inspiration, coughing, and movement. In contrast to chest wall pain, it is usually not localized by palpation.

Spontaneous Pneumothorax. Spontaneous pneumothorax occasionally affects the exercising individual and occurs without obvious preceding trauma or infection. Peak incidence in adults is 20 to 40 years of age. Patients frequently present with the acute onset of pleuritic chest pain localized to the side of the pneumothorax. The pain may be referred to the shoulder or scapula. Any chest pain accompanied by a persistent cough (whether dry or productive) or other constitutional symptoms, such as vomiting, fever, hemoptysis, dizziness, dyspnea (with or without exertion), and night sweats must be medically diagnosed (Strauss, 1984).

Cardiac Causes

There are many causes of chest pain, both cardiac and noncardiac in origin. Cardiac-related pain may arise secondary to angina, myocardial infarction, pericarditis, or dissecting aortic aneurysm. Cardiac-related chest pain can also occur when there is normal coronary circulation, such as in the case of patients with pernicious anemia (chronic, progressive reduction of erythrocytes and subsequent loss of oxygen). These patients may have chest pain (angina) on physical exertion because of the lack of nutrition to the myocardium. (For more detailed information on cardiac causes of chest pain, the reader is referred to Chapter 3.)

Noncardiac causes of chest pain include pleuropulmonary disorders, musculoskeletal disorders, neurologic disorders, GI disorders, breast pain, and anxiety states. Both cardiac- and noncardiac-related causes of chest pain are discussed in detail in Chapter 3 and are not repeated here.

Epigastric Causes

Epigastric pain is typically characterized by substernal or upper abdominal (just below the xyphoid process) discomfort. This may occur with radiation posteriorly to the back secondary to long-standing ulcers. Lesions of the upper esophagus may cause pain in the (anterior) neck, whereas lesions of the lower esophagus are more likely to be characterized by pain originating from the xyphoid process, radiating around the thorax to the middle of the back. Epigastric pain or discomfort may occur in association with disorders of the liver, gallbladder, common bile duct, and pancreas with referral of pain to the interscapular, subscapular, or middle/low back regions.

Breast Pain

Although more typical with women, both men and women can have chest, back, scapular, and shoulder pain referred by pathology of the breast. The typical referral pattern for breast pain is around the chest into the axilla, to the back at the level of the breast, occasionally into the neck and posterior aspect of the shoulder girdle (see Fig. 3–12). The pain may continue along the medial aspect of the ipsilateral arm to the fourth and fifth digits. Pain in the upper inner arm may arise from outer quadrant breast tumors, but pain in the local chest wall may point to any breast pathology, such as abscess, mastitis (inflammation of the breast), or lactation (breast feeding) problems.

Any recently discovered or changing lumps or nodules must be examined by a physician. Any suspicious finding by report, on observation, or by palpation should be checked by a physician, especially in the case of the woman with a previous personal or family history of breast cancer. A previous history of cancer is always cause to question the patient further regarding the onset and pattern of current symptoms. This is especially true for women with a previous history of breast cancer or cancer of the reproductive system now presenting with shoulder, chest, back, hip, or SI pain of unknown etiology. Removal of a breast due to primary cancer may seem so far remote from symptoms of these body locations that the patient may not volunteer this essential information (Cyriax, 1982; Wedge, 1983).

One of the most extensive patterns of pain from irritable trigger points is the complex one from the anterior scalene muscle. This pattern may produce ipsilateral sternal pain, anterior chest wall pain, or breast pain and vertebral border of the scapula, shoulder, shawl, and arm pain radiating to the thumb and index finger (Zohn, 1988). Trigger points in the pectoral muscles can also cause pain in the anterior chest wall.

Special Questions to Ask: Chest/Thoracic

Musculoskeletal

- □ Have you strained a muscle from coughing?
- □ Have you ever injured your chest?
- □ Does it hurt to touch your chest or to take a deep breath (e.g., coughing, sneezing, sighing or laughing)? **(Myalgia, fractured rib, costochondritis, myofascial trigger point)**
- □ Do you have frequent attacks of heartburn, or do you take antacids to relieve heartburn or acid indigestion? **(Noncardiac cause of chest pain, abdominal muscle trigger point, GI disorder)**

Neurologic

- □ Do you have any trouble taking a deep breath? **(Weak chest muscles secondary to polymyositis, dermatomyositis, myasthenia gravis)**
- □ Does your chest pain ever travel into your armpit, arm, neck, or wing bone (scapula)? **(Thoracic outlet syndrome)**

  If yes, do you ever feel burning, pricking, numbness, or unusual sensation in any of these areas?

Pulmonary

- □ Have you ever been treated for a lung problem?

  If yes, please describe what this problem was, when it occurred, and how it was treated.
- □ Do you think your chest or thoracic (upper back) pain is caused by a lung problem?
- □ Have you ever had trouble with breathing?
- □ Are you having difficulty with breathing now?
- □ Do you ever have shortness of breath, breathlessness, or can't quite catch your breath?

  If yes, does this happen when you rest; lie flat; walk on level ground; walk up stairs; or when you are under stress or tension?

  How long does it last?

  What do you do to get your breathing back to normal?
- □ How far can you walk before you feel breathless?
- □ What symptom stops your walking (e.g., shortness of breath, heart pounding, or weak legs)?

Subjective Exam

Special Questions to Ask

- □ Do you have any breathing aids (e.g., oxygen, nebulizer, humidifier, or intermittent positive pressure breathing [IPPB])?
- □ Do you have a cough? (Note whether the patient smokes, for how long and how much: Do you have a smoker's hack?)

  If yes to having a cough, distinguish it from a smoker's cough. Ask when it started.

  Does coughing increase or bring on your symptoms?

  Do you cough anything up? If yes, please describe the color, amount, and frequency.

  Are you taking anything for this cough? If yes, does it seem to help?
- □ Do you have periods when you can't seem to stop coughing?
- □ Do you ever cough up blood?

  If yes, what color is it? (Bright red = fresh; brown or black = older)

  If yes, has this been treated?
- □ Have you ever had a blood clot in your lungs? If yes, when and how was it treated?
- □ Have you had a chest x-ray taken during the last 5 years? If yes, when and where did it occur? What were the results?
- □ Do you work around asbestos, coal, dust, chemicals, or fumes? If yes, please describe.

  Do you wear a mask at work? If yes, approximately how much of the time do you wear a mask?
- □ If the patient is a farmer, ask what kind of farming: Some agricultural products may cause respiratory irritation.
- □ Have you ever had tuberculosis or a positive skin test for tuberculosis?

  If yes, when did it occur and how was it treated? What is your current status?
- □ When was your last test for tuberculosis? Was the result normal?

Cardiac

- □ Has a physician ever told you that you have heart trouble?
- □ Have you ever had a heart attack? If yes, when? Please describe.

  If yes to either question: Do you think your current symptoms are related to your heart problems?
- □ Do you have angina (pectoris)?

  If yes, please describe the symptoms and tell me when it occurs.

  If no, pursue further with the following questions.
- □ Do you ever have discomfort or tightness in your chest **(angina)?**
- □ Have you ever had a crushing sensation in your chest with or without pain down your left arm?

Subjective Exam

Special Questions to Ask

- □ Do you have pain in your jaw, either alone or in combination with chest pain?
- □ If you climb a few flights of stairs fairly rapidly, do you have tightness or pressing pain in your chest?
- □ Do you get pressure or pain or tightness in the chest if you walk in the cold wind or face a cold blast of air?
- □ Have you ever had pain or pressure or a squeezing feeling in the chest that occurred during exercise, walking, or any other physical or sexual activity?
- □ Do you ever have bouts of rapid heart action, irregular heart beats, or palpitations of your heart?

Epigastric

- □ Have you ever been told that you have an ulcer?
- □ Does the pain under your breast bone radiate (travel) around to your back or do you ever have back pain at the same time that your chest hurts?
- □ Have you ever had heartburn or acid indigestion?

  If yes, how is this pain different?

  If no, have you noticed any association between when you eat and when this pain comes on?

Breast

- □ Do you have any discharge from your breasts or nipples?

  If yes, do you know what is causing this discharge?

  Have you received medical treatment for this problem?
- □ Are you lactating (nursing a baby)?
- □ Have you examined yourself for any lumps or nodules and found any thickening or lump?

  If yes, where was it and how long was it present?

  Has your physician examined this lump?

  If no (for women), do you examine your own breasts?

  If yes, when was the last time that you did a self-breast examination?
- □ Have you been involved in any activities of a repetitive nature that could cause sore muscles (e.g., painting, washing walls, push-ups or other calisthenics, heavy lifting or pushing, overhead movements, prolonged running, or fast walking)?
- □ Have you recently been coughing excessively?

Table 12–6. SHOULDER PAIN

Right Shoulder		**Left Shoulder**	
Systemic Origin	***Location***	***Systemic Origin***	***Location***
Peptic ulcer	Lateral border, R scapula	Ruptured spleen	L shoulder
Myocardial ischemia	R shoulder, down arm	Myocardial ischemia	L pectoral/L shoulder
Hepatic/biliary		Pancreas	L shoulder
Acute cholecystitis	R shoulder; between scapulae; R subscapular area		
Liver abscess	R shoulder		
Gallbladder	R upper trapezius		
Liver disease (hepatitis, cirrhosis, metastatic tumors)	R shoulder, R subscapula		

SHOULDER PAIN

Systemic disease may also present itself clinically as shoulder pain (Table 12–6). Pain is commonly referred to one or the other shoulder joint from diseased viscera in the chest and in the upper abdomen, including pathologic conditions in the neck, cervical spine, axilla, thorax, thoracic spine, and chest wall (Table 12–7). Pain of cardiac and diaphragmatic origin is often experienced in the shoulder, because the heart and diaphragm are supplied by the C5–C6 spinal segment, and the visceral pain is referred to the corresponding somatic area (Heimer and Scharf, 1983). Differential diagnosis of shoulder pain is sometimes especially difficult, because any pain that is felt in the shoulder will affect the joint as though the pain was originating in the joint (Mennell, 1964).

Many visceral diseases are notorious for presenting as unilateral shoulder pain. Esoph-

Table 12–7. SYSTEMIC CAUSES OF SHOULDER PAIN*

Shoulder pain may be referred from the neck, chest (thorax or thoracic spine), abdomen, and from systemic diseases. The following have been diagnosed as having the onset or origin of presenting symptoms in the shoulder:

Neck	**Chest**	**Abdomen**	**Systemic Disease**
Bone tumors	Angina/myocardial infarct	Liver disease	Collagen vascular disease
Metastases	Pericarditis	Ruptured spleen	Gout
Tuberculosis	Aortic aneurysm	Spinal metastases	Syphilis/Gonorrhea
Nodes in neck (from metastases, leukemia, and Hodgkin's disease)	Empyema and lung abscess	Dissecting aortic aneurysm	Sickle cell anemia
	Pulmonary tuberculosis	Diaphragmatic irritation	Hemophilia
	Pancoast's tumor	Peptic ulcer	Rheumatic disease
Cervical cord tumors	Lung cancer (bronchogenic carcinoma)	Gallbladder disease	Metastatic cancer
		Subphrenic abscess	Breast
	Spontaneous pneumothorax	Hiatal hernia	Prostate
	Nodes in mediastinum/axilla	Pyelonephritis	Kidney
	Metastases in thoracic spine	Diaphragmatic hernia	Lung
	Breast disease	Upper urinary tract	Thyroid
	Primary or secondary cancer		
Mastodynia	Hiatal hernia		

* Adapted from Zohn, D.A.: Musculoskeletal Pain: Diagnosis and Physical Treatment, 2nd ed. Boston, Little, Brown, 1988, p. 178.

ageal, pericardial, or myocardial diseases, aortic dissection, and diaphragmatic irritation from thoracic or abdominal diseases can all present as unilateral shoulder pain. Usually with referred pain from the thoracic or abdominal viscera, the history will present sufficient symptoms in the chest or abdomen to indicate a systemic problem (Riggins, 1986).

Shoulder pain with any of the following features should be approached as a manifestation of systemic visceral illness, even if the pain is exacerbated by shoulder movement or if there are objective findings at the shoulder (Hadler, 1987):

- Pleuritic component
  - Persistent dry, hacking, or productive cough
  - Blood-tinged sputum
  - Musculoskeletal symptoms aggravated by respiratory movements, such as coughing, laughing, deep breathing
  - Chest pain
- Exacerbation by recumbency
- Coincident diaphoresis
- Coincident nausea, vomiting, dysphagia
- Other GI complaints
  - Anorexia
  - Early satiety
  - Epigastric pain or discomfort and fullness
- Exacerbation by exertion unrelated to shoulder movement
- Urologic complaints
- Jaundice

Extensive disease may occur in the periphery of the lung without occurrence of pain until the process extends to the parietal pleura. Pleural irritation then results in sharp, localized pain that is aggravated by any respiratory movement. Patients usually note that the pain is alleviated by lying on the affected side, which diminishes the movement of that side of the chest ("autosplinting") (Heimer and Scharf, 1983).

Hepatic and Biliary Diseases and Shoulder Pain

As with many of the organ systems in the human body, the hepatic and biliary organs (liver, gallbladder, and common bile duct) can develop diseases that mimic primary musculoskeletal lesions. The musculoskeletal symptoms associated with hepatic and biliary pathology are generally confined to the midback, scapular, and right shoulder regions. These musculoskeletal symptoms can occur alone (as the only presenting symptom) or in combination with other systemic signs and symptoms. Fortunately, in most cases of shoulder pain referred from visceral processes, shoulder motion is not compromised and local tenderness is not a prominent feature.

Referred shoulder pain may be the only presenting symptom of hepatic or biliary disease. Sympathetic fibers from the biliary system are connected through the celiac and splanchnic plexuses to the hepatic fibers in the region of the dorsal spine. These connections account for the intercostal and radiating interscapular pain that accompanies gallbladder disease (see Fig. 8–5). Although the innervation is bilateral, most of the biliary fibers reach the cord through the right splanchnic nerves, producing pain in the right shoulder, (Given and Simmons, 1979; Way, 1983).

Rheumatic Diseases and Shoulder Pain

A number of systemic rheumatic diseases can present as shoulder pain, even as unilateral shoulder pain. The HLA-B27 associated spondyloarthropathies (disease of the joints of the spine), such as ankylosing spondylitis, most frequently involve the sacroiliac joints and spine. Involvement of large central joints, such as the hip and shoulder, is common, however. Rheumatoid arthritis and its variants likewise frequently involve the shoulder girdle. These systemic rheumatic diseases are suggested by the details of the shoulder examination, by coincident systemic complaints of malaise and easy fatigability, and by complaints of discomfort in other joints either coincidental with the presenting shoulder complaint or in the past (Hadler, 1987).

Other systemic rheumatic diseases with major shoulder involvement include polymyalgia, rheumatica, and polymyositis (inflammatory disease of the muscles). Both may be somewhat asymmetric, but almost always present with bilateral involvement and impressive systemic symptoms (Hadler, 1987).

Neoplasm (Cyriax, 1982)

Questions about visceral function are relevant when the pattern for malignant invasion at the shoulder emerges. Invasion of the upper humerus and glenoid area by secondary malignant deposits affects the joint and the adjacent muscles.

CLINICAL SIGNS AND SYMPTOMS OF NEOPLASM

- Marked limitation of movement at the shoulder joint
- Severe muscular weakness and pain with resisted movements

The muscle wasting is greatly in excess of any attributable to arthritis and follows a bizarre pattern, which does not conform to any one neurologic lesion or to any one muscle. Localized warmth felt at any part of the scapular area may prove to be the first sign of a malignant deposit eroding bone. Within at most 1 or 2 weeks after this observation, a palpable tumor will have appeared and erosion of bone will be visible on radiograph.

Primary Neoplasm

This neoplasm occurs chiefly in young patients in whom a causeless limitation of movement of the shoulder should lead the physician to a study of the radiographic appearances. If the tumor originates from the shaft of the humerus, the first symptoms may be a feeling of "pins and needles" in the hand, associated with fixation of the biceps and triceps muscles and leading to limitation of movement at the elbow.

Pulmonary (Secondary) Neoplasm

Occasionally, there is the patient who requires medical referral because there is shoulder pain referred from metastatic lung cancer. When the shoulder is examined, the patient is unable to lift the arm beyond the horizontal position. Muscles respond with spasm that limits joint movement. If the neoplasm interferes with the diaphragm, diaphragmatic pain (C3, C4, C5) is often felt at the shoulder at each breath (at the fourth cervical dermatome [i.e., at the deltoid area]), in correspondence with the main embryologic derivation of the diaphragm. Pain arising from the part of the pleura that is not in contact with the diaphragm is also brought on by respiration, but is felt in the chest. Although the lung is insensitive, large tumors invading the chest wall set up local pain and cause spasm of the pectoralis major muscle, with consequent limitation of elevation of the arm. If the neoplasm encroaches on the ribs, stretching the muscle attached to the ribs leads to sympathetic spasm (i.e., of the pectoralis major).

By contrast, the scapula is mobile, and a full range of passive movement is present at the shoulder joint. The same signs are found in contracture of the pectoral scar after radical mastectomy, but there is no pain.

Pancoast's tumors of the lung apex usually do not cause symptoms while confined to the pulmonary parenchyma. They can extend into the surrounding structures, infiltrating the chest wall into the axilla, presenting with shoulder pain and occasionally with brachial plexus (eighth cervical and first thoracic nerve) involvement. This nerve involvement produces (sharp) neuritic pain in the axilla, shoulder, and subscapular area on the affected side with eventual atrophy of the upper extremity muscles. Bone pain is aching, exacerbated at night, and is a cause of restlessness and musculoskeletal movement. These features are not found in any regional musculoskeletal disorder, including such disorders of the shoulder (Hadler, 1987). There are usually associated general systemic signs and symptoms present (Cailliet, 1981).

Painful Shoulder-Hand Syndrome

The shoulder-hand syndrome is a poorly understood condition of the upper extremity and is believed to be caused by a malfunction of the autonomic nervous system. The patient has severe and bizarre pains in the extremity associated with excessive sweating and coolness. There is glossiness of the skin with a loss of normal skin texture and associated joint stiffness. This syndrome occurs more commonly in people who are emotionally unstable and who have extremely low pain thresholds (Riggins, 1986).

The initiating factor may be trauma, often quite minor, or it may result from remote disease of the thoracic or abdominal viscera that causes referred pain to the shoulder and arm (Riggins, 1986). A painful shoulder-hand syndrome may follow a myocardial infarction or cerebral vascular accident ([CVA] or stroke). This syndrome can occur from 1 to 3 months after the infarction or CVA. It was a more common complication of myocardial infarctions when patients were treated with strict, prolonged bed rest and immobilization. The change from prolonged bed rest to early ambulation has almost eliminated this problem (Hurst, 1986).

This syndrome occurs with equal frequency in either or both shoulders and, except when caused by coronary occlusion, is most frequent in women. The shoulder is generally involved first, but the painful hand may precede the shoulder. Regardless of the site or source of the pain sensation, the syndrome follows a specific pattern.

Pain Pattern

Three stages of the complex are recognized (Table 12–8). First the shoulder becomes "stiff," limited in range of motion, and may proceed to a "frozen shoulder." Even in cases after a myocardial infarction, the shoulder initially resembles the pericapsulitis from other causes. Tenderness about the shoulder is diffuse and is not localized to a specific tendon or bursal area. The duration of the initial shoulder stage, before the hand component begins, is extremely variable.

The shoulder may be "stiff" for several months before the hand becomes involved, or both may occur simultaneously. The hand and fingers become diffusely swollen. At first, the edema is pitting and may be relieved by prolonged elevation of the arm. This edema is noted predominantly on the dorsum of the hand and is usually observed over the meta-

Table 12–8. STAGES OF SHOULDER-HAND SYNDROME*

Stage 1	Stage 2	Stage 3
Limited shoulder range of motion with or without pain Swelling of the dorsum of the hand Full flexion of the fingers and joints Wrist assumes a flexed posture Skin is usually moist with small bubbles of perspiration, and the hand may be pale and cool or assume a pink hue	Shoulder pain subsides, and shoulder range may even increase Edema of the hand may subside, but fingers will become even stiffer Sensitivity decreases No change in skin appearance—pale, atrophic	Progressive atrophy of the bones, skin, and muscles Limitation of hands, wrists, and fingers increases, leaving the hand painless but in a useless, atrophied, clawed position

* From Cailliet, R.: Shoulder Pain, 2nd ed. Philadelphia, F.A. Davis, 1981.

carpophalangeal and proximal interphalangeal joints. The skin over the knuckles becomes puffy and loses the normal creases. The hand becomes boggy and painful. As the edema forms under the extensor tendons, flexion becomes increasingly more limited. The collateral ligaments, which must elongate to permit flexion of the metacarpophalangeal joints, become shortened and thus prevent or limit full flexion.

Limited shoulder action prevents elevation of the arm above shoulder level so that lymphatic and vascular pumping actions are restricted. The skin gradually becomes shiny and atrophic. The edema containing protein converts into a diffuse, cobweblike tissue that adheres to the tendons and joint capsules and prevents further movement. The joints undergo disuse atrophy of the cartilage, and the capsule thickens. The bones become osteoporotic (Cailliet, 1981).

Special Questions to Ask: Shoulder

General Systemic

□ Does your pain ever wake you at night from a sound sleep? **(Cancer)**

Can you find any way to relieve the pain and get back to sleep?

If yes, how? **(Cancer: nothing relieves it)**

□ Have you sustained any injuries in the last week during a sports activity, car accident, etc? **(Ruptured spleen associated with pain in the left shoulder: positive Kehr's sign)**

□ Since the beginning of your shoulder problem, have you had any unusual perspiration for no apparent reason, night sweats, or fever?

□ Have you had any unusual fatigue (more than usual with no change in life style), joint pain in other joints, or general malaise? **(Rheumatic disease)**

Pulmonary

□ Do you currently have a cough?

If yes, is this a smoker's cough?

If no, how long has this been present?

Is this a productive cough (can you bring up sputum?) and is the sputum tinged with blood?

□ Does your shoulder pain increase when you cough, laugh, or take a deep breath?

□ Do you have any chest pain?

□ What effect does lying down or resting have on your shoulder pain?

Subjective Exam

Special Questions to Ask

(Pulmonary problem may be made worse, whereas the musculoskeletal problem may experience some relief; on the other hand, pain may be relieved when the patient lies on the affected side, which diminishes the movement of that side of the chest)

Cardiac

□ Do you ever notice sweating, nausea, or chest pain when the pain in your shoulder occurs?

□ Have you noticed your shoulder pain increasing with exertion that does not necessarily cause you to use your shoulder (e.g., climbing stairs)?

Gastrointestinal

□ Have you ever had an ulcer?

If yes, when? Do you still have any pain from your ulcer?

Have you noticed any association between when you eat and when your symptoms increase or decrease?

□ Does eating relieve your pain? **(Duodenal or pyloric ulcer)**

How soon is the pain relieved after eating?

□ Does eating aggravate your pain? **(Gastric ulcer, gallbladder inflammation)**

□ Does your pain occur 1 to 3 hours after eating or between meals? **(Duodenal or pyloric ulcers, gallstones)**

□ Have you ever had gallstones?

□ Do you have a feeling of fullness after only one or two bites of food? **(Early satiety: stomach and duodenum or gallbladder)**

□ Have you had any nausea, vomiting, difficulty in swallowing, loss of appetite, or heartburn since the shoulder started bothering you?

HIP PAIN

Regional pain referred from disorders affecting the low back, abdomen, or retroperitoneal region (with irritation of the psoas muscle), nerve roots, peripheral nerves, or overlying soft-tissue structures may all present as "hip pain." These disorders may include both primary musculoskeletal lesions as well as disorders affecting the organs within the pelvic cavity and other diseases. A careful history and physical examination usually differentiate these entities from true hip disease (Hadler, 1987). Systemic causes of hip pain follow.

- Spinal metastases
- Bone tumors
    - Osteoid osteoma
    - Chondroblastomas
    - Chondrosarcoma
    - Giant cell tumor
    - Ewing's sarcoma
- Iliopsoas abscess

- Appendicitis
- PID
- Crohn's disease (regional enteritis)
- Femoral hernia
- Ureteral colic
- Reiter's syndrome
- Ankylosing spondylitis
- Tuberculosis
- Sickle cell anemia
- Hemophilia

Normal rotations in extension in the reproduction of hip pain should alert one to consider an extra-articular cause. Pain in the lumbrosacral region of any etiology may be referred to the hip. The classic example of this is referred pain along the course of T12 to L1 secondary to prolapsed intervertebral disk. However, pain originating from such diverse causes as simple low back strain or metastatic carcinoma to the vertebrae may also cause referred pain to the hip. Hip pain referred from the lower lumbar vertebrae and sacrum are usually felt in the gluteal region, with radiation down the back or outer aspect of the thigh. Lesions in the upper lumbar vertebrae often refer pain into the anterior aspect of the thigh (Hadler, 1987).

Systemic Causes of Hip Pain

Spinal Metastases

Spinal metastases to the femur or lower pelvis may present as hip pain. Although it may be said that any metastatic tumor may appear in bone, this is true for many tumors only when they have existed long enough and are in the terminal stage. Tumors have usually been recognized much earlier and no longer present a diagnostic problem (D'Ambrosia, 1986). With the exception of myeloma and a rare lymphoma, metastasis to the synovium is unusual, so that joint motion is not compromised by these bone lesions. Although any tumor of the bone, cartilage, or soft tissue may present at the hip, there are some benign and malignant neoplasms that have a propensity to occur in this location (Hadler, 1987).

Osteoid Osteoma

Osteoid osteoma, a small, benign but painful tumor, is relatively common with 20% of lesions occurring in the proximal femur and 10% in the pelvis. The patient usually presents in the second decade of life complaining of chronic dull, hip, knee, or thigh pain that is worse at night and alleviated by activity and aspirin. A physical examination usually reveals an antalgic gait and may demonstrate point tenderness over the lesion and restriction of hip motion. The physician's diagnosis takes into consideration the typical pain pattern, the patient's age, response to aspirin, and radiographic findings (Hadler, 1987).

Other Bone Tumors

There are a great many varieties of benign and malignant tumors that may present differently depending on the age of the patient, the site, and the duration of the lesion (D'Ambrosia, 1986). Other bone tumors, such as chondroblastomas, chondrosarcoma, giant cell tumors, and Ewing's sarcoma causing hip pain, are discussed in greater detail in Chapter 10. In each case, the patient's age and location of symptoms are used in conjunction with radiographs by the physician to make a positive diagnosis.

Inflammatory Diseases

Abdominal or intraperitoneal inflammation, which leads to irritation of the psoas muscle, may present as hip pain. Chronic inflammation, such as *psoas abscess* or persistent *appendicular* or *pelvic inflammation* (PID), may provoke psoas spasm producing a flexion contracture of the hip. Pain in the right hip, which may also involve the medial aspect of the thigh and femoral triangle area, may be caused by iliopsoas abscess, Crohn's disease, and appendicitis. These systemic causes of hip pain are usually associated with a loss of appetite, fever, and night sweats.

Other Causes of Hip Pain

Referred symptoms from *femoral hernia* or *ureteral colic* are less likely to be confused with hip pain by the history, presence of systemic symptoms, and pattern of pain. There have been reports of Reiter's syndrome or ankylosing spondylitis presenting as referred pain to the hip (Hadler, 1987).

Although *ankylosing spondylitis* is primarily an arthritis of the spine, one fifth of the patients notice the first symptoms in the peripheral joints and approximately one third of these patients ultimately develop hip disease. Late in the disease, marked hip flexion contractures are present and bony ankylosis of the hip may occur (D'Ambrosia, 1986).

In the developed countries, *tubercular disease* of the hip is rare, but can occur. The patient usually presents with a chronic limp and pain in the hip that persists at rest. Approximately 60% of patients do not have constitutional symptoms, although the tuberculin skin test is usually positive and radiographs are similar to those for septic arthritis (Hadler, 1987).

Sickle cell anemia resulting in avascular necrosis (death of cells due to lack of blood supply) of the hip and hemarthrosis (blood in joint) associated with *hemophilia* are two of the most common hematologic diseases to cause pain in the hip.

CLINICAL SIGNS AND SYMPTOMS ASSOCIATED WITH HIP AVASCULAR NECROSIS

- Pain in the groin or thigh
- Tenderness to palpation over the hip joint
- Antalgic gait with a limp
- Hip motion decreased in flexion, internal rotation, and abduction

CLINICAL SIGNS AND SYMPTOMS ASSOCIATED WITH HIP HEMARTHROSIS

- Pain in the groin and thigh
- Fullness in the hip joint both anterior in the groin and over the greater trochanter
- Limited motion in hip flexion, abduction, and external rotation (allows most room for the blood in the joint capsule)

Special Questions to Ask: Hip

Because hip pain can be caused by referred pain from disorders of the low back, abdomen, and reproductive and urologic structures, special questions should include consideration of the following:

- Special questions for women
- Special questions for men
- Special questions for back patients:
  - General systemic questions
  - GI questions
  - Urologic questions

These questions are fully outlined elsewhere in this chapter and are not repeated here.

GROIN PAIN

The physical therapist is not likely to be faced with a patient complaining of just groin pain or symptoms. It is more typical to see a patient who has low back, hip, or SI problems and who has a secondary complaint of groin pain. However, on examination, the physical therapist may palpate enlarged lymph nodes in the groin area, or the patient may indicate these nodes to the examiner.

Painless, progressive enlargements of lymph nodes that persist for more than 4 weeks or that involve more than one area are an indication of a need for a medical referral. *Hodgkin's disease* arises in the lymph glands most commonly on one side of the neck or groin, but lymph nodes also enlarge in response to infections throughout the body, thus the patient must seek medical diagnosis to be certain of the cause of enlarged lymph nodes.

As always, the physical therapist must question the patient further regarding the onset of symptoms and the presence of any associated symptoms, such as fever, weight loss, bleeding, and skin lesions.

Causes of Groin Pain

Primary and secondary spinal cord tumors may initially present with discomfort in the thoracolumbar area in a beltlike distribution. The pain may extend to the groin or legs and may be constant or intermittent; a dull ache; or a sharp, knifelike sensation (Snyder, 1986). The location of the pain can be primarily at the site of the lesion or may refer to the ipsilateral groin and down the ipsilateral extremity with radicular involvement (nerve root compression or irritation).

Ureteral pain is felt in the groin and genital area (see Fig. 7–3) with radiation forward around the flank into the lower abdominal quadrant. Abdominal muscle spasm with rebound tenderness can occur on the same side as the source of pain. The pain can also be generalized throughout the abdomen with nausea, vomiting, and impaired intestinal motility present. Abdominal rebound tenderness results when the adjacent peritoneum becomes inflamed (Perlmutter and Blacklow, 1983). Active trigger points along the upper rim of the pubis and the lateral half of the inguinal ligament may lie in the lower internal oblique muscle and possibly in the lower rectum abdominis. These trigger points can cause increased irritability and spasm of the detrusor and urinary sphincter muscles, producing urinary frequency, retention of urine, and groin pain (Travell and Simons, 1983).

Ascites, an abnormal accumulation of serous (edematous) fluid within the peritoneal cavity, can also cause low back pain or groin pain. This condition is associated with liver disease and alcoholism. The patient presents with a distended abdomen, lumbar lordosis, and possible edema bilaterally in the ankles.

Hemophilia may involve GI bleeding accompanied by low abdominal and groin pain due to bleeding into the wall of the large intestine or iliopsoas muscle. This retroperitoneal hemorrhage produces a muscle spasm of the iliopsoas muscle with a subsequent hip flexion contracture. Other symptoms may include melena, hematemesis, and fever.

Special Questions to Ask: Groin

Refer to the *Special Questions To Ask: Sacroiliac/Sacrum section*

SUMMARY

Throughout this text, the physical therapist has been encouraged to assess musculoskeletal complaints of unknown origin affecting the back, shoulder, chest, thorax, hip, groin, or sacroiliac joint with the idea that systemic origin of symptoms must be considered. A carefully taken medical history, review of systems, and appropriate questions asked during the physical therapy interview must be correlated with the objective findings. These tools will help the physical therapist in making a physical therapy diagnosis or in making the decision to refer the patient to another health care practitioner.

This chapter has specifically compared the possible systemic versus musculoskeletal causes of pain associated with the back, shoulder, chest, thorax, hip, groin, or sacroiliac joint. Special questions to ask have been provided to assist the physical therapist in identifying the potential presence of signs and symptoms associated with systemic disease. Additionally, special questions appropriate for women and men have been outlined, depending on the presenting musculoskeletal complaints.

In discussing musculoskeletal versus systemic symptoms, we have attempted to provide the physical therapist with important information needed when making an assessment of the patient, including:

- Patient's history and systems review
- Types of pain
    - Signs and symptoms of systemic pain
    - Signs and symptoms of musculoskeletal pain
    - Classifications of back pain
- Systemic causes of back pain
    - Cervical
    - Thoracic
    - Scapular
    - Lumbar (low back pain)
    - Sacroiliac joint/sacrum
- Systemic causes of chest pain

- Systemic causes of shoulder pain
- Systemic causes of hip pain
- Systemic causes of groin pain
- Special questions to ask by anatomic location

SYSTEMIC SIGNS AND SYMPTOMS

Systemic signs and symptoms generally follow patterns characteristic of the organ or system involved. Constitutional (i.e., systemic) symptoms that are characteristic of multisystems should serve as "red flags" to alert the physical therapist to the possibility of a patient's complaints that are more than just musculoskeletal in nature. The following signs and symptoms are the most common.

Systemic Signs and Symptoms Requiring Physician Referral

Abdominal pain	Dysphagia	Night pain
Anorexia	Dyspnea	Night sweats
Bilateral symptoms	Early satiety	Palpitations
Bowel/bladder changes	Fatigue	Paresthesia
Chills	Fever	Persistent cough
Constipation	Headaches	Skin rash
Diaphoresis	Heartburn	Vision changes
Diarrhea	Hemoptysis	Vomiting
Dizziness	Hoarseness	Weakness
Dysesthesia	Indigestion	Weight loss/gain
	Jaundice	
	Nausea	

PHYSICIAN REFERRAL

A careful history and close observation of the patient is important in determining whether a person may need a medical referral for possible systemic origin of pain or symptoms masquerading as musculoskeletal involvement. Any patient presenting with back (cervical, thoracic, scapular, lumbar, SI), hip, or shoulder pain without a history of trauma (including forceful movement of the spine, repetitive movements of the shoulder or back, or easy lifting) should be screened for possible systemic origin of symptoms.

It is not the physical therapist's responsibility to differentiate diagnostically among the various causes of systemic signs and symptoms, but rather to identify when the patient's history, subjective report, and objective findings do not support the presence of a musculoskeletal problem, thus requiring a medical follow-up.

Each of the visceral systems reviewed in this text have specific patterns of pain referral with accompanying signs and symptoms or history to assist the physical therapist in making a thorough investigation of the presenting problem. Familiarity with these patterns and the appropriate follow-up questions is essential when considering medical referral for possible visceral involvement.

Physical therapists are often the health care representatives to whom patients describe problems or concerns that are most appropriately reported to the physician. Conversations of this nature are not unusual when considering the consistent daily or weekly contact that physical therapists may have with patients. The knowledgeable physical therapist who can recognize this information may also be able to guide the patient effectively in seeking the necessary medical attention.

Additionally, exercise may be the precipitating or aggravating factor for the onset of some conditions, such as angina, asthma, vascular or migraine headaches, spontaneous pneumothorax, or dehydration secondary to the use of diuretic medications, requiring that the physical therapist communicate and collaborate with the physician. Knowledge of the correct information to give the physician can facilitate the communication process.

CASE STUDY

Referral

A 65-year-old retired railroad engineer has come to you with a left "frozen shoulder." During the course of the subjective examination, he also tells you that he is taking two cardiac medications.

What questions should you ask that might help you to relate these two problems (shoulder/cardiac) or to rule out any relationship?

Onset/History

What do you think is the cause of your shoulder problem?

When did it occur or how long have you had this problem (sudden or gradual onset)?

Can you recall any specific incident when you injured your shoulder, for example, by falling, being hit by someone or something, automobile accident?

Did you ever have a snapping or popping sensation just before your shoulder started to hurt? **(Ligamentous or cartilagenous lesion)**

Did you injure your neck in any way before your shoulder developed these problems?

Have you had a recent heart attack? Have you had nausea, fatigue, sweating, chest pain, or pressure with or without pain in your neck, jaw, left shoulder, or down your left arm?

Has your left hand ever been stiff or swollen? **(Shoulder-hand syndrome after myocardial infarction)**

Do you associate the symptom relating to your shoulder with your heart problems?

Shortly before you first noticed difficulty with your shoulder, were you involved in any kind of activities that would require repetitive movements, such as painting, gardening, playing tennis or golf?

Medical History

Have you had any surgery during the past year?

How has your general health been? **(Shoulder pain is a frequent site of referred pain from other internal medical problems, such as diabetes, arthritis, cancer)**

Did you ever have rheumatic fever when you were a child?

What is your typical pattern of chest pain or angina?

Has this pattern changed in any way since your shoulder started to hurt? For example, does the chest pain last longer, come on with less exertion, and feel more intense?

Do your heart medications relieve your shoulder symptoms, even briefly?

If so, how long after you take the medications, do you notice a difference?

Does this occur every time that you take your medications?

CASE STUDY

Medical Testing

Have you had any recent x-rays taken of the shoulder or your neck?

Have you received medical or physical therapy treatment for shoulder problems before?

If so, where, when, why, who, and what (see *The Physical Therapy Interview* for specific questions)?

Have you had any (extensive) medical testing during the past year?

Pain/Symptoms

Is your shoulder painful?

If yes, how long has the shoulder been painful?

Follow the usual line of questioning regarding the pattern, frequency, intensity, and duration outlined in *The Physical Therapy Interview* to establish necessary information regarding pain.

Aggravating/relieving activities

How does rest affect your shoulder symptoms? **(True muscular lesions are relieved with prolonged rest [i.e., more than 1 hour], whereas angina is usually relieved more immediately by cessation of activity or rest [i.e., usually within 2 to 5 minutes, up to 15 minutes].**

Does your shoulder pain occur during exercise (e.g., walking, climbing stairs, mowing the lawn) or any other physical or sexual activity? (Evaluate the difference between total body exertion causing shoulder symptoms versus just movements of the upper extremities reproducing symptoms. Total body exertion causing shoulder pain may be secondary to angina or myocardial infarction; whereas, movements of just the upper extremities causing shoulder pain are more indicative of a primary musculoskeletal lesion.)

Subacute/acute/chronic musculoskeletal lesion versus systemic pain pattern (see *The Physical Therapy Interview* for specific meaning to the patient's answers to these questions):

Can you lie on that side?

Does the shoulder pain awaken you at night?

If so, is this because you have rolled onto that side?

Do you notice any chest pain, night sweats, fever, or heart palpitations when you wake up at night?

Have you ever noticed these symptoms (e.g., chest pain, heart palpitations) with your shoulder pain during the day?

Do these symptoms wake you up separate from your shoulder pain or does your shoulder pain wake you up and you have these additional symptoms? (As always when asking questions about sleep patterns, the patient may be unsure of the answers to the questions. In such cases, the physical therapist is advised to ask the patient to pay attention to what happens related to sleep during the next few days up to 1 week and report back to the therapist with more definitive information.)

References

Aach, R.D.: Abdominal pain. *In* Blacklow, R.S. (ed.): MacBryde's Signs and Symptoms, 6th ed. Philadelphia, J.B. Lippincott, 1983, pp. 165–179.

Bauwens, D.B., and Paine, R.: Thoracic pain. *In* Blacklow, R.S. (ed): MacBryde's Signs and Symptoms, 6th ed. Philadelphia, J.B. Lippincott, 1983, pp. 139–164.

Blacklow, R.S.: The study of symptoms. *In* Blacklow, R.S. (ed): MacBryde's Signs and Symptoms, 6th ed. Philadelphia, J.B. Lippincott, 1983, pp. 1–16.

Cailliet, R.: Shoulder Pain, 2nd ed. Philadelphia, F.A. Davis, 1981.

Cyriax, J.: Textbook of Orthopaedic Medicine, Vol. 1, 8th ed. London, Bailliere Tindall, 1982.

D'Ambrosia, R.: Musculoskeletal Disorders: Regional Examination and Differential Diagnosis, 2nd ed. Philadelphia, J.B. Lippincott, 1986.

Engel, G.L.: Pain. *In* Blacklow, R.S. (ed): MacBryde's Signs and Symptoms, 6th ed. Philadelphia, J.B. Lippincott, 1983, pp. 41–60.

Given, B.A., and Simmons, S.J.: Gastroenterology in Clinical Nursing. Baltimore, C.V. Mosby, 1979.

Hadler, N.M. (ed): Clinical Concepts in Regional Musculoskeletal Illness. Orlando, FL, Grune & Stratton, 1987.

Hadler, N.M.: Medical Management of Regional Musculoskeletal Diseases: Backache, Neck Pain, Disorders of the Upper and Lower Extremities. Orlando, FL, Grune & Stratton, 1984.

Hadler, N.M.: The patient with low back pain. Hosp. Pract., Oct. 30, 1987, pp. 17–22.

Hall, A.: Back pain. *In* Blacklow, R.S. (ed): MacBryde's Signs and Symptoms, 6th ed. Philadelphia, J.B. Lippincott, 1983, pp. 195–210.

Heimer, D., and Scharf, S.M.: History and physical examination. *In* Baum, G.L., and Wolinsky, E. (eds): Textbook of Pulmonary Diseases, 3rd ed. Boston, Little, Brown, 1983, pp. 223–233.

Hurst, J.W. (ed): The Heart, Vols. 1 and 2. New York, McGraw-Hill, 1986.

Kirkaldy-Willis, W.H. (ed): Managing Low Back Pain. New York, Churchill Livingstone, 1983.

McKenzie, R.A.: The Lumbar Spine: Mechanical Diagnosis and Therapy. New Zealand, Spinal Publications, 1981.

McNab, I.: Backache. Baltimore, Williams & Wilkins, 1977.

Mennell, J.M.: Joint pain: Diagnosis and Treatment Using Manipulative Techniques. Boston, Little, Brown, 1964.

Perlmutter, A. and Blacklow, R.: Urinary tract pain, hematuria and pyuria. *In* Blacklow, R.S. (ed): MacBryde's Signs and Symptoms, 6th ed. Philadelphia, J.B. Lippincott, 1983, pp. 181–192.

Riggins, R.S.: The shoulder. *In* D'Ambrosia, R.: Musculoskeletal Disorders: Regional Examination and Differential Diagnosis, 2nd ed. Philadelphia, J.B. Lippincott, 1986, pp. 367–393.

Rodnan, G.P., and Schumacher, H.R. (eds): Primer on the Rheumatic Diseases, 8th ed. Atlanta, GA, Arthritis Foundation, 1983.

Snyder, C.C.: Oncology Nursing. Boston, Little, Brown, 1986.

Strauss, R.H. (ed): Sports Medicine. Philadelphia, W.B. Saunders Company, 1984.

Travell, J.G., and Simons, D.G.: Myofascial Pain and Dysfunction: The Trigger Point Manual. Baltimore, Williams & Wilkins, 1983.

Way, L.W.: Abdominal pain. *In* Sleisenger, M.H., and Fortran, J.S. (eds): Gastrointestinal Disease, 2nd ed. Philadelphia, W.B. Saunders Company, 1983, pp 207–221.

Wedge, J.H.: Differential diagnosis of low back pain. *In* Kirkaldy-Willis, W.H. (ed): Managing Low Back Pain. New York, Churchill Livingstone, 1983, pp. 129–143.

Zohn, D.A.: Musculoskeletal Pain: Diagnosis and Physical Treatment, 2nd ed. Boston, Little, Brown, 1988.

Zohn, D.A., and Mennell, J.: Musculoskeletal Pain: Principles of Physical Diagnosis and Physical Treatment, 2nd ed. Boston, Little, Brown, 1988.

Bibliography

Amendola, M., and Gordon, R.: Diagnosis of Uterine Disorders. Philadelphia, W.B. Saunders Company, 1988.

Azzopardi, J.G.: Problems in Breast Pathology. Philadelphia, W.B. Saunders Company, 1979.

Benson, D.R.: The back: Thoracic and lumbar spine. *In* D'Ambrosia, R.: Musculoskeletal Disorders: Regional Examination and Differential Diagnosis, 2nd ed. Philadelphia, J.B. Lippincott, 1986, pp. 287–365.

Buchsbaum, H.J., and Schmidt, J.D.: Gynecologic and Obstetric Urology, 2nd ed. Philadelphia, W.B. Saunders Company, 1986.

Danforth, D.S. (ed): Obstetrics and Gynecology. Philadelphia, J.B. Lippincott, 1986.

Haagensen, C.D.: Diseases of the Breast, 3rd ed. Philadelphia, W.B. Saunders Company, 1986.

Hacker, N., and Moore, J.G.: Essentials of Obstetrics and Gynecology. Philadelphia, W.B. Saunders Company, 1986.

Henderson, D.E., and Shaffer, T.E.: The gastrointestinal system. *In* Strauss, R.H. (ed): Sports Medicine. Philadelphia, W.B. Saunders Company, 1984, pp. 140–148.

Kase, N.G., and Weinhold, A.B.: Principles and Practice of Clinical Gynecology. New York, John Wiley, 1983.

Layzer, R.B.: Neuromuscular Manifestations of Systemic Disease. Philadelphia, F.A. Davis, 1985.

Pitkin, R., and Scott, J. (eds): Clinical Obstetrics and Gynecology. Philadelphia, J.B. Lippincott, 1986.

Puhl, I., and Brown, C.H. (eds): The Menstrual Cycle and Physical Activity. Champaign, IL, Human Kinetics Publications, 1986.

GLOSSARY

Acetylcholine: An acetic acid ester of choline, normally present in many parts of the body, having important physiologic functions; it is a neurotransmitter at cholinergic synapses

Achalasia: Failure to relax the smooth muscle fibers of the gastrointestinal tract at any junction of one part with another; especially failure of the lower esophagus to relax with swallowing

Acidosis: A pathologic condition resulting from accumulation of acid or depletion of the alkaline reserve (bicarbonate content) in the blood and body tissues and characterized by an increase in hydrogen ion concentration (decrease in pH); the opposite of alkalosis

Acquired immunodeficiency syndrome (AIDS): Suppression or deficiency of the cellular immune response, acquired by exposure to the human T-cell lymphotrophic virus (HIV); infection by the virus and the consequent suppression of the immune response predisposes the infected person to opportunistic infections and malignancies

Acroparesthesia: An abnormal sensation, such as tingling, numbness, pins and needles in the digits

Adenoma: A benign epithelial tumor in which the cells form recognizable glandular structures or in which the cells are derived from glandular epithelium

Agglutination: Aggregation of separate particles into clumps or masses, especially the clumping together of bacteria by the action of a specific antibody directed against a surface antigen

Albumin: A plasma protein formed principally in the liver and responsible for much of the colloidal osmotic pressure of the blood

Alkalosis: A pathologic condition resulting from an accumulation of base or from a loss of acid without comparable loss of base in the body fluids, characterized by a decrease in hydrogen ion concentration (increase in pH)

Allergen: A substance, protein or nonprotein, capable of inducing allergy or specific hypersensitivity

Allergy: A state of abnormal and individual hypersensitivity acquired through exposure to a particular allergen; re-exposure revealing a heightened capacity to react

Alopecia: Loss of hair, baldness

Alveoli: Air sac or thin-walled chamber in the lungs, surrounded by networks of capillaries through whose walls exchange of carbon dioxide and oxygen takes place

Amebiasis: Infection with amebas, especially *Entamoeba histolytica;* amebic dysentery

Amyloidosis: The disposition in various tissues of amyloid, a protein resembling starch that causes tissues to become waxy and nonfunctioning

Anabolism: The constructive phase of metabolism in which the body cells synthesize protoplasm for growth and repair; the opposite of catabolism

Anaplasia: Loss of differentiation of cells; a characteristic of tumor cells

Anastomoses: Connecting channels between blood vessels

Androgens: Any steroid hormone that promotes male characteristics; the two main androgens are androsterone and testosterone

Anemia: A reduction below normal in the number of erythrocytes (red blood cells or RBCs) or in the quantity of hemoglobin in the blood

Aneurysm: A sac formed by the dilatation of the wall of an artery, a vein, or the heart

Angina (pectoris): Spasmodic, choking, suffocating chest pain usually due to a lack of adequate blood supply (oxygen) to the heart muscle

Angiodysplasia: Small vascular abnormalities, especially of the intestinal tract

Angioma (spider): Branched dilatation of the superficial capillaries resembling a spider

Angiotensin: A vasoconstrictive principle formed in the blood when renin is released from the juxtaglomular apparatus in the kidney

Anicteric: Without jaundice

Anisocytosis: The presence in the blood of erythrocytes showing abnormal variations in size

Ankylosis: Immobility and consolidation or fusion of a joint due to disease, injury, or surgical procedure; ankylosis may be caused by destruction of the membranes that line the joint or by faulty bone structure

Anorexic: Loss of appetite due to emotional state

Antibody: An immunoglobulin molecule having a specific amino acid sequence that gives each antibody the ability to adhere to and interact with only the antigen that induced its synthesis; this antigen-specific property of the antibody is the basis of the antigen-antibody reaction that is essential to an immune response

Antigen: Any substance that is capable, under appropriate conditions, of inducing a specific immune response and of reacting with the products of that response; that is, with specific antibody or specifically sensitized T-lymphocytes, or both. Antigens may be soluble substances, such as toxins and foreign proteins, or particulate, such as bacteria and tissue cells

Anuria: Complete suppression of urine formation by the kidney

Aplastic anemia: A deficiency of circulating erythrocytes because of the arrested development of erythrocytes within the bone marrow

Arrhythmia: Any irregularity of the heartbeat; any variation from the normal regular rhythm of the heart

Arteriosclerosis: A group of diseases characterized by the thickening and hardening of the usually supple arterial walls; it comprises three distinct forms: atherosclerosis, Mönckeberg's arteriosclerosis, and arteriolosclerosis

Arteriosclerosis obliterans: Atheroscleromas (plaques) of the intima (innermost structure) of small vessels has caused complete obliteration of the lumen (cavity or channel within a tube) of the artery; effects the aorta and its branches to the extremities

Arteritis: Inflammation of an artery

Arthralgia: Pain in a joint

Ascites: Effusion and accumulation of serous (clear liquid) fluid that accumulates in the peritoneal (abdominal) cavity

Aspirate: To inhale vomitus, mucus, or food into the respiratory tract

Asterixis: A motor disturbance marked by intermittent lapses of an assumed posture as a result of intermittency of sustained contraction of groups of muscles; called liver flap because of its occurrence in liver disease

Atheroma: Slow deterioration of arteries in which fatty deposits called plaque (lipids such as triglycerides and cholesterol) are laid down in the (intima) inner lining of the arteries occurring in atherosclerosis, a form of arteriosclerosis

Atherosclerosis: An extremely common form of arteriosclerosis in which deposits of yellow plaques (atheromas) containing cholesterol, lipoid material, and lipophages are formed within the intima and inner media of large and medium-sized arteries

Atopy: A clinical hypersensitivity state or allergy with a hereditary predisposition

Atrial septal defect: Hole between the atria of the heart

Autoantibody: An antibody formed in response to, and reacting against, an antigenic constituent of the individual's own tissues

Autoimmune disease: Disease due to immunologic action of one's own cells or antibodies on components of the body

Autonomic: Not subject to voluntary control; the branch of the nervous system that works without conscious control

Avascular necrosis: Death of cells due to a lack of blood supply

Bacteriuria: Bacteria in the urine

Basophilia: Abnormal increase of basophilic leukocytes in the blood

Basophils: A granular leukocyte with an irregularly shaped, relatively pale-staining nucleus that is partially constricted into two lobes, and with cytoplasm containing coarse blue-black granules of variable size; basophils contain vasoactive amines, for example, histamine and serotonin that are released on appropriate stimulation

B-cells: B-lymphocytes, white blood cells of the immune system derived from bone marrow and involved in the production of antibodies; associated with humoral mediated immunity

Bile: A clear yellow or orange fluid produced by the liver; it is concentrated and stored in the gallbladder and is poured into the small intestine via the bile ducts when needed for digestion; bile helps in alkalinizing the intestinal contents and plays a role in the emulsification, absorption, and digestion of fat

Bilirubin: A bile pigment produced by the breakdown of heme and reduction of biliverdin; failure of the liver cells to excrete bile (or obstruction of the bile ducts) can cause an increased amount of bilirubin in the body fluids and lead to obstructive jaundice

Biliverdin: A green bile pigment formed by catabolism of hemoglobin and converted to bilirubin in the blood.

Bradycardia: Slowness of the heart beat, which is shown by slowing of the pulse rate to less than 60 beats/min

Bradykinin: A nonpeptide kinin formed from a plasma protein, high-molecular-weight (HMW) kininogen by the action of kallikrein (enzyme that releases kinins); it is a very powerful vasodilator that increases capillary permeability and, in addition, constricts smooth muscle and stimulates pain receptors

Bronchiectasis: Chronic dilatation of the bronchi and bronchioles with secondary infection, usually involving the lower lobes of the lung

Bronchus (pl. bronchi): Any of the larger passages conveying air to and within the lungs

Buerger's disease: See thromboangiitis obliterans

Bulemic: Eating disorder characterized by episodic binge eating followed by purging behavior, such as self-induced vomiting and laxative abuse

Calcinosis: A condition characterized by abnormal deposition of calcium salts in the tissues

Calculus (pl. calculi): Stones either in the kidney or gallbladder, composed of mineral salts

Caliculus (pl. caliculi): Small cup or cup-shaped structure

Canaliculi: An extremely narrow tubular passage or channel

Cancellous: Of a lattice, sponge-like structure; referring to bone

Cancer: Any malignant, cellular tumor; this term encompasses a group of neoplastic diseases in which there is a transformation of normal body cells into malignant ones

Carcinoma: A malignant new growth made up of epithelial cells tending to infiltrate surrounding tissues and give rise to metastases

Carcinoma in situ: A neoplastic entity in which the tumor cells have not invaded the basement membrane but are still confined to the epithelium of origin

Carcinomatous neuromyopathy: There are many types of carcinomatous neuromyopathy; however, pertinent to the physical therapist, presentation may be as idiopathic weakness of the proximal muscles that may be accompanied by the diminution of two or more deep tendon reflexes

Catabolism: Any destructive process by which complex substances are converted by living cells into simpler compounds, with release of energy; the opposite of anabolism

Celiac plexus: A network of ganglia and nerves supplying the abdominal viscera; also called solar plexus

Chemotaxis: Force or movement in response to the influence of chemical stimulation; for example, the attraction of neutrophils to the immune complex

Cholangiocarcinoma: A primary (fatal) cancer of the liver that develops in the bile ducts

Cholecystectomy: Excision of the gallbladder

Cholecystitis: Inflammation of the gallbladder, acute or chronic

Cholecystokinin: A polypeptide hormone secreted in the small intestine that stimulates gallbladder contraction and secretion of pancreatic enzymes

Choledocholithiasis: Calculi in the common duct

Cholelith: Gallstone

Cholelithiasis: The presence or formation of gallstones

Chondrodynia: Pain in a cartilage

Chondromas: A tumor or tumorlike growth of cartilage cells; it may remain in the interior or substance of a cartilage or bone (true chondroma or enchondroma), or it may develop on the surface of a cartilage and project under the periosteum of bone (ecchondroma or ecchondrosis)

Chondrosarcoma: A malignant tumor derived from cartilage cells or their precursors

Chordoma: A malignant tumor arising from embryonic remains of the notochord (cylindrical cord of cells on the dorsal aspect of an embryo, marking its longitudinal axis; it is the center of development of the axial skeleton)

Chyme: The semifluid material produced by action of the gastric juice on ingested food and discharged through the pylorus into the duodenum

Cirrhosis: A liver disease characterized by the loss of the normal microscopic lobular architecture and regenerative replacement of necrotic parenchymal tissue with fibrous bands of connective tissue that eventually constrict and partition the organ into irregular nodules

Claudication: Limping or lameness caused by ischemia or insufficient blood flow in occlusive arterial disease of the limbs. If claudication is intermittent, this represents a complex of symptoms characterized by the absence of pain or discomfort in a limb when at rest, the commencement of pain, tension, and weakness after walking is begun with intensification of the condition until walking is impossible, requiring rest until the symptoms have disappeared.

Clearance: Complete removal by the kidneys of a solute or substance from a specific volume of blood per unit of time

Closed-ended question: Question that requires only a "yes" or "no" answer

Clotting factors: Factors essential to normal blood clotting whose absence, diminution, or excess may lead to abnormality of the clotting; there are 12 factors, commonly designated by Roman numerals

Clubbing: Bulbous swelling of the terminal phalanges of the fingers and toes, giving them a "club" appearance

Coagulation: Formation of a clot

Coccygodynia: Pain in the coccyx and neighboring region

Collagen: A fibrous structural protein that constitutes the protein of the white fibers (collagenous fibers) of skin, tendon, bone, cartilage, and all other connective tissues

Colloid osmotic pressure (oncotic): Pressure exerted by proteins in the blood to pull fluid from the interstitial space back into the vascular area

Complement: A term originally used to refer to the heat-labile factor in serum that causes immune cytolysis, the lysis of antibody-coated cells, and now refers to the entire functionally related system, consisting of at least 20 distinct serum proteins, that is the effector of immune cytolysis and other biologic functions

Congestive heart failure: The heart's inability to pump enough blood for the body to function well; the heart muscles gradually fail to contract vigorously enough to adequately cycle the total volume of circulating blood

Conjugate: In biochemistry, the joining of a toxic substance with some natural substance of the body to form a detoxified product for elimination from the body

Constipation: A condition in which waste matter in the bowel is too hard to pass easily or in which bowel movements are so infrequent that discomfort and other symptoms interfere with one's usual daily activities and sense of well-being; constipation can be said to exist when a person reports a frequency of bowel elimination that is less than the usual pattern or when defecation occurs less than three times a week, stools are hard and well-formed and possibly less than the usual amount. Straining at stool occurs regularly and the person experiences headache, abdominal pain, a feeling of fullness in the abdomen or rectum, and either diminished appetite or nausea

Constitutional symptoms: Affecting the whole constitution of the body, not local; systemic

Conversion symptoms: A mental disorder in which a patient "converts" the anxiety caused by a psychologic conflict into physical symptoms

COPD: Chronic obstructive pulmonary disease

Coronary thrombosis: Sudden blockage of coronary artery

Cor pulmonale: Heart disease (enlargement of the right ventricle) secondary to pulmonary disease

Costochondritis: Inflammation of the costal cartilage or rib and rib cartilage

Cretinism: Arrested physical and mental development with dystrophy of bones and soft tissues, due to congenital lack of thyroid gland secretion from hypofunctioning or absence of the gland

Crohn's disease: Inflammation of the terminal portion of the ileum; also called regional enteritis and regional ileitis; it can affect any segment of the intestinal tract, although it is more commonly located in the terminal ileum

Cutaneous: Pertaining to the skin

Cyanosis: Blue discoloration of the skin and mucous membranes due to excessive concentration of reduced hemoglobin in the blood

Cystine: A naturally occurring amino acid, the chief sulfur-containing component of the protein molecule; it is sometimes found in the urine and in the kidneys in the form of minute hexagonal crystals frequently forming cystine calculus (stones) in the bladder

Cystitis: Inflammation of the bladder

Cystocele: Herniation of the urinary bladder into the vagina

Cytology (cytologic): The study of cells, their origin, structure, function, and pathology

Cytolysis: Cell lysis produced by antibody with the participation of complement

Cystoscopy: Examination of the bladder by means of a scope especially designed for passing through the urethra into the bladder to permit visual inspection of the interior of that organ

Dactylitis: Inflammation of a finger or toe

Demyelinization (or demyelination): Destruction, removal, or loss of the myelin sheath of a nerve or nerves

Dependent edema: Edema (abnormal accumulation of fluid in the intercellular spaces of the body) affecting most severely the lowermost parts of the body that are maintained in a dependent (unsupported) position

Depolarization: The rapid reversal of the resting membrane potential that results from a sequence of events in which the cell membrane permeability to sodium increases spontaneously (e.g., in pacemaking cells) or in response to a stimulus, then a rapid influx of sodium occurs and potassium moves out of the cell; this movement of ions across the membrane creates an electrical current or impulse that spreads as a wave of depolarization to adjacent cells

Diaphoresis: Perspiration, especially excessive or profuse perspiration

Diarrhea: Rapid movement of fecal matter through the intestine, resulting in poor absorption of water, nutritive elements, and electrolytes and producing abnormally frequent evacuation of watery stools

Diastole: The phase of the cardiac cycle in which the heart relaxes between contractions; specifically, the period when the two ventricles are dilated by the blood flowing into them

Differentiation: The process of acquiring completely individual characteristics, such as occurs in the progressive diversification of cells and tissues

Diffuse lymphoma: A malignant lymphoma in which the neoplastic cells infiltrate the entire lymph node without any organized pattern; this unorganized infiltration is called effacement

Diffusion: Movement of solutes of particles from an area of greater concentration to an area of lesser concentration through a semipermeable membrane

Diplopia: Double vision; the perception of two images of a single object

Disseminated: Scattered; distributed over a considerable area

Disseminated intravascular coagulation: Widespread formation of thromboses in the microcirculation, mainly within the capillaries; it is a secondary complication of a diverse group of obstetric, surgical, infectious, hemolytic, and neoplastic disorders, all of which intrinsically affect the coagulation sequence

Diuresis: Increased excretion of the urine

Dyesthesias: Impairment of any sense, especially the sense of touch; a painful, persistent sensation induced by a gentle touch of the skin

Dysphagia: Difficulty in swallowing

Dysplasia (dysplastic): Alteration in size, shape, and organization of adult cells

Dyspnea: Labored or difficult breathing; it is a symptom of a variety of disorders and is primarily an indication of inadequate ventilation or insufficient amounts of oxygen in the circulating blood

Dysuria: Painful or difficult urination

Ecchymosis: Hemorrhagic spot, larger than a petechia, in the skin or mucous membrane, forming a nonelevated, rounded or irregular, blue or purple patch; a bruise

Ectopic: Pertaining or characterized by displacement or malposition, especially if congenital

Ectopic pregnancy: Pregnancy in which the fertilized ovum becomes implanted outside the uterus instead of in the wall of the uterus; also called extrauterine pregnancy

Effusion: Escape of fluid into a body part

Embolism: The sudden blocking of an artery by a clot of foreign material (embolus) that has been brought to its site of lodgment by the blood current; may also be a fat globule, air bubble, piece of tissue, or clump of bacteria

Embolus (pl. emboli): Part or all of a clot that breaks away and circulates through the bloodstream

Emphysema: A pathologic accumulation of air in tissues or organs. The term is generally used to designate chronic pulmonary emphysema, a lung disorder in which the terminal bronchioles become plugged with mucus. Eventually, there is a loss of elasticity in the lung tissue so that inspired air becomes trapped in the lungs, making breathing difficult, especially during the expiratory phase

Empyema: Accumulation of pus in a body cavity

Endemic: Present in a community at all times

Endocarditis: Inflammation of the endocardium (lining covering the heart and valves)

Endocardium: The endothelial lining membrane of the cavities of the heart and the connective tissue bed on which it lies; the innermost layer lining the heart

Endometriosis: A condition in which tissue more or less perfectly resembling the endometrium (the mucous membrane lining the uterus) occurs aberrantly in various locations in the pelvic cavity and elsewhere

(Cardiac) Endothelium: Layer of cells lining the cavities of the heart and blood vessels

Enuresis: Involuntary discharge of urine, usually referring to involuntary discharge of urine during sleep at night; bed-wetting beyond the age when bladder control should have been achieved

Eosinophilia: The formation and accumulation of an abnormally large number of eosinophils in the blood

Eosinophils: A granular leukocyte with a nucleus that usually has two lobes connected by a thread of chromatin, and cytoplasm containing coarse, round granules of uniform size

Epicardium: The serous pericardium (visceral pleura) or layer on the surface of the heart that immediately envelopes the heart

Epigastric: Upper middle region of the abdomen and lower sternum

Epigastrium: The upper and middle region of the abdomen, located within the sternal angle

Epistaxis: Hemorrhage from the nose; nosebleed

Epitope: A characteristic shape or marker on an antigen's surface

Eructation: Belching

Erythema: Redness of the skin caused by congestion of the capillaries in the lower layers of the skin; it occurs with any skin injury, infection, or inflammation

Erythema nodosum: Red bumps/purple knots over the ankles and shins

Erythrocytes: A red blood cell or corpuscle; one of the formed elements of the peripheral blood; the functions of erythrocytes include transportation of oxygen and carbon dioxide; they are important in the maintenance of a normal acid-base balance, and because they help to determine the viscosity of the blood, they also influence its specific gravity

Erythropoiesis: The formation of erythrocytes

Erythropoietin: A glycoprotein hormone secreted by the kidney in the adult and by the liver in the fetus, which acts on stem cells of the bone marrow to stimulate red blood cell production

Esophageal varices: Varicosities (distentions) of branches of the azygous vein that anastomose (connection between two normally distinct structures) with tributaries of the portal vein in the lower esophagus; due to portal hypertension in cirrhosis of the liver

Esophagitis: Inflammation of the esophagus

Exogenous: Developed or originating outside the organism

Extracellular fluid (ECF): Fluid found outside body cells

Extramedullary: Outside of the spinal cord but still within the spinal canal

Fiberoptic endoscopy: Visual examination of the interior structures of the body with an instrument (endoscope) used for direct visual inspection of the hollow organs or body cavities

Fibrillations: Involuntary twitching or contraction of the heart muscle fibrils, but not the muscle as a whole

Fibrin: An insoluble protein that is essential to clotting of blood, formed from fibrinogen by action of thrombin

Fibrinogen: A high-molecular-weight protein in the blood plasma that, by the action of thrombin, is converted into fibrin; also called clotting factor I; in the clotting mechanism, fibrin threads form a meshwork for the basis of a blood clot; most of the fibrinogen in the circulating blood is formed in the liver

Fibroids: Having a fibrous structure, fibroma; tumor consisting mainly of fibrous or fully developed connective tissue

Fibrosis: Formation of fibrous tissue

Flatulence: Excessive formation of gases in the intestine or stomach

Frequency: Referring to urinary or bowel frequency: increased number of times urination or defecation occurs without an increase in the daily volume or output, due to reduced bladder or colon capacity

Funnel technique: Moving from an open-ended line of questions to the closed-ended questions

Giant cell tumor: A bone tumor, ranging from benign to malignant, consisting of cellular spindle cell stroma (tissue containing the ground substance, framework, or matrix of an organ) containing multinucleated giant cells resembling osteoclasts

Gliosis: Fibrous cells (astrocytes) in damaged areas of the central nervous system

Glomerular filtration rate (GFR): The amount of fluid filtered by the glomerular capillaries in 1 minute (approximately 125 ml/min)

Glomerulonephritis: A variety of nephritis (inflammation of the kidney) characterized by inflammation of the capillary loops in the glomeruli of the kidney; it occurs in acute, subacute, and chronic forms and is usually secondary to an infection

Glucagon: A polypeptide hormone secreted by the alpha cells of the islets of Langerhans in response to hypoglycemia or to stimulation by growth hormone; it increases blood glucose concentration by stimulating glycogenolysis in the liver and is administered to relieve hypoglycemic coma from any cause, especially hyperinsulinism

Glucocorticoids: Any corticoid substance that increases gluconeogenesis, raising the concentration of liver glycogen and blood sugar (i.e., cortisol [hydrocortisone], cortisone, and corticosterone)

Glycosuria: The presence of glucose in the urine

Goiter: Enlargement of the thyroid gland, causing a swelling in the front of the neck

Gout: The manifestation of an inherited inborn error of purine metabolism, characterized by an elevated serum uric acid (hyperuricemia); may cause gouty arthritis or renal disease due to the deposition of urate crystals in tissues

Granulocytes: Any cell containing granules, especially a granular leukocyte; a cell of the immune system filled with granules of toxic chemicals that enable them to digest microorganisms; basophils, neutropils, eosinophils, and mast cells are examples of granulocytes

Gynecomastia: Excessive development of mammary glands in the male, even to the functional state

Helper T-cells (T_h): A subset of T-cells that initiates antibody production

Hemangioma: Benign tumor made up of newly formed blood vessels, clustered together

Hemarthrosis: Blood in the cavity of the joint

Hematemesis: Vomiting blood

Hematogenous: Disseminated by the bloodstream or by the circulation

Hematoma: A localized collection of extravasated (escaped) blood, usually clotted, in an organ, space, or tissue

Hematopoiesis: The formation and development of blood cells, usually taking place in the bone marrow

Hematopoietic: Pertaining to or affecting the formation of blood cells; an agent that promotes the formation of blood cells

Hematuria: The discharge of blood in the urine;

the urine may be slightly blood-tinged, grossly bloody, or a smoky brown color

Heme: The nonprotein, insoluble, iron protoporphyrin (a prophyrin, which in combination with iron, forms hemes) constituent of hemoglobin of various other respiratory pigments and of many cells, both animal and vegetable; it is an iron compound or protoporphyrin and thus constitutes the pigment portion or protein-free part of the hemoglobin molecule and is responsible for its oxygen-carrying properties

Hemoglobin: A protein found in the erythrocytes (red blood cells) that transports molecular oxygen (O_2) in the blood; symbol Hb

Hemolysis: Rupture of erythrocytes (red blood cells) with the release of hemoglobin into the plasma

Hemoptysis: Coughing and spitting of blood as a result of bleeding from any part of the respiratory tract

Hemorrhoids: An enlarged (varicose) vein in the mucous membrane inside or just outside of the rectum; also called "piles"

Hemostasis: The arrest of the escape of blood by either natural (clot formation or vessel spasm) or artificial (compression or ligation) methods, or the interruption of blood flow to a part

Hepatic encephalopathy: A condition, usually occurring secondarily to advanced liver disease, marked by disturbances of consciousness that may progress to deep coma (hepatic coma), psychiatric changes of varying degree, flapping tremor, and fetor hepaticus (characteristic breath odor)

Hepatomegaly: Enlargement of the liver

HLA-B27: A genetic marker: human leukocyte antigen

Homan's sign: Slight pain or discomfort at the back of the knee or calf when the ankle is forcibly dorsiflexed, indicative of thrombus in the veins of the leg

Hormone: A chemical transmitter substance produced by cells of the body and transported by the bloodstream to the cells and organs on which it has a specific regulatory effect

Hydrarthrosis: Accumulation of watery fluid in the cavity of a joint

Hydrostatic pressure: Pressure exerted by a stationary fluid

Hyperalgesia: Excessive sensitivity to pain

Hyperalimentation: A program of parenteral administration of all nutrients for patients with gastrointestinal dysfunction; also called total parenteral alimentation (TPA) and total parenteral nutrition (TPN)

Hyperbilirubinemia: An excess of bilirubin in the blood as a result of liver or biliary tract dysfunction, or with excessive destruction of erythrocytes

Hypercalcemia: An excess of calcium in the blood

Hyperesthesia: Increased sensitivity to touch or other sensory stimulation

Hyperfunction: Excessive functioning of a part or a gland

Hyperglycemia: An excess of glucose in the blood

Hyperkalemia: Abnormally high potassium concentration in the blood, most often due to defective renal excretion, such as in kidney disease, severe and extensive burns, intestinal obstruction, and Addison's disease

Hyperkeratosis: Hypertrophy of the horny layer of the skin (e.g., nails, soles of the feet), or any disease characterized by it

Hyperkinesis: Abnormal increase in motor function or activity

Hyperlipidemia: A general term for elevated concentrations of any or all of the lipids in the plasma

Hyperosmolar: A solution that consists of a large amount of solute and a small amount of water

Hyperplasia: Abnormal increase in the volume of tissue or organ caused by the formation and growth of new normal cells

Hypersplenism: A condition characterized by exaggeration of the hemolytic function (rupture of the erythrocytes with the release of hemoglobin into the plasma) of the spleen, resulting in deficiency of peripheral blood elements

Hypertension: Persistent elevation of blood pressure

Hypertonic: Same as hyperosmolar

Hypertrophy: Increase in volume of a tissue or organ produced entirely by enlargement of existing cells

Hyperuricemia: An excess of uric acid or urates in the blood

Hyperuricosuria: An excess of uric acid excreted in the urine

Hypesthesia (hypoesthesia): Abnormal decrease in sensitivity to sensory stimulation

Hypochromia: Decrease of hemoglobin in the erythrocytes so that the erythrocytes are abnormally pale

Hypofunction: Diminished functioning of a part or gland

Hypo-osmolar: A solution that consists of a large amount of water and a small amount of solute

Hypotonic: Same as hypo-osmolar

Hypoxia: A broad term meaning diminished availability of oxygen to the body tissues

Hypovolemic shock: Abnormally decreased volume of circulating fluid (plamsa) in the body

Icteric: Pertaining to or affected with jaundice, yellowed

IgE: Immunoglobulin E, a protein of animal origin with known antibody activity

Ileum: The distal portion of the small intestine, extending from the jejunum to the cecum

Immune complex: Large molecules formed when antigen and antibody bind together

Immunocompetence: The capacity to develop an immune response after exposure to antigen

Immunodeficient: Deficiency of immune response or a disorder characterized by deficient immune response

Immunoglobulin: There are five classes of immunoglobulins: IgM, IgG, IgA, IgE, and IgD; each immunoglobulin is a protein of animal origin with known antibody activity; immunoglobulins are major components of what is called the humoral immune response system; they are synthesized by lymphocytes and plasma cells and are found in the serum and in other body fluids and tissues, including the urine, spinal fluid, lymph nodes, and spleen

Incontinence: Inability to control excretory functions (may be bowel or urinary)

Induration: The quality of being hard

Infarction: Irreversible tissue damage (necrosis) due to lack of oxygen resulting from obstruction of an artery, most commonly by a thrombus or embolus

Insulin: A double-chain protein hormone formed in the beta cells of the pancreatic islets of Langerhans; the major fuel-regulating hormone, it is secreted into the blood in response to a rise in concentration of blood glucose or amino acids

Interferon: A natural glycoprotein released by cells invaded by viruses; it is not itself an antiviral agent, but acts instead as a stimulant to noninfected cells causing them to synthesize another protein with antiviral characteristics

Internuncial: Neurons connecting other neurons

Interstitial compartment: Space between cells

Intracellular fluid (ICF): Fluid found inside body cells

Intradural: Within or beneath the dura mater, the outermost, toughest, and most fibrous of the three membranes (meninges) covering the brain and spinal cord

Intramedullary: Within the spinal cord

Intravascular compartment: Vascular spaces; spaces within the blood vessels

Iridocyclitis: Inflammation of the iris and ciliary body of the eye

Iritis: Inflammation of the iris, the circular pigmented membrane behind the cornea of the eye

Ischemia: Loss of blood supply in an area, usually caused by a functional constriction or mechanical obstruction of a blood vessel

Isotonic: A solution that contains both water and solutes in the same concentration as that of the fluid in the body

Jaundice: Yellowness of the skin, sclerae, mucous membranes, and excretions due to hyperbilirubinemia and deposition of bile pigments; also called icteric

Kernicterus: A condition in the newborn marked by severe neural symptoms associated with high levels of bilirubin in the blood

Ketonuria: An excess of ketone bodies (normal metabolic products of lipid and pyruvate within the liver) in the urine

Kussmaul's respiration: A distressing dyspnea characterized by increased respiratory rate (above 20/min), increased depth of respiration, panting, and labored respiration typical of air hunger; seen in metabolic acidosis, especially diabetic ketoacidosis and renal failure

Lactation: The secretion of milk by the breast; also describes the period of weeks or months during which a child is nursed at the breast

Leukocytes: A colorless blood corpuscle capable of ameboid movement, whose chief function is to protect the body against microorganisms causing disease; classified into two main groups: granular (basophils, neutrophils, eosinophils) and nongranular (lymphocytes, monocytes)

Leukocytosis: A transient increase in the number of leukocytes in the blood, due to various causes

Leukopenia: Also known as leukocytopenia; a reduction in the number of leukocytes in the blood, the count being 5,000 or less

Leukopoiesis: Production of leukocytes

Leukopoietin: Any factor or agent promoting leukopoiesis

Lumen: The cavity or channel within a tube or tubular organ, such as a blood vessel or the intestine

Lymph: A transparent, usually slightly yellow liquid found within the lymphatic vessels and collected from tissues in all parts of the body and returned to the blood via the lymphatic system

Lymphadenopathy: Disease of the lymph nodes

Lymphedema: An excessive accumulation of fluid in tissue spaces

Lymph nodes: Any of the accumulations of lymphoid tissue organized as definite lymphoid organs along the course of lymphatic vessels; they are the main source of lymphocytes in the peripheral blood and act as a defense mechanism by removing noxious agents (e.g., bacteria, toxins)

Lymphocytes: Any of the mononuclear, nonphagocytic leukocytes found in the blood, lymph, and lymphoid tissues that comprise the body's immunologically competent cells and their precursors; they are divided into two classes: B-lymphocytes, responsible for humoral and cellular immunity, respectively

Lymphoid cells: Cells pertaining to lymph or to tissue of the lymphatic system, specifically lymphocytes and plasma cells

Lymphokines: A general term for soluble protein mediators released by sensitized lymphocytes on contact with antigen; believed to play a role in macrophage activation, lymphocyte transformation, and cell-mediated immunity

Lymphomas: Any neoplastic disorder of lymphoid tissue, including Hodgkin's disease; often used to denote malignant lymphoma, classifications of which are based on predominant cell type and degree of differentiation. Various categories may be subdivided into nodular and diffuse types depending on the predominant pattern of cell arrangement.

Lysis: Destruction or decomposition, especially by enzymatic digestion

Macrophage: Any of the large, mononuclear, highly phagocytic cells derived from monocytes that occur in the walls of blood vessels and in loose connective tissue; they function in phagocytosis, presentation of antigens to T-lymphocytes and B-lymphocytes, and secretion of a variety of products, including enzymes, several complement components and coagulation factors, some prostaglandins, and several regulatory molecules

Mast cells: A connective tissue cell capable of releasing basophilic granules that contain histamine, heparin, hyaluronic acid, and slow-reacting substance of anaphylaxis (SRS-A); in some species, capable of releasing serotonin

Mastitis: Inflammation of the breast occurring in a variety of forms and in various degrees of severity

Mastodynia: Mammary neuralgia of the intercostal nerves of the upper dorsal branches on one side

Mediastinum: The mass of tissues and organs separating the sternum in front and the vertebral column behind, containing the heart and its large vessels, trachea, esophagus, thymus, and lymph nodes

Melanoma: A tumor arising from the skin; refers to malignant melanoma

Melena: Blood in stool characterized by a dark, tarry color

Menarche: Establishment or beginning of the menstrual function

Menorrhagia: Excessive menstruation

Metaplasia: The change in the type of adult cells in a tissue to a form abnormal for that tissue

Metastases: The transfer of cancer cells from one organ or part to another not directly connected with the original organ

Mineralocorticoids: Any of a group of hormones elaborated by the cortex of the adrenal gland, so-called because of their effects on sodium, chloride, and potassium concentrations in the extracellular fluid to regulate fluid and electrolyte balance; the primary mineralocorticoid is aldosterone

Monoarthritis: Asymmetric presentation of arthritis, affecting one joint at a time

Monocytes: A mononuclear, phagocytic leukocyte derived from promonocytes in the bone marrow; they circulate in the blood for about 24 hours before migrating to the tissues, such as in the lung and liver, where they develop into macrophages

Monokines: A general term for soluble mediators of immune responses that are not antibodies or complement components and that are produced by mononuclear phagocytes (monocytes or macrophages)

Morbidity: A condition of being diseased (sickness or illness)

Morphea: A condition in which there is a connective tissue replacement of the skin and sometimes of the subcutaneous tissue, marked by the formation of ivory white or pink patches, bands, or lines that are sometimes bordered by a purple areola. The lesions are firm, but not hard, and are usually depressed; they may remain localized or may involute, leaving atrophy and scarring; also called localized scleroderma

Multiparity: Woman who has had two or more pregnancies resulting in viable offspring

Multiple myeloma: A malignant neoplasm of plasma cells in which the plasma cells proliferate and invade the bone marrow, causing destruction of the bone and resulting in pathologic fracture and bone pain

Myalgia: Muscular pain

Myelin: Lipid substance forming a sheath around the axons of certain nerve fibers

Myelofibrosis: Replacement of bone marrow by fibrous tissue

Myocardial infarct: Necrosis of the cells of an area of the heart muscle (myocardium) occurring as a result of oxygen deprivation, which in turn is caused by obstruction of the blood supply; commonly referred to as a "heart attack"

Myocardium: The middle and thickest layer of the heart wall consisting of cardiac muscle

Myoedema: Localized knot or edema of contracting muscle induced by direct percussion or by some other form of mechanical irritation of the muscle

Myokymia: A benign condition in which there is persistent quivering of the muscles

Myopathy: Any disease of a muscle

Myositis: Inflammation of a voluntary muscle

Myxedema: A condition resulting from advanced hypothyroidism or a deficiency of thyroxine

Necrosis: Morphologic changes indicative of cell death caused by enzymatic degradation; death of tissue

Neoplasm: Tumor; any new and abnormal growth, specifically one in which cell multiplication is uncontrolled and progressive. Neoplasms may be benign or malignant.

Nephrolithiasis: A condition marked by the presence of renal calculi or kidney stones

Neuraxis: Axon; central nervous system

Neuritis: Constant irritation of nerve endings; inflammation of a nerve

Neurogenic: Forming nervous tissue or originating in the nervous system

Neurohormones: A hormone stimulating the neural mechanism

Neutrophils: A granular leukocyte that has a nucleus with three to five lobes connected by threads of chromatin and cytoplasm containing very fine granules; neutrophils have the property of chemotaxis, adherence to immune complexes, and phagocytosis; also called polymorphonuclear, polynuclear, or neutrophilic leukocytes

Night sweats: Gradual increase in body temperature followed by a sudden drop in temperature that usually occurs during sleep; the person affected may awaken when the sudden reduction of body temperature results in profuse sweating

Nitroglycerin: Medication used as a coronary artery vasodilator

Nocturia: Excessive urination at night

Nodular lymphoma: Malignant lymphoma in which the lymphomatous cells are clustered into identifiable nodules within the lymph nodes that somewhat resemble the germinal centers of lymph node follicles

Nystagmus: Involuntary, rapid, rhythmic movement (horizontal, vertical, rotatory, or mixed) of the eyeball

Obstipation: Intractable (not easily relieved) constipation

Occult: Hidden from view, obscure

Odynophagia: Painful swallowing of food

Oliguria: Diminished urine secretion in relation to fluid intake

Oncogene: A gene found in the chromosomes of tumor cells whose activation is associated with the initial and continuing conversion of normal cells into cancer cells

Oncogenesis: The production or causation of tumors

Onycholysis: Loosening or separation of a nail from its bed

Oophorectomy: Removal of one or both ovaries; also called ovariectomy

Open-ended question: Question that elicits more than a one-word response

Orthopnea: Difficult breathing except in the upright position; the person must sit or stand to breathe

Orthostatic hypotension: Excessive fall (20 or more mm Hg) in blood pressure on assuming the erect position

Osmolality: The concentration of a solution in terms of osmoles of solutes per kilogram of solvent

Osmosis: Movement of water from an area of high concentration of water to an area of low concentration of water through a semipermeable membrane

Osmotic diuresis: Rapid loss of sodium and water through the inhibition of their reabsorption in the kidney tubules and the loop of Henle

Osteoblastomas: A benign, painful, vascular tumor of bone marked by the formation of osteoid tissue and primitive bone

Osteochondromas: A benign bone tumor consisting of projecting adult bone capped by cartilage

(Renal) Osteodystrophy: Demineralization of bones related to decreased calcium absorption and resultant calcium/phosphorus imbalance

Osteogenic sarcoma (osteosarcoma): A malignant primary tumor of bone consisting of a malignant connective tissue stroma (tissue forming the framework, ground substance of matrix of an organ)

Osteoid osteoma: A benign hemarthromatous (blood filled) lesion of cortical bone in young individuals

Osteolytic lesions: Dissolution of bone; removal or loss of calcium from the bone

Osteomalacia: Softening of the bones, resulting from impaired mineralization with excess accumulation of osteoid (bone that has not calcified), caused by vitamin D deficiency in adults

Osteomyelitis: Inflammation of bone, localized

or generalized, due to a pyogenic (producing pus) infection; it may result in bone destruction and in stiffening of joints if the infection spreads to the joints

Osteoporosis: Decreased mass per unit volume of normally mineralized bone compared with age and sex-matched controls

Palpitations: Subjective sensation of throbbing, fluttering, skipping, rapid, or forcible pulsation of the heart; may be regular or irregular

Pannus: An inflammatory exudate overlying synovial cells on the inside of a joint capsule, usually occurring in rheumatoid arthritis; fatty, bloody, edematous mass within the synovial membrane

Papilloma: A benign tumor derived from epithelium; papillomas may arise from skin, mucous membranes, or glandular ducts

Paraneoplastic syndrome: A collective term for disorders arising from metabolic effects of cancer on tissues remote from the tumor; such syndromes may appear as primary endocrine, hematologic, or neuromuscular disorders

Paraphrasing technique: Repeating information presented by the patient for clarification

Parenchyma: The essential or functional elements of an organ; for example, the kidney itself

Parenteral: Not through the alimentary canal, but by subcutaneous, intramuscular, intrasternal, or intravenous injection

Paresthesias: Abnormal sensation, such as burning or prickling without a loss of objective neurologic findings

Parietal: Of or pertaining to the walls of an organ or cavity

Parietal pericardium: The serous membrane between the (fibrous) pericardium and the epicardium (or visceral surface) of the heart

Parietal pleura: The serous membrane lining the walls of the thoracic cavity

Paroxysmal: A sudden, recurrent, intensification of symptoms; a spasm

Paroxysmal nocturnal dyspnea: Acute dyspnea occurring suddenly at night, usually waking the patient after a few hours of sleep; caused by pulmonary congestion and edema that result from left-sided heart failure; varies in severity from nocturnal restlessness or anxiety to extreme respiratory distress

Patent ductus arteriosus: Shunt caused by an opening between the aorta and the pulmonary artery

Pericardial: Related to the pericardium; the fibroserous sac enclosing the heart and the roots of the great vessels

Pericardium: The fibrous sac enveloping the entire heart consisting of two layers: the epicardium (visceral layer immediately surrounding the heart) and the serous parietal pericardium

Peristalsis: The wormlike movement by which the alimentary canal or other tubular organs with both longitudinal and circular muscle fibers propel their contents, consisting of a wave of contraction passing along the tube

Petechiae: Minute, pinpoint, nonraised, perfectly round, purple-red spot caused by intradermal or submucous hemorrhage that later turns blue or yellow

Peyer's patches: White, oval, elevated patches of closely packed lymph follicles in mucous and submucous layers of the small intestine

pH: The negative logarithm of the hydrogen ion concentration $[H^+]$, a measure of the degree to which a solution is acidic or alkaline

Phagocytes: Any cell capable of ingesting particulate matter; the term refers to two types of phagocytes: polymorphonuclear leukocytes and mononuclear phagocytes (macrophages and monocytes); these cells ingest microorganisms and other particulate antigens that are coated with antibody or complement, a process that is mediated by specific cell-surface receptors

Phagocytosing: The process of ingesting particulate matter by phagocytes

Phagocytosis: The engulfing of microorganisms or other cells and foreign material

Phlebitis: Inflammation of a vein

Phlebotomy: Incision of a vein and removal of blood

Phrenic nerve: A major branch of the cervical plexus that extends through the thorax to provide innervation of the diaphragm; nerve impulses from the inspiratory center in the brain travel down the phrenic nerve, causing contraction of the diaphragm and inspiration occurs

Piloerection: Erection of the hair

Pitting edema: Edema in which pressure leaves a persistent depression in the tissues

Platelet: A small disk or platelike structure, the smallest of the formed elements in blood; also called thrombocytes. These disk-shaped, nonnucleated blood elements are very fragile and tend to adhere to uneven or damaged surfaces; their rate of formation is governed by the amount of oxygen in the blood and the presence of nucleic acid derivatives from injured tissue. The functions of platelets are related to coagulation and the clotting of blood; because of their adhesion and aggregation capabilities, platelets can occlude small breaks in blood vessels and prevent blood from escaping. Platelets are also able to take up, store, transport, and release serotonin and platelet factor III

Pleura: A thin, transparent, moist, serous membrane enveloping the lungs (pulmonary pleura) and lining the thoracic cavity (parietal pleura), completely enclosing a potential space known as the pleural cavity

Pleural space: The potential space between the parietal pleura and the pulmonary pleura (visceral pleura of the lungs)

Pleurisy: Inflammation of the pleura; it may be caused by infection, injury, or tumor; it may be a complication of lung diseases, particularly of pneumonia or sometimes tuberculosis, lung abscess, or influenza

Pleuropulmonary: Pertaining to the pleura (serous membrane around the lungs and lining the thoracic cavity enclosing the pleural cavity) and the lungs

Pneumothorax: Accumulation of gas or air in the pleural cavity resulting in the collapse of the lung on the affected side

Poikilocytosis: The presence of abnormally shaped red blood cells in the blood

Polyarthritis: Inflammation of several joints

Polycythemia: An increase in the total red cell mass of the blood

Polydypsia: Excessive thirst

Polymyositis: A chronic, progressive inflammatory disease of skeletal muscle, occurring in both children and adults

Polyp: Any growth or mass protruding from a mucous membrane

Polyphagia: Excessive ingestion of food

Polyuria: Excessive excretion of urine

Portal hypertension: Abnormally increased pressure in the portal circulation (i.e., circulation from the gastrointestinal tract and spleen through the portal vein to the liver) due to narrowing of the capillary branches of the portal vessels; the result is impairment of the liver's ability to detoxify wastes and transport nutrients, resulting in hepatic encephalopathy, anorexia, and metabolic acidosis. The increased pressure can lead to escape of fluid through the liver capsule and into the abdominal cavity (ascites).

Precordia(ium): The region over the heart and lower part of the thorax; sometimes the diaphragm is referred to as the precordium

Prolapse: The falling down or downward displacement of a part or organ

Prostaglandins: A group of naturally occurring, chemically related, long-chain hydroxy fatty acids that stimulate contractility of the uterine and other smooth muscles and have the ability to lower blood pressure, regulate acid secretion of the stomach, regulate body temperature and platelet aggregation, and control inflammation and vascular permeability. They also affect the action of certain hormones.

Proteinuria: An excess of serum proteins in the urine; may cause foamy urine

Pruritus: Itching common in many skin disorders, especially allergic inflammation and parasitic infestation; systemic diseases that may cause pruritus include diabetes mellitus and liver disorders with jaundice

Ptosis: Drooping of the upper eyelid (caused by extraocular muscle weakness in the context of this chapter)

Pulmonary infarct: Localized necrosis of lung tissue due to obstruction of the arterial blood supply

Pulmonary pleura: Membrane enveloping the lungs

Purkinje's fibers: Modified cardiac muscle fibers in the subendothelial tissue, concerned with conducting impulses to the heart

Purpura: A hemorrhagic disease characterized by extravasation of blood into the tissues, under the skin and through the mucous membranes, and producing spontaneous ecchymoses (bruises) and petechiae (small red patches) on the skin

Pyelonephritis: Inflammation of the kidney and renal pelvis (funnel-shaped expansion of the upper end of the ureter into which the renal cavities open, usually the renal sinus); also called nephropyelitis

Pyoderma: Any purulent (containing or forming pus) skin disease; deep ulcers or canker sores

Raynaud's disease: Vasospasm of digital arteries with blanching and numbness of fingers

Raynaud's phenomenon: Intermittent spasm of the digital arteries with blanching and numbness of the fingers or toes, bilaterally

Rectocele: Hernial protrusion of part of the rectum into the vagina

Referred: Related to a remote origin

Reflux: A backward or return flow

Regional enteritis: See Crohn's disease

Relaxin: A hormone that produces relaxation of the symphysis pubis and dilation of the uterine cervix

Renin: A proteolytic enzyme synthesized, stored, and secreted by the juxtaglomerular cells of the kidney; it plays a role in the regulation of blood pressure by catalyzing the conversion of the plasma glycoprotein angiotensinogen to angiotensin I

Reticuloendothelial: Pertaining to the reticuloendothelium or to the reticuloendothelial system that is a network of cells and tissues found throughout the body, especially in the blood, general connective tissue, spleen, liver, lungs, bone marrow, and lymph nodes. Reticuloendothelial cells are concerned with blood cell formation and destruction, storage of fatty materials, and metabolism of iron and pigment; they play a role in inflammation and immunity. Some of the cells are motile (capable of motion) and phagocytic, ingesting and destroying unwanted foreign material. The reticuloendothelial cells of the spleen possess the ability to dispose of disintegrated erythrocytes, but do not destroy hemoglobin that is liberated in the process.

Retinopathy: Noninflammatory disease of the retina

Retrosternum: Behind the sternum

Retroversion: Tipping backward of an entire organ, specifically the uterus

Sacroiliitis: Inflammation of the sacroiliac joint

Sarcoma: A tumor, often highly malignant, consisting of cells derived from connective tissue, such as bone and cartilage, muscle, blood vessel, or lymphoid tissue; these tumors usually develop rapidly and metastasize through the lymph channels

Satiety: State or condition of satisfaction, as full gratification of appetite or thirst with abolition of the desire to ingest further food or liquids

Sclerae: The tough, white outer coat of the eyeball

Sclerodactyly: Chronic hardening and shrinking of the fingers and toes

Scotomas: An area of lost or depressed vision within the visual field; perceived as black spots before the eyes

Septic (sepsis): The presence of blood or other tissues of pathogenic microorganisms or their toxins

Septicemia: Blood poisoning

Signs: Any objective evidence of disease or dysfunction; an observable physical phenomenon

Sinoatrial node: The cardiac pacemaker located in the right atrium of the heart

Sinusitis: Inflammation of one or more of the paranasal sinuses, often occurring during an upper respiratory infection when the infection in the nose spreads to the sinuses

Sinusoids: Resembling a sinus; a form of terminal blood channel consisting of large, irregular, anastomosing vessel with a lining of reticuloendothelium

Somatic: Pertaining to or characteristic of the body (soma); the body as distinguished from the mind; the body tissue as distinguished from the germ cells

Spider angiomas: Branched dilatation of the superficial capillaries resembling a spider

Splenectomy: Excision of the spleen

Splenomegaly: Enlargement of the spleen

Spondylitis: Inflammation of the vertebrae

Spondyloarthropathy: Disease of the joints of the spine

Spondylotic bars: A union of the bones of a joint by proliferation of bone cells in the shape of a bar extending between two bones (or vertebrae)

Spontaneous pneumothorax: Accumulation of air or gas in the pleural cavity, resulting in collapse of the lung on the affected side

Stem cells: Any precursor cell; a mother cell with the capacity for replication and differentiation

Stenosis: Narrowing or stricture of a duct, canal, body passage, or opening

Stress incontinence: Involuntary escape of urine due to strain on the orifice of the bladder, such as in coughing or sneezing

Stricture: An abnormal narrowing of a duct or passage

Suppressor T-cells (T_s): Subset of T-cells that "turn off" antibody production

Surfactant: A mixture of phospholipids secreted by the alveolar cells into the alveoli and respiratory passages that reduce the surface tension of pulmonary fluids and thus contributes to the elastic properties of pulmonary disease

Symptoms: Any indication of disease as perceived by the patient

Syncope: Episodes of fainting or loss of consciousness due to generalized cerebral ischemia

Syndesmophyte: Ossification of connective tissue other than bone, such as ligaments, tendons, or outer margins of the intervertebral disk

Systole: The contraction, or period of contraction, of the heart, especially of the ventricles during which blood is forced into the aorta and pulmonary artery

Tachycardia: Rapid beating of the heart; the term is usually applied to a heart rate above 100 beats/min

Tachypnea: Very rapid, shallow breathing; respiratory rate greater than 20 breaths/min

Target gland: Glands in the body that are specifically affected by pituitary hormones

T-cells: White blood cells that are processed in the thymus and then produce lymphokines; responsible in part for carrying out the immune response; also called T-lymphocytes

Telangiectasia: Vascular lesion formed by dilation of a group of small blood vessels

Tenesmus: Ineffective and painful straining at stool or in urinating

Tetralogy of Fallot: A combination of congenital cardiac defects, consisting of pulmonary stenosis, interventricular septal defect, displacement of the aorta so that it overrides the interventricular septum and receives venous as well as arterial blood, and right ventricular hypertrophy

Thrombin: An enzyme resulting from the activation of prothrombin that catalyzes the conversion of fibrinogen to fibrin

Thromboangiitis obliterans: (Buerger's disese): An intense inflammatory and obliterative disease of the blood vessels of the extremities, primarily the lower extremities; also called Buerger's disease

Thrombocyte: A blood platelet

Thrombocytopenia: Decrease in the number of platelets in circulating blood resulting from decreased or defective platelet production or from accelerated platelet destruction.

Thrombocytosis: Increase in the number of platelets in the circulating blood

Thrombophlebitis: Inflammation of a vein accompanied by thrombus formation

Thrombopoiesis: Thrombogenesis; clot formation

Thrombopoietin: Any agent or factor involved in thrombopoiesis (clot formation)

Thromboxanes: An intermediate in the metabolic pathway of arachidonic acid, formed from prostaglandin endoperoxides and released from suitably stimulated platelets; the unstable form, thromboxane A_2 is a potent inducer of platelet aggregation and constrictor of arterial smooth muscle

Thrombus (pl. thrombi): A blood clot formed within a blood vessel or cavity of the heart that remains attached to the site at which it formed; an aggregation of blood factors, primarily platelets and fibrin with entrapment of cellular elements, frequently causing vascular obstruction at the point of its formation. Some experts differentiate a thrombus from a blood clot

Thymectomy: Excision of the thymus

Thymus: A ductless glandlike body lying in the upper mediastinum beneath the sternum, which plays an immunologic role throughout life; a lymphoid organ

Tophus (tophi): A chalky deposit of sodium urate occurring in gout; tophi form most often around the joints in cartilage, bone, bursae, and subcutaneous tissue producing a chronic, foreign-body inflammatory response

Total parenteral nutrition (TPN): See hyperalimentation

Transient ischemia attacks (TIAs): Temporary disruption of blood supply to part of the brain lasting 5 to 20 minutes; an early warning signal of possible impending CVA or stroke

Trigger point: Hypersensitive spot in the skeletal musculature that produces pain that can be referred to other parts of the body

Ulcerative colitis: A recurrent acute and chronic disorder characterized by extensive inflammatory ulceration in the colon, chiefly of the mucosa and submucosa

Urate salts: Salt of uric acid

Uremia: An excess in the blood of urea, creatinine, and other nitrogenous end-products of protein and amino acid metabolism; referred to more correctly as azotemia and, in current medical usage, the entire complex of signs and symptoms of chronic renal failure

Uremic breath: Characteristic urinelike odor of breath secondary to a build-up and release of uremic toxins

Urethritis: Inflammation of the urethra, a tubular passage through which urine is discharged from the bladder to the exterior of the body

Urgency: Referring to bowel and bladder urgency: the sudden compelling desire to urinate or defecate

Urgency incontinence: Inability to hold back urination when feeling the urge to void; a major complaint of patients with urinary tract infections

Urinary urgency: The sudden compelling desire to urinate

Urticaria: A vascular reaction of the skin marked by the transient appearance of slightly elevated patches (wheals) that are redder or paler than the surrounding skin and are often attended by severe itching; also called hives

Uveitis: Inflammation of part or all of the middle (vascular) tunic of the eye (uvea)

Varicose: Dilated or distended

Vasodilatory: Capable of opening up the blood vessels

Ventricular septal defect: Hole between the ventricles of the heart

Vertical transmission: Method of transmission by which an infant is infected with hepatitis by its mother either during pregnancy or after birth

Vertigo: An illusion of movement; a sensation as if the external world were revolving around the patient; the term is sometimes erroneously used to mean any form of dizziness, but the patient will usually use the word "dizzy" to describe the symptom

Viscera: Plural of viscus; any large interior organ in any of the great body cavities, especially those in the abdomen

Visceral: Pertaining to a viscus or any large interior organ in any of the great body cavities, especially those in the abdomen

Visceral peritoneum: The serous membrane lining the organs

Visceral pleura: The membrane enveloping an organ

Viscus: Any large interior organ in any of the great body cavities, especially those in the abdomen

Xanthine: A purine compound found in most body tissues and fluids; it is a precursor of uric acid

*Appendix: Universal Precautions to Prevent Transmission of HIV**

The increasing prevalence of HIV increases the risk that health care workers will be exposed to blood from patients infected with HIV, especially when blood and body-fluid precautions are not followed for all patients. The Centers for Disease Control emphasize the need for health care workers to consider *all* patients as being potentially infected with HIV or other blood-borne pathogens and to adhere rigorously to infection control precautions for minimizing the risk of exposure to blood and body fluids of all patients (Centers for Disease Control, 1987a).

Universal precautions do not apply to feces, nasal secretions, sputum, sweat, tears, urine, and vomitus unless they contain visible blood. The risk of transmission of HIV from these fluids and materials is extremely low or is nonexistent (Centers for Disease Control, 1988).

- All health care workers should routinely use appropriate barrier precautions to prevent skin and mucous-membrane exposure when contact with blood or other body fluids of any patient is anticipated. Gloves should be worn for touching:
    - Blood and body fluids
    - Mucous membranes
    - Nonintact skin of all patients
    - Handling items or surfaces soiled with blood or body fluids
- Gloves should be changed after contact with each patient.
- Masks and protective eyewear or face shields should be worn during procedures that are likely to generate droplets of blood or other body fluids to prevent exposure of mucous membranes of the mouth, nose, and eyes.
- Gowns or aprons should be worn during procedures that are likely to generate splashes of blood or other body fluids.
- Hands and other skin surfaces should be washed immediately and thoroughly if contaminated with blood or other body fluids. Hands should be washed immediately after gloves are removed.
- All health care workers should take precautions to prevent injuries:
    - Caused by sharp instruments, such as scissors or scalpels during procedures
    - When handling sharp instruments after procedures
    - When cleaning used instruments
    - During disposal of used needles

- Dispose of needles and sharp instruments in a puncture-resistant container
- Although saliva has not been implicated in the transmission of HIV to minimize the need for emergency mouth-to-mouth resuscitation, mouthpieces, resuscitation bags, or other ventilation devices should be available for use in areas in which the need for resuscitation is predictable.
- Health care workers who have exudative lesions or weeping dermatitis should refrain from all direct patient care and from handling patient-care equipment until the condition resolves.
- Pregnant health care workers are not known to be at a greater risk of contracting HIV infection than health care workers who are not pregnant; however, if a health care worker develops HIV infection during pregnancy, the infant is at risk of infection resulting from perinatal transmission. Because of this risk, pregnant health care workers should be especially familiar with and strictly adhere to precautions to minimize the risk of HIV transmission.

Physical therapists are encouraged to evaluate each patient's treatment in order to determine when these precautions are indicated. Open wounds, wound dressing, whirlpools, patients with pulmonary problems, and catheterized patients are some examples of commonly encountered situations requiring adherence to these precautions.

---

* Adapted from Centers for Disease Control: Recommendations for prevention of HIV transmission in health-care settings. MMWR, *36*:2S, 1987.

Index

Page numbers in boldface indicate clinical signs and symptoms.
Page numbers in *italics* indicate illustrations.
Page numbers followed by *t* indicate tables.

C

F

M

N

O

P

R

T

U